Beth L. Adams
Edward B. Kuvlesky
Craig N. Story

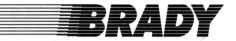

Prehospital Emergency Care

FIFTH EDITION

BRENT Q. HAFEN, Ph.D.
Professor, Department of Health Sciences
Brigham Young University
Provo, Utah

KEITH J. KARREN, Ph.D.
Chairperson, Department of Health Sciences
Brigham Young University
Provo, Utah

JOSEPH J. MISTOVICH, M.Ed., NREMT-P
Assistant Professor of Allied Health
Director of Emergency Medical Technology
Youngstown State University
Youngstown, Ohio

MEDICAL EDITOR
HOWARD A. WERMAN, M.D.

BRADY
Prentice Hall
Upper Saddle River, New Jersey, 07458

ABOUT THE WRITERS

Beth Lothrop Adams, MA, RN, NREMT-P, is ALS Coordinator, EMS Degree Program, and Adjunct Assistant Professor of Emergency Medicine at The George Washington University.
Edward B. Kuvlesky, NREMT-P, is Captain, Indian River County EMS, Indian River County, Florida.
Craig N. Story, EMT-P, is EMS Program Director, Polk Community College, Winter Haven, Florida.

PUBLISHER: Susan Katz
MARKETING MANAGER: Judy Streger
MANAGING PRODUCTION EDITOR: Patrick Walsh
PRODUCTION AND COMPOSITION: Navta Associates
MANAGING DEVELOPMENT EDITOR: Lois Berlowitz
PROJECT EDITOR: Sandra Breuer
COVER PHOTOGRAPHS: Ken Kerr (left), Richard Logan (right)
DIRECTOR OF MANUFACTURING & PRODUCTION: Bruce Johnson
MANUFACTURING BUYER: Ilene Sanford
EDITORIAL ASSISTANT: Carol Sobel
PRINTER/BINDER: Banta, Harrisonburg, VA

Prentice-Hall International (UK) Limited, *London*
Prentice-Hall of Australia Pty. Limited, *Sydney*
Prentice-Hall Canada Inc., *Toronto*
Prentice-Hall Hispanoamericana, S.A., *Mexico*
Prentice-Hall of India Private Limited, *New Delhi*
Prentice-Hall of Japan, Inc., *Tokyo*
Simon & Schuster Asia Pte. Ltd., *Singapore*
Editora Prentice-Hall do Brasil, Ltda., *Rio de Janeiro*

NOTICE ON CARE PROCEDURES

This workbook reflects current EMS practices based on the 1994 U.S. Department of Transportation's EMT-Basic National Standard Curriculum. It is the intent of the authors and publisher that this workbook be used as part of a formal Emergency Medical Technician education program taught by qualified instructors and supervised by a licensed physician. The procedures described in this workbook are based upon consultation with EMS and medical authorities. The authors and publisher have taken care to make certain that these procedures reflect currently accepted clinical practice; however, they cannot be considered absolute recommendations.

The material in this workbook contains the most current information available at the time of publication. However, federal, state, and local guidelines concerning clinical practices, including, without limitation, those governing infection control and body substance isolation precautions, change rapidly. The reader should note, therefore, that new regulations may require changes in some procedures.

It is the responsibility of the reader to familiarize himself or herself with the policies and procedures set by federal, state, and local agencies as well as the institution or agency where the reader may be employed. The authors and the publisher of this workbook disclaim any liability, loss, or risk resulting directly or indirectly from the suggested procedures and theory, from any undetected errors, or from the reader's misunderstanding of the text. It is the reader's responsibility to stay informed of any new changes or recommendations made by any federal, state, or local agency as well as by his or her employing institution or agency.

If when reading this workbook you find an error, have an idea for how to improve it, or simply want to share your comments with us, please send your letter to the authors at

Brady Marketing Department
c/o Judy Streger
Prentice Hall
One Lake Street
Upper Saddle River, NJ 07458

CONTENTS

MODULE 6:
INFANTS AND CHILDREN

MODULE 7:
OPERATIONS

MODULE 8:
ADVANCED AIRWAY
ELECTIVE

INTRODUCTION

Welcome to the workbook that accompanies *Prehospital Emergency Care, 5th Edition*. This is a self-instructional workbook, written to follow up on key concepts presented in the textbook. You can work on the chapters at your own pace and monitor your progress and understanding by checking the answer key and rereading the text pages indicated in the key.

Each chapter is divided into five major sections. The first section, ***Cognitive Objectives***, lists the cognitive objectives from the U.S. Department of Transportation's 1994 *Emergency Medical Technician-Basic: National Standard Curriculum* that relate to that chapter. (These objectives are also listed at the beginning of the corresponding textbook chapter.) The second section, ***Key Ideas***, summarizes the chapter and lists key concepts. The third section, ***Terms and Concepts***, reviews major terms that were introduced in bold type in the textbook chapter and are listed at the end of the textbook chapter. The fourth section, ***Content Review***, asks a series of questions to review and reinforce your understanding of key information and concepts from the chapter. The final section, ***Case Study***, presents one or more realistic scenarios, situations like those you may encounter on real emergency calls, and requires you to apply chapter information to solving patient management problems.

The emphasis is on multiple-choice questions (with a few fill-ins here and there) because this is the format of most standardized tests, such as a state or national exam. The Course Review Self Test (150 items covering all of the chapters in the text) is entirely in multiple-choice format. The test items for the various chapters are in scrambled order (not the same order as the chapters in the text) as they might be on a major standardized or national test. However, the chapter each item comes from and the page on which the information was covered is, again, identifiable by consulting the answer key for the Self Test.

The authors and the publisher welcome any comments you may have regarding this workbook or ideas for improving it. We ask that you please address your comments to the publisher. Good luck with your studies as you train to be an EMT-B.

Beth Lothrop Adams
Ed Kuvlesky
Craig Story

COGNITIVE OBJECTIVES

Numbered objectives are from the United States Department of Transportation 1994 EMT-Basic National Standard Curriculum. Asterisked objectives, if any, pertain to material that is supplemental to the DOT curriculum.

1-1.1   Define Emergency Medical Services (EMS) systems.

1-1.2   Differentiate the roles and responsibilities of the EMT-Basic from other prehospital care providers.

1-1.3   Describe the roles and responsibilities related to personal safety.

1-1.4   Discuss the roles and responsibilities of the EMT-Basic toward the safety of the crew, the patient, and bystanders.

1-1.5   Define quality improvement and discuss the EMT-Basic's role in the process.

1-1.6   Define medical direction and discuss the EMT-Basic's role in the process.

1-1.7   State the specific statutes and regulations in your state regarding the EMS system.

KEY IDEAS

This chapter describes the EMS system and the roles and responsibilities of the EMT-Basic. Emphasis is placed upon the personal safety of the EMT-Basic and the safety of other rescuers.

▶ Prehospital care is provided by the EMS (Emergency Medical Services) system. Each state manages its EMS system in its own way but using federal guidelines.

▶ EMS, fire, and law enforcement services may be accessed in many areas by the universal access number 9-1-1, in other areas by non-9-1-1 numbers.

▶ The four levels of emergency medical technician training are: First Responder, EMT-Basic, EMT-Intermediate, and EMT-Paramedic.

▶ The health care system includes the EMS system, hospital emergency departments, and specialized critical care facilities such as trauma or burn centers.

CHAPTER

1

INTRODUCTION TO EMERGENCY MEDICAL CARE

▶ The responsibilities of the EMT-B include personal safety, the safety of others, patient assessment and emergency medical care, safe lifting and moving, transport and transfer, record keeping and data collection, and patient advocacy. Your first priority is your own safety, then the safety of other rescuers. Once the scene is safe, the patient's needs are your priority.

▶ The professional attributes required of the EMT-B are knowledge and skills, a professional appearance, good health, a pleasant temperament, leadership abilities, good judgment, moral character, stability, and adaptability.

▶ Every EMS system must have a physician medical director who is legally responsible for the clinical and patient care aspects of the system.

▶ The goal of quality improvement is to identify aspects of the system that can be improved and to implement programs to improve identified shortcomings.

TERMS AND CONCEPTS

1. **Write the number of the correct term next to each definition.**

    1. EMS system
    2. EMT-Basic
    3. EMT-Intermediate
    4. EMT-Paramedic
    5. First Responder
    6. prehospital care

    _____ **a.** One who is trained in all aspects of prehospital care including intravenous lines, administering medications, decompressing chest injuries, reading electrocardiograms, and manual defibrillation

    _____ **b.** The first person on the scene who has emergency care training

    _____ **c.** An organization that coordinates emergency care as part of the continuum of health care

    _____ **d.** Care provided prior to transport to the hospital

    _____ **e.** One who is certified to perform some (but not all) advanced prehospital emergency care skills

    _____ **f.** One who performs skills in three areas: controlling life threatening situations, stabilizing non-life threats, and non-medical skills such as driving. Has completed a 110-hour course and is certified by the state EMS Division

CONTENT REVIEW

1. The roles and responsibilities of the EMT-B include
    a. Insertion of intravenous lines
    b. Controlling life-threatening situations
    c. Decompressing the chest cavity
    d. Reading and interpreting electrocardiograms

2. The EMT-B's responsibilities for scene safety include
   a. Personal safety first, then other rescuers'/bystanders' safety, then patient safety
   b. Other rescuers'/bystanders' safety first, then personal safety, then patient safety
   c. Personal safety first; the EMT-B has no responsibility for the safety of others
   d. Patient safety first, then other rescuers'/bystanders' safety, then personal safety

3. From the following list, select the items that are potential hazards that may be present at an emergency scene.

   1. A poorly lit, high traffic area
   2. A car leaking gasoline
   3. A chemical spill
   4. A crime scene

   a. 2, 3
   b. 2, 4
   c. 1, 2, 3, 4
   d. 1, 2, 3

4. List two ways the EMT-B can reduce the risk of being struck by traffic at nighttime scenes.

   a.

   b.

5. You are responding to the scene of a shooting. The dispatcher advises you that law enforcement is also responding. On arrival you observe a large crowd of people who appear to be fighting. The patient is lying next to the crowd. Law enforcement has not yet arrived. You should next
   a. Be alert to any threat and approach the patient
   b. Retreat to a safe area and await law enforcement arrival
   c. Exit the vehicle and await law enforcement arrival
   d. Remain in the vehicle and await law enforcement arrival

6. A process of internal and external reviews and audits of all aspects of an emergency medical system is called
   a. Chart review
   b. Quality improvement
   c. Medical command
   d. Medical control

7. The EMT-B must wear protective equipment to decrease the risks of infectious disease exposure. The protective clothing most commonly worn for this purpose includes
   a. Leather gloves, hard hat, eye protection, boots
   b. Latex gloves, eye protection, mask, gown
   c. Turnout gear, helmet, boots, mask
   d. Leather gloves, helmet, boots, and self-contained breathing apparatus

8. During a routine physical examination, your personal physician informs you that he is interested in becoming the medical director for the service that you work for. He asks you to describe the medical director's responsibilities. List two of the important responsibilities.

   a.

   b.

9. Which of the following statements best describes the relationship between the EMT-B and the EMS system medical director?
   a. The prehospital care rendered by the EMT-B is not governed or controlled by the medical director.
   b. All care rendered by the EMT-B is considered an extension of the medical director's authority.
   c. The in-hospital care rendered by the EMT-B is considered an extension of the medical director's authority.
   d. The medical director advises the on-scene paramedic who guides the EMT-B.

10. To be effective as an EMT-B you must have the personality characteristics that are listed below. Using a 1–5 ranking system (5 is the highest), rate your own personality characteristics.

    Personal rank:

    _____ Pleasant personality (ability to get along with others, reassuring calming voice and manner)

    _____ Leadership ability (takes control, sets priorities, able to give clear directions)

    _____ Good judgment (able to make appropriate decisions quickly in unsafe or stressful conditions)

    _____ Good moral character (high ethical standards)

    _____ Stability (able to deal with feelings openly and honestly)

    _____ Adaptability (able to adapt to change quickly)

11. The EMT-B is responsible for the patient's privacy and valuables. The EMT-B should also honor patient requests as possible. The term that best describes these responsibilities is
    a. EMS advocacy
    b. Patient's rights
    c. EMS rights
    d. Patient advocacy

12. 9-1-1 is frequently called the "Universal Number." What services can generally be accessed by calling 9-1-1?
    a. Law enforcement and fire services only
    b. Law enforcement and EMS only
    c. Law enforcement, EMS, and fire services
    d. Fire services and EMS only

CASE STUDY

▼

It's 1 o'clock in the morning and you have been dispatched to a single-vehicle auto crash. You wipe the sleep from your eyes and prepare to respond to the call. The dispatcher informs you that law enforcement is on scene and there is one patient who has a possible head injury. A fire/rescue truck is also responding to the call. The car has struck a power pole just over the top of a steep hill.

1. Which has the primary responsibility for traffic control at this scene?
   a Fire/rescue department
   b. EMS/ambulance service
   c. Power company
   d. Law enforcement

2. Which has the primary responsibility for extrication/rescue at this scene?
   a Fire/rescue department
   b. EMS/ambulance service
   c. Power company
   d. Law enforcement

3. Which has the primary responsibility for patient care and transport?
   a. Fire/rescue department
   b. EMS/ambulance service
   c. Power company
   d. Law enforcement

   Law enforcement is on scene controlling traffic as you arrive. The fire/rescue crew and power company have stabilized potential hazards. You evaluate the patient and determine that he has minor injuries and is in stable condition. While you are transporting the patient to the hospital, the patient asks you to please call his wife and let her know he is "OK." The patient is stabilized and prepared for transport to a local hospital.

4. Which statement best describes the most appropriate action to take in response to the patient's request to call his wife and explain what has happened?
   a. Contact the police and let them call his wife.
   b. Contact your supervisor and let the supervisor call his wife.
   c. Explain that this is not a part of your responsibilities.
   d. Call the patient's wife and explain what has happened.

5. What information could be used by the EMS system administration for quality improvement audits on this call?
   a. Prehospital care report of call
   b. Feedback from crews on scene
   c. Feedback from the patient involved
   d. a, b, and c

6. Which of the following is a potential hazard (or hazards) at this scene?
   a. Highway traffic
   b. Gasoline leak
   c. Power lines
   d. a, b, and c

CHAPTER 2

THE WELL-BEING OF THE EMT-BASIC

COGNITIVE OBJECTIVES

Numbered objectives are from the United States Department of Transportation 1994 EMT-Basic National Standard Curriculum. Asterisked objectives, if any, pertain to material that is supplemental to the DOT curriculum.

1-2.1   List possible emotional reactions that the EMT-Basic may experience when faced with trauma, illness, death, and dying.

1-2.2   Discuss the possible reactions that a family member may exhibit when confronted with death and dying.

1-2.4   State the steps in the EMT-Basic's approach to the family confronted with death and dying.

1-2.4   State the possible reactions that the family of the EMT-Basic may exhibit due to their outside involvement in EMS.

1-2.5   Recognize the signs and symptoms of critical incident stress.

1-2.6   State possible steps that the EMT-Basic may take to help reduce/alleviate stress.

1-2.7   Explain the need to determine scene safety.

1-2.8   Discuss the importance of body substance isolation (BSI).

1-2.9   Describe the steps the EMT-Basic should take for personal protection from airborne and bloodborne pathogens.

1-2.10 List the personal protective equipment necessary for each of the following situations:

—— Hazardous materials

—— Rescue operations

—— Violent scenes

—— Crime scenes

—— Exposure to bloodborne pathogens

—— Exposure to airborne pathogens

KEY IDEAS

This chapter provides an overview of ways you can safeguard your emotional and physical well-being while providing emergency care.

▶ Your ability to recognize and effectively deal with stressful situations is as essential for your well-being as it is for that of your patients and their family members.

► The highly charged environment of emergency care requires that you recognize the warning signs of stress and remedy them before stress results in burnout.

► Scene safety includes practicing body substance isolation to protect yourself from infectious disease and following proper rescue techniques to prevent accidental injury.

TERMS AND CONCEPTS

1. Write the number of the correct term next to each definition.

   1. burnout
   2. critical incident stress debriefing (CISD)
   3. body substance isolation (BSI)
   4. sterilization
   5. personal protective equipment

   _____ a. State of exhaustion, irritability, and fatigue
   _____ b. Strict infection control measures based on the presumption that all blood and body fluids are infectious
   _____ c. Session in which a team of counselors help rescuers deal with an emotionally difficult experience
   _____ d. Items worn to guard against injury or disease transmission
   _____ e. Use of chemical or physical substances to kill all surface microorganisms

CONTENT REVIEW

1. Generally, patients and their families may cope with death or dying by experiencing the following five emotional stages: _____, anger, bargaining, _____, and acceptance.

2. You are at the scene with a patient who is dying. Describe three things you might do to help the patient and family members cope.

3. As an EMT-Basic, you should be alert to recognize warning signs of stress. Which of the following may signal stress?
   a. Irritability, loss of appetite, loss of interest in work
   b. Desire to be left alone, difficulty sleeping, indecisiveness
   c. Anxiety, guilt, loss of sexual desire
   d. All of these are signs of stress.

4. _____ is a session held prior to a critical incident stress debriefing for rescuers most directly involved to provide an opportunity to vent emotions.

5. Microorganisms (such as bacteria or viruses) that can spread disease by contact with blood, inhalation of airborne droplets, or contaminated objects are called

_____.

6. Which of the following is considered to be the single most important way to prevent the spread of infection?
   a. Handwashing
   b. Sterilizing reusable equipment
   c. Bagging contaminated laundry
   d. Placing sharp objects in a container

7. You should usually call for assistance from _____ before attempting rescue or patient care in a situation involving a life-threatening danger.

8. Arrange the following steps in logical and proper order (1–5) for providing emergency care at a scene involving possible hazardous materials.

_____   a. Provide patient assessment and emergency care.

_____   b. Look for and compare placards or signs to the *DOT Hazardous Materials: The Emergency Response Guidebook.*

_____   c. Make sure the scene is controlled by a specialized hazardous materials team before you enter.

_____   d. Use binoculars to try to identify hazards before approaching the scene.

_____   e. Put on appropriate protective clothing, such as a self-contained breathing apparatus and a "hazmat" suit.

9. If you suspect potential violence at an emergency scene, you should
   a. Request law enforcement assistance before entering the scene
   b. Enter cautiously and call for law enforcement assistance if needed
   c. First remove patients from the scene and then call for police assistance
   d. First secure the scene and then begin patient assessment and care

10. If you are providing emergency care at a crime scene, you should take precautions to preserve the chain of evidence by
   a. Waiting to start treatment until all evidence has been collected by police
   b. Avoiding disturbing the scene unless necesssary to provide care
   c. Immediately removing the patient from the scene to begin care
   d. Contacting medical direction for permission to enter the scene

CASE STUDY

You have been called to a scene at a railroad yard where one of the workmen is trapped from the waist down between two rail cars. Specialty rescue teams are en route and the patient's wife, who has been called by his co-worker, has just arrived at the scene. Your patient is responsive and in stable condition. He tells you that he knows that as soon as they separate the cars he will die. He asks that you leave him alone with his wife and that you do nothing heroic to try to intervene.

1. Of the five stages of emotional response to death and dying, which stage does your patient seem to be exhibiting to his imminent death?

2. What should you do now?

As predicted, as soon as the cars are separated, your patient rapidly loses responsiveness and becomes pulseless and apneic. He has sustained massive open crush injuries to his abdomen and pelvis. There is nothing that can be done to save his life and he dies. In the days following this incident, you begin to have trouble sleeping and often have nightmares. You are having trouble concentrating, and your heart pounds every time you get dispatched on a call.

3. What should you do?

COGNITIVE OBJECTIVES

Numbered objectives are from the United States Department of Transportation 1994 EMT-Basic National Standard Curriculum. Asterisked objectives, if any, pertain to material that is supplemental to the DOT curriculum.

1-3.1 Define the EMT-Basic scope of practice.

1-3.2 Discuss the importance of Do Not Resuscitate (DNR) (advance directives) and local or state provisions regarding EMS application.

1-3.3 Define consent and discuss the methods of obtaining consent.

1-3.4 Differentiate between expressed and implied consent.

1-3.5 Explain the role of consent of minors in providing care.

1-3.6 Discuss the implications for the EMT-Basic in patient refusal of transport.

1-3.7 Discuss the issues of abandonment, negligence, and battery and their implications to the EMT-Basic.

1-3.8 State the conditions necessary for the EMT-Basic to have a duty to act.

1-3.9 Explain the importance, necessity, and legality of patient confidentiality.

1-3.10 Discuss the considerations of the EMT-Basic in issues of organ retrieval.

1-3.11 Differentiate the actions that an EMT-Basic should take to assist in the preservation of a crime scene.

1-3.12 State the conditions that require an EMT-Basic to notify local law enforcement.

KEY IDEAS

The EMT-Basic provides patient care in an increasingly complex legal and ethical environment. Important ethical and legal concepts are described in this chapter.

▶ The EMT-Basic's scope of practice is determined by the National Standard Curriculum, state law, and the EMS system's medical director.

▶ The EMT-Basic's legal right to function is contingent upon medical direction.

▶ An advance directive is also known as a living will or Do Not Resuscitate (DNR) order. As a general rule you should begin resuscitative efforts when you are unsure as to the validity of an advance directive.

▶ Permission to care for a patient is called consent. You must obtain consent from every patient prior to treatment. There are three forms of consent: expressed, implied, and minor/mentally incompetent consent.

▶ A competent adult has the right to refuse treatment. The competent adult must be informed of and understand potential risks in refusing treatment or transportation.

▶ Document refusals of care completely and accurately. Make sure the patient is competent and not under the influence of drugs or alcohol, consult medical direction, and try again to persuade the patient to accept treatment prior to departing the scene.

▶ Your obligation to provide care for a patient is called the "duty to act."

▶ Four items must be demonstrated in a successful negligence action. (1) The EMT-Basic had a duty to act. (2) A patient was injured. (3) The EMT-Basic provided an inappropriate standard of care. (4) The EMT-Basic's action (or inaction) caused or contributed to the injury.

▶ Information obtained when treating a patient must be kept confidential.

▶ Appropriate crime scene actions include: Touch/move only what is required to care for the patient, document anything unusual, do not cut through knots or bullet or stab holes in the patient's clothing, and preserve evidence in sexual assault cases.

▶ Law enforcement should be notified in cases of abuse, injuries related to a crime, and drug-related injuries. Follow your state laws.

▶ When dealing with difficult legal or ethical issues, always put the welfare of the patient first.

TERMS AND CONCEPTS

1. **Write the number of the correct term next to each definition.**
    1. scope of practice
    2. advance directive
    3. duty to act
    4. minor consent
    5. expressed consent
    6. implied consent

_____ **a.** Permission obtained from a parent or legal guardian for emergency treatment of a patient who is under legal age or who is a mentally incompetent adult

_____ **b.** Assumes an unresponsive patient would agree to emergency treatment

_____ **c.** Permission which must be obtained from every conscious, mentally competent adult before emergency treatment may be provided

_____ **d.** Written instructions regarding future resuscitation and care, such as living wills and DNR orders

_____ **e.** The obligation to care for a patient who requires it

_____ **f.** The actions and care that are legally allowed to be provided by an EMT-Basic

CONTENT REVIEW

1. The EMT-Basic's scope of practice is determined by all of the following EXCEPT
   a. Local and/or state laws
   b. Federal laws
   c. National Standard Curriculum
   d. System medical director

2. On a call, you begin to dress the severely bleeding wound of a patient who has told you to go away and leave her alone. You can legally be charged with
   a. Rape
   b. Negligence
   c. Abandonment
   d. Battery

3. A law that provides some protection from liability for emergency care performed in good faith is called a
   a. Code of ethics
   b. Malpractice act
   c. Good Samaritan law
   d. Emergency care statute

4. Emergency care that is expected of any EMT-Basic under similar circumstances is known as
   a. Standard of care
   b. Code of care
   c. Patient care guidelines
   d. Emergency care guidelines

5. Under the law, to care for a patient you must receive
   a. Consent from the wife or husband of the patient
   b. The patient's expressed or implied consent
   c. Prior consent from medical direction
   d. Consent that is written and witnessed

6. A 10-year-old is critically injured. The parents cannot be located. Treatment can be initiated under which form of consent?
   a. Implied consent
   b. Expressed consent
   c. Minor consent
   d. Incapacitated person consent

7. Under the law, in order to refuse treatment a *patient* must meet which of the following requirements?

   1. Be mentally competent
   2. Be informed of and understand the risks and consequences of refusal
   3. Be free of any life-threatening injuries or conditions
   4. Sign a form releasing the EMT-Basic from liability
   5. Have a witness to the refusal of treatment

a. 1, 2, and 4
b. 1, 2, 3, 4, and 5
c. 1 and 2
d. 2, 4, and 5

8. Which of the following is considered a valid indication of refusal of care?
   a. Shaking the head no before treatment begins
   b. Pushing you away after treatment has begun
   c. Both a and b
   d. Neither a nor b

9. Stopping care without ensuring that another health care professional with equivalent or better training will take over is called
   a. Neglect
   b. Abandonment
   c. Refusal
   d. Battery

10. Confidential patient information may be released only under certain circumstances. Which of the follow is NOT one of these circumstances?
    a. While off-duty, another EMT-Basic asks you about patient care information.
    b. You are requested to provide patient information by the police as part of a potential criminal investigation.
    c. The information is required on a third-party insurance billing form.
    d. A health care provider needs to know in order to continue medical care.

CASE STUDY 1

It's 4 o'clock in the morning, and you have been dispatched to care for a patient complaining of chest pain. Upon arrival you observe a male patient who appears to be in his mid 60s. He looks pale and sweaty. However, he appears to be alert and is able to give you his name, address, day of the week, and time of day. He describes his pain as severe but refuses to be treated or transported to the hospital. You describe the need for medical care to the patient. While you are explaining this information to him he repeatedly cups his hand behind his ear and asks, "What? What are you telling me?" Unexpectedly, your partner asks the patient to sign a refusal-of-care release form. The patient signs the form quickly and hands it back. Your partner looks at you and says, "Let's go!"

1. What are the important concerns you should have relating to this patient's refusal of treatment?
   1. The patient's mental competence
   2. The patient's understanding of the possible consequences of refusal
   3. The patient's signing the release without reading it
   4. Lack of professional courtesy if you "second-guess" your partner's suggestion to go

a. 1 and 2
b. 2 and 3
c. 3 and 4
d. 1, 2, 3, and 4

2. Your next action in the situation described above should be to
   a. Leave as soon as the refusal form has been signed
   b. Encourage the patient to seek help if additional symptoms develop
   c. Have a witness sign the refusal form along with the patient
   d. Try again to persuade the patient to accept treatment

CASE STUDY 2

You are employed as an EMT-Basic for a public EMS agency. Your partner, Joe, and you are dispatched to a call for a child who is choking. You are dispatched at 3:00 PM. You have about a 10-block response to the scene. En route, your unit runs out of gas. You look at Joe. Joe gives you a blank stare and says, "I guess I forgot to fill it up!" A secondary unit responds to the call and arrives in 10 minutes. You learn later that the secondary unit arrived on scene and quickly removed a piece of hot dog from the child's airway. The child suffered permanent brain damage as a result of this incident.

1. Listed below are four items that must be demonstrated to be successful in a negligence action. Place a Y for yes or an N for no next to each item to determine if negligence occurred in this case.

   _____ a. The EMT-Basics had a duty to act.

   _____ b. The patient was injured.

   _____ c. The EMT-Basics violated the standard of care reasonably expected of an EMT-Basic with similar background and training.

   _____ d. The EMT-Basics' action or lack of action in violating the standard of care caused or contributed to the patient's injury.

COGNITIVE OBJECTIVES

▼

Numbered objectives are from the United States Department of Transportation 1994 EMT-Basic National Standard Curriculum. Asterisked objectives, if any, pertain to material that is supplemental to the DOT curriculum.

1-4.1 Identify the following topographic terms: medial, lateral, proximal, distal, superior, inferior, anterior, posterior, midline, right and left, midclavicular, bilateral, and midaxillary.

1-4.2 Describe the anatomy and function of the following major body systems: respiratory, circulatory, musculoskeletal, nervous, and endocrine.

* Identify and define other common descriptive anatomical terms.

* Describe the anatomy and function of the skin.

KEY IDEAS

▼

This chapter introduces basic terminology and concepts of the anatomy and physiology of the human body — information you will need to help you determine when the body is functioning normally and when it is not, and to help you communicate with other health care providers.

▶ The EMT-B must be able to identify the following positions: *normal anatomical position, supine, prone, lateral recumbent, Fowler's,* and *Trendelenburg.*

▶ The EMT-B must be able to define descriptive terms such as *midline, midclavicular line, midaxillary line, plantar,* and *palmar.*

▶ The EMT-B must be able to define the terms *anterior, superior, dorsal, lateral, distal* and their opposites, *posterior, inferior, ventral, medial,* and *proximal.*

▶ The EMT-B must be able to understand and describe the anatomy and physiology of the following body systems: musculoskeletal, respiratory, circulatory, nervous, endocrine, and the skin.

▶ The EMT-B must be able to identify and locate the central and peripheral pulse points.

THE HUMAN BODY

TERMS AND CONCEPTS

1. In each space, write the term described by the statement. Not all terms will be used.

anterior   midline

distal   normal anatomical position

inferior   posterior

lateral   prone

medial   superior

midaxillary   transverse line

midclavicular

_____ a. An imaginary line drawn horizontally through the waist to divide the body into superior and inferior planes

_____ b. The back or toward the back

_____ c. Lying on the stomach

_____ d. Above, toward the head

_____ e. Position in which the patient is standing erect, facing forward, with arms down at the sides and palms forward

_____ f. Refers to the center of the armpit

_____ g. Below, toward the feet

_____ h. Refers to the side, left or right of the midline, or away from the midline of the body

_____ i. The front or toward the front

_____ j. Distant or far from the point of reference

_____ k. An imaginary line drawn vertically through the middle of the patient's body, dividing it into right and left planes

CONTENT REVIEW

1. When you are describing an injury to the right chest, *right* refers to
   a. Your right, while facing the patient
   b. Your right, while facing away from the patient
   c. The patient's right, regardless of position
   d. None of the above

2. Fill in each term of direction on the appropriate line.

anterior   midline
distal   palmar
inferior   plantar
lateral   posterior
medial   proximal
midaxillary   superior

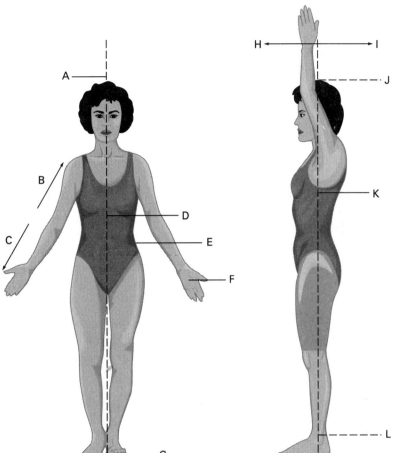

A _____

B _____

C _____

D _____

E _____

F _____

G _____

H _____

I _____

J _____

K _____

L _____

3. The emergency department physician confirms that your patient has sustained *bilateral femur* fracture. This would indicate
   a. Both right and left thigh bones are fractured
   b. Both right and left forearm bones are fractured
   c. There are two fractures of one forearm bone
   d. There are two fractures of one thigh bone

4. Describing the location of your patient's burns as *posterior thigh* would indicate
   a. The back of the thigh
   b. The front of the thigh
   c. On the inner side of the thigh
   d. On the outer side of the thigh

5. You place a patient on his side so fluids can drain from his mouth. In what position have you placed him?
   a. Supine
   b. Prone
   c. Lateral recumbent or recovery position
   d. Fowler's position

6. The section of the spinal column that the ribs are attached to is the
   a. Cervical spine
   b. Lumbar spine
   c. Sacral spine
   d. Thoracic spine

7. Which section of the spine is most prone to injury?
   a. Cervical spine
   b. Lumbar spine
   c. Sacral spine
   d. Thoracic spine

8. Shoulder and hip joints are _____, the kind of joint that permits the widest range of motion.
   a. Hinged joints
   b. Condyloid joint
   c. Gliding joints
   d. Ball and socket joints

9. Which muscle type is responsible for deliberate movements such as walking and chewing?
   a. Cardiac muscles
   b. Involuntary muscles
   c. Voluntary muscles
   d. Smooth muscles

10. In the unresponsive patient what anatomical structure may not work properly, permitting vomit or other liquids to enter the trachea?
    a. Diaphragm
    b. Epiglottis
    c. Bronchi
    d. Larynx

11. What occurs when the diaphragm and the intercostal muscles contract, increasing the size of the thoracic cavity?
    a. Air flows out of the lungs; exhalation.
    b. Air flows into the lungs; inhalation.
    c. Air flows rapidly in, then out in a sneeze.
    d. Air flows out in an involuntary cough.

12. Which of the following is NOT true about infants and young children as compared to adults?
    a. The infant or child's trachea is narrower.
    b. The infant or child's tongue takes up proportionately less space in the pharynx.
    c. Infants and children rely more heavily on the diaphragm for breathing.
    d. The infant or child's head is larger in proportion to the body.

13. Inadequate breathing for the adult patient may be characterized by
    a. Warm, dry skin
    b. Rate of 12 to 20 breaths per minute
    c. Equal chest expansion
    d. Use of accessory muscles during breathing

14. Fill in each skeletal term on the appropriate line.

A _____
B _____
C _____
D _____
E _____
F _____
G _____
H _____
I _____
J _____
K _____
L _____
M _____
N _____
O _____
P _____
Q _____
R _____
S _____
T _____
U _____
V _____
W _____
X _____
Y _____
Z _____
AA _____
BB _____
CC _____
DD _____
EE _____
FF _____
GG _____
HH _____
II _____

calcaneus	frontal bone	occipital bone	sternum
carpals	greater trochanter	patella	symphysis pubis
cervical vertebra	humerus	parietal bone	tarsals
clavicle	iliac crest	pelvic girdle	temporal bone
coccyx	ilium	phalanges	tibia
cranium	maxilla	radius	ulna
elbow	mandible	ribs	xiphoid process
femur	metacarpals	sacrum	zygomatic bone
fibula	metatarsals	scapula	

15. Carbon dioxide is exchanged for oxygen through the walls of the capillaries at the
    a. Alveoli and cells
    b. Alveoli and bronchi
    c. Arteries and veins
    d. Bronchi and cells

16. The heart is comprised of four chambers. The two upper chambers, called (1) _____, receive blood from the veins. The two lower chambers, called (2) _____, pump blood out to the arteries.
    a. (1) pericardium, (2) myocardium
    b. (1) arterioles, (2) venules
    c. (1) aortas, (2) valves
    d. (1) atria, (2) ventricles

17. Which component of the blood is responsible for defending against infection?
    a. Platelets
    b. Plasma
    c. Red blood cells
    d. White blood cells

18. Pulses felt at different points on the body are classified as central or peripheral. Which of the following is considered to be a central pulse?
    a. Radial
    b. Brachial
    c. Carotid
    d. Tibial

19. The delivery of oxygen and other nutrients to the cells, through adequate circulation of blood through the capillaries, is known as
    a. Diastolic circulation
    b. Systolic circulation
    c. Hypoperfusion
    d. Perfusion

20. The central nervous system consists of which of the following?
    a. Brain and spinal cord
    b. Brain and heart
    c. Heart and lungs
    d. Spinal cord and vertebrae

21. Which is considered to be the master gland, located at the base of the brain?
    a. Adrenal
    b. Pituitary
    c. Thyroid
    d. Parathyroid

22. Which of the following is true concerning the skin?
    a. The epidermis contains the blood vessels, sweat glands, oil glands, and nerves.
    b. The skin consists of three layers with the epidermis consisting of mostly fatty tissue.
    c. The skin is the second largest organ of the body and consists of two layers, the epidermis being the thickest layer.
    d. The skin is the largest organ of the body, protects the body against bacteria, and regulates temperature.

CASE STUDY

You are a student EMT-B riding with an ambulance unit. At 1400 hours the unit is dispatched to a car-versus-tree crash. As you approach the scene, you notice a heavily damaged auto. The scene appears to be under control by police and rescue personnel. The experienced EMT-Bs remind you to wear your body substance isolation gear. You find the patient lying supine with a police officer supporting his neck.

1. Define the supine position.

The patient appears to be unresponsive. The senior EMT-B states he has conducted the initial assessment and will manage the airway while his partner retrieves the equipment to stabilize the spine. "You need to do a rapid trauma assessment (head-to-toe exam for obvious injuries)," he tells you. He supervises as you examine the head and neck. Then, as you cut away the patient's shirt, you note a large laceration to the center of the chest area above the nipple on the patient's right, your left as you face him. Further examination reveals a deformity to the upper arm (patient's left, your right) close to the shoulder.

2. How would you describe the lacerated chest?
   a. Large laceration to the right midclavicular line superior to the right nipple
   b. Large laceration to the right midaxillary line superior to the right nipple
   c. Large laceration to the right midclavicular line inferior to the right nipple
   d. Large laceration to the left midclavicular line superior to the left nipple

3. How would you describe the arm injury?
   a. Deformity to the proximal end of the left humerus
   b. Deformity to the proximal end of the right radius/ulna
   c. Deformity to the proximal end of the left calcaneus
   d. Deformity to the distal end of the left humerus

   After exposing the lower body you find that both right and left thighs are grossly deformed. A puncture wound is found on the left thigh away from the midline and close to the knee.

4. How would you describe the injuries?
   a. Right and left thigh area deformity with a puncture wound to the left medial thigh proximal to the patella
   b. Bilateral femoral region deformity with a puncture wound to the left lateral thigh proximal to the patella
   c. Bilateral femoral region deformity with a puncture wound to the left ventral area distal to the greater trochanter
   d. Bilateral femoral region deformity with a puncture wound to the left dorsal area distal to the patella

After the patient is secured to a spine immobilization device and loaded onto the wheeled stretcher, the senior EMT-B asks you to place the patient into a Trendelenburg position.

5. Describe the Trendelenburg position.

While transporting the patient to the hospital the senior EMT-B commends you on your knowledge of anatomy and anatomical terms.

COGNITIVE OBJECTIVES

CHAPTER 5

BASELINE VITAL SIGNS AND HISTORY TAKING

Numbered objectives are from the United States Department of Transportation 1994 EMT-Basic National Standard Curriculum. Asterisked objectives, if any, pertain to material that is supplemental to the DOT curriculum.

1-5.1   Identify the components of vital signs.

1-5.2   Describe the methods to obtain a breathing rate.

1-5.3   Identify the attributes that should be obtained when assessing breathing.

1-5.4   Differentiate between shallow, labored, and noisy breathing.

1-5.5   Describe the methods to obtain a pulse rate.

1-5.6   Identify the information obtained when assessing a patient's pulse.

1-5.7   Differentiate between a strong, weak, regular, and irregular pulse.

1-5.8   Describe the methods to assess the skin color, temperature, and condition (capillary refill in infants and children).

1-5.9   Identify the normal and abnormal skin colors.

1-5.10 Differentiate between pale, blue, red, and yellow skin color.

1-5.11 Identify the normal and abnormal skin conditions.

1-5.12 Differentiate between hot, cool, and cold skin temperature.

1-5.13 Identify normal and abnormal skin conditions.

1-5.14 Identify normal and abnormal capillary refill in infants and children.

1-5.15 Identify the methods to assess the pupils.

1-5.16 Identify normal and abnormal pupil size.

1-5.17 Differentiate between dilated (big) and constricted (small) pupil size.

1-5.18 Differentiate between reactive and nonreactive pupils and equal and unequal pupils.

1-5.19 Describe the methods to assess blood pressure.

1-5.20 Define systolic pressure.

1-5.21 Define diastolic pressure.

1-5.22 Explain the difference between auscultation and palpation for obtaining a blood pressure.

1-5.23 Identify the components of the SAMPLE history.

1-5.24 Differentiate between a sign and a symptom.

1-5.25 State the importance of accurately reporting and recording the baseline vital signs.

1-5.26 Discuss the need to search for additional medical information.

KEY IDEAS

This chapter focuses on the critical EMT-Basic skills of obtaining a patient history and taking vital signs. These skills are key elements of patient assessment, measuring the patient's response to prehospital emergency care, and providing essential information for hospital personnel.

▶ Baseline vital sign measurements are your first assessments related to breathing; pulse; skin color, condition, and temperature; pupils; and blood pressure. All subsequent measurements of these "signs of life" will be compared to your initial baseline.

▶ Breathing assessments include rate, which is assessed by observing the number of inhalations and exhalations per minute, and quality. Breathing quality refers to how much air is moving in and out with each breath, as well as how well it is moving.

▶ Pulses are pressure waves generated by each heartbeat which can be felt in an artery that is near the skin surface. Pulses are assessed for rate (the number of heartbeats per minute) and quality (strength and regularity).

▶ Skin provides many important clues about the patient's status. When assessing the patient's skin you should note its color, condition, and temperature.

▶ Capillary refill is considered a reliable sign of circulatory status only in infants and children.

▶ The size, equality, and reactivity of the patient's pupils can provide helpful information about what might be wrong with your patient.

▶ Blood pressure is assessed by using a sphygmomanometer to measure the amount of pressure exerted against the arterial walls when the left ventricle of the heart contracts (systolic pressure) and when the left ventricle of the heart is at rest (diastolic pressure). Blood pressure is measured in millimeters of mercury (mmHg).

▶ Vital signs should be taken and recorded as often as necessary to provide proper care. Generally, reassessing vital signs every 15 minutes is reasonable for a stable patient, but an unstable patient should have vital signs taken every 5 minutes.

▶ Obtaining a medical history for your patient can be done easily using the SAMPLE history. SAMPLE is an acronym to remind you to ask about and record information about signs and symptoms, allergies, medications, pertinent past history, last oral intake, and events leading to the injury or illness.

▶ Assessment activities may embarrass your patients or make them anxious, so it is important that you reassure them and make every effort to maintain their dignity.

TERMS AND CONCEPTS

1. **Write the number of the correct term next to each definition.**

   1. auscultation
   2. diastolic blood pressure
   3. palpation
   4. signs
   5. stridor
   6. symptoms
   7. systolic blood pressure

   _____ **a.** A harsh, high pitched airway sound

   _____ **b.** Assessment by listening with a stethoscope

   _____ **c.** Assessment by feeling

   _____ **d.** Conditions that you can observe

   _____ **e.** Pressure in the arteries when the heart's left ventricle contracts

   _____ **f.** Pressure in the arteries when the heart's left ventricle rests

   _____ **g.** Conditions that must be described by the patient

CONTENT REVIEW

1. List the components of vital sign assessment.

2. Breathing is usually assessed by counting the number of respirations
   a. In a 15-second period and multiplying by 4
   b. In a 20-second period and multiplying by 3
   c. In a 30-second period and multiplying by 2
   d. In a 60-second period

3. Normal respiration is characterized by
   a. The use of accessory muscles
   b. Slight motion of the chest or abdominal wall
   c. Increased effort of breathing
   d. Inhalations and exhalations of about the same length

4. Assessing the quality of breathing tells you how much air is moving as well as how well it is moving. An abnormal quality of breathing may be
   a. Shallow
   b. Labored
   c. Noisy
   d. All of these

5. Fill in the name of each pulse on the appropriate line.

brachial

carotid

dorsalis pedis

femoral

posterior tibial

radial

A _____

B _____

C _____

D _____

E _____

F _____

6. To assess your patient's pulse, palpate the artery and count the number of beats
   a. For 15 seconds and multiply by 4
   b. For 20 seconds and multiply by 3
   c. For 30 seconds and multiply by 2
   d. For 60 seconds

7. To assess the pulse of your 6-month-old patient, you should check the _____ pulse.
   a. Carotid
   b. Brachial
   c. Radial
   d. Femoral

8. For the 6-month-old patient, what would be considered a normal pulse rate?
   a. 60 beats per minute
   b. 80 beats per minute
   c. 100 beats per minute
   d. 120 beats per minute

9. In terms of pulse quality, which of the following would be considered normal for an adult?
   a. Weak and irregular at 60 beats per minute
   b. Full and regular at 60 beats per minute
   c. Bounding and irregular at 60 beats per minute
   d. Thready and regular at 60 beats per minute

10. _____ may be a sign of extreme vasoconstriction or blood loss.
   a. Pale conjunctiva
   b. Red nail beds
   c. Blue-gray oral mucosa
   d. Yellow skin

11. To assess the skin of an infant or young child, check color, temperature, condition, and

    _____.

12. Relative skin temperature is assessed by placing _____
    against the patient's skin.

13. Normal skin condition is described as being _____.

14. Normal capillary refill time is _____.

15. To assess the pupils, briefly shine your penlight into your patient's eyes to determine

    _____, _____, and

    _____.

16. Blood pressure is a reflection of the pressure in the
    a. Ventricles
    b. Arteries
    c. Veins
    d. Capillaries

17. Define systolic blood pressure and explain what "sound" determines the systolic pressure.

18. Define diastolic blood pressure and explain what "sound" determines the diastolic pressure.

19. When measuring a patient's blood pressure by auscultation, you need
    a. A sphygmomanometer and your fingertips
    b. A sphygmomanometer and a penlight
    c. A syphygmomanometer and a stethoscope
    d. Only a sphygmomanometer

20. After selecting and applying the proper size sphygmomanometer, arrange the following steps
    for measuring a patient's blood pressure in the proper sequence (1–5).

    _____ Apply the stethoscope to the brachial pulse and deflate the cuff at approximately 2
            mmHg per second.

    _____ Leave the deflated cuff in place so you can take additional readings.

    _____ When you hear two or more consecutive beats, this is the systolic pressure. Record it.

    _____ Continue releasing air until you hear the last sound or until the sound changes from clear
            tapping to soft, muffled tapping. This is the diastolic pressure. Record it.

    _____ Inflate the cuff to 30 mmHg above the point where you no longer feel the radial pulse.

21. In a stable patient, vital signs should be taken and recorded every _____ minutes. In an unstable patient, vital signs should be taken and recorded every _____ minutes.

22. Identify which element of the SAMPLE history applies to each statement below by writing S, A, M, P, L, or E, according to the key.

S sign or symptom

A allergies

M medications

P pertinent past history

L last oral intake

E events leading to the illness or injury

_____ **a.** Medic Alert tag notes "reacts to penicillin."

_____ **b.** Ate large meal two hours ago

_____ **c.** Patient complains of nausea.

_____ **d.** Requires insulin daily to control diabetes

_____ **e.** Diagnosed with emphysema 10 years ago

_____ **f.** Patient has chest pain that radiates down the left arm.

_____ **g.** Mother reports that patient gets rashes from poison ivy.

_____ **h.** Patient was outside shoveling snow.

_____ **i.** Obvious deformity noted in right lower leg.

_____ **j.** Has taken only small amounts of liquids since early morning

_____ **k.** Takes aspirin two to three times each day for pain of arthritis

_____ **l.** Husband says patient has had epilepsy since head injury last year.

CASE STUDY

As you read the following scenario, remember that baseline vital signs and the SAMPLE history are key elements of patient assessment and provide essential information for hospital personnel.

At 10:30 PM, you are dispatched on a call for difficulty breathing. You find your 60-year-old male patient sitting up in bed with his wife at his bedside. Mr. Baker is in obvious distress and reports that he can't breathe. He is breathing at a rate of 26 breaths per minute. He is using accessory muscles, and you hear wheezing and gurgling with each breath. You find that his radial pulse is weak and irregular at a rate of 50 beats per minute. His skin is slightly cyanotic, cool, and moist. Using your penlight, you assess his pupils and find them to be equal, reactive, and of normal size. You auscultate his blood pressure at 80/50 mmHg.

1. How would you describe this patient's respiratory status?

2. What is the significance of his skin color, temperature, and condition?

3. What do his pulse and blood pressure tell you about his circulatory status?

While your partner starts Mr. Baker on high flow oxygen therapy, you begin to get his history from his wife. Mrs. Baker is upset and very worried about her husband. She tells you that he had a heart attack 5 years ago and takes Digoxin (a medication to strengthen his heart's contractions) and Lasix (a water pill) daily. Mr. Baker also occasionally takes nitroglycerin for episodes of chest pain, but she says he denied having chest pain today. Although she told him that he shouldn't, he shoveled snow this morning and since then has been increasingly short of breath. He did not eat supper and only ate a bowl of soup at lunch. Mrs. Baker says that her husband has no allergies.

4. Identify the elements of the SAMPLE history found in this scenario.

5. Based on his status, how frequently should you reassess Mr. Baker's vital signs? Why?

COGNITIVE OBJECTIVES

Numbered objectives are from the United States Department of Transportation 1994 EMT-Basic National Standard Curriculum. Asterisked objectives, if any, pertain to material that is supplemental to the DOT curriculum.

1-6.1 Define body mechanics.

1-6.2 Discuss the guidelines and safety precautions that need to be followed when lifting a patient.

1-6.4 Describe the guidelines and safety precautions for carrying patients and/or equipment.

1-6.5 Discuss one-handed carrying techniques.

1-6.6 Describe correct and safe carrying procedures on stairs.

1-6.7 State the guidelines for reaching and their applications.

1-6.8 Describe correct reaching for log rolls.

1-6.9 State the guidelines for pushing and pulling.

KEY IDEAS

This chapter presents proper methods of lifting and moving patients and equipment. It is not enough to know this material. You need to continuously use the information every day and on every response.

▶ Proper use of body mechanics can greatly decrease injuries. The four basic principles of body mechanics are: (1) Keep the weight of the object close to the body. (2) To lift a heavy object, use leg, hip, and gluteal muscles plus contracted abdominal muscles. (3) "Stack" shoulders over hips, hips over feet. (4) Reduce the height or distance an object must be lifted.

▶ Poor posture can fatigue your back and promote injury.

▶ Communication and teamwork are essential to safe lifting and moving.

▶ It is important to be able to perform the following techniques: power lift, squat lift, one-handed carrying technique, stair-chair technique, reaching techniques, and pushing and pulling techniques.

TERMS AND CONCEPTS

1. **Define each of the following terms.**

   a. body mechanics

   b. power grip

   c. power lift

CONTENT REVIEW

1. You are much more likely to injure your back when performing which task?
   a. Reaching a great distance to lift a light object
   b. Reaching a short distance to lift a heavy object
   c. Reaching up to shoulder height to lift a light object
   d. Lifting a light object while keeping it close to you

2. When moving heavy objects, which muscles will provide the most power with the greatest degree of safety?
   a. Leg, hip, and gluteal muscles
   b. Back and shoulder muscles
   c. Chest and arm muscles
   d. All of the above

3. The body mechanics principle called "stacking" means
   a. Stacking objects to be lifted one on top of the other
   b. Keeping your shoulders, hips, and feet in vertical alignment
   c. Eliminating curvature from your spine
   d. Staying under an object being lifted overhead

4. To help prevent injury and manage stress you should follow a physical fitness program that includes which four ingredients?

5. If you are performing a power lift, which of the following is correct?
   a. Stand to side of object and lift hips before upper body
   b. Turn feet inward, lock knees, and lift hips before upper body
   c. Lock the back and lift upper body before hips
   d. Bend forward at the waist and lift upper body before hips

6. When performing the squat lift with a weak leg or ankle, you should
    a. Place the weaker leg slightly behind your good leg
    b. Place the weaker leg slightly forward of the good leg
    c. Place the weaker leg beside and parallel to the good leg
    d. The squat lift should not be used with a weak leg

7. When using the one-handed carrying technique, avoid
    a. Leaning to the opposite side
    b. Bending your knees
    c. Locking your back
    d. Bending at the hips

8. When you are navigating stairs using a stair chair, you should
    a. Tilt the stair chair forward
    b. Position the patient facing the stairs
    c. Keep one hand on the railing
    d. Use a spotter to direct and navigate

9. If you have to reach for an object that is greater than _____ from your body, you should
   reposition yourself closer to the object.
    a. 5 inches
    b. 10 inches
    c. 20 inches
    d. 3 feet

10. When you need to push or pull an object, which of the following is correct?
    a. Push rather than pull and keep the load at knee level.
    b. Push rather than pull and keep the load between hips and shoulders.
    c. Pull rather than push and keep the load at shoulder level.
    d. Pull rather than push and keep the load at hip level.

CASE STUDY

▼

You and your partner Kyle work in an East coast community and are dispatched to a guarded beach for an injured surfer. As you and Kyle approach the scene, you are met by lifeguard captain Vicky. She explains that the patient has deeply lacerated his leg and will need to be carried across the beach and over the dune line to the parking lot. Fortunately there is a ramp that leads to a boardwalk. A set of stairs connects the boardwalk with the parking lot. Vicky says she has three lifeguards who can assist with moving the patient. Kyle suggests a four-corner carry with the wheeled stretcher in the up position (legs fully extended), thus reducing the chance of dropping the patient. If the carriers need a break, this position will allow the stretcher to be rested on the extended wheels without lowering the patient to ground level, thus reducing the chance of injury. You commend Kyle for his foresight and planning.

1. After the patient has been loaded and you are ready to move him, you instruct the rescuers on the corners of the stretcher to
   a. Keep their backs leaning to the opposite side of the patient to compensate the weight
   b. Keep their backs locked and stay as close to the stretcher as possible, avoiding leaning
   c. Relax their back muscles and bend at the waist to keep the stretcher moving forward
   d. Grip the stretcher handles with only their fingers, avoiding contact between palms and handles

2. As you and the team reach the boardwalk, you instruct them to
   a. Continue to carry the stretcher, because once you are in motion stopping will result in fatigue
   b. Continue to carry the stretcher, because it is important that the patient receive a smooth ride
   c. Lower the stretcher onto its wheels so the stretcher does part of the work, with the rescuers at the back pushing it along the boardwalk
   d. Lower the stretcher onto its wheels so the stretcher does part of the work, with the rescuers at the front pulling it along the boardwalk

3. As you reach the stairs, your team takes a brief break. You instruct your team to lower the stretcher (legs retracted) so the wheels won't catch on the stairs. You should also instruct them to
   a. Have a spotter at the bottom to help guide them
   b. Flex the body at the hips and not the waist
   c. Keep the weight and arms close to the body
   d. All of the above

4. You and Kyle will use the power lift technique to lift the stretcher into the up position. Regarding the power lift, all of the following are correct EXCEPT
   a. This technique is not recommended for use with heavy patients.
   b. This technique offers you the best defense against injury.
   c. This technique protects the patient with a safe and stable move.
   d. This technique is useful for rescuers with weak knees or thighs.

MODULE 1 REVIEW
PREPARATORY: CHAPTERS 1-6

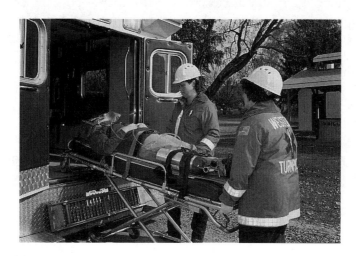

The U.S. Department of Transportation *Emergency Medical Technician-Basic: National Standard Curriculum* is divided into eight modules. The *Prehospital Emergency Care* textbook is divided into modules that correspond to the DOT curriculum modules.

The first module, "Preparatory," is an introduction to the EMS system and some basic concerns, including your safety and well-being as an EMT-B, certain legal and ethical issues, fundamental anatomy and physiology, and essential skills of measuring vital signs and taking a patient history.

Q **The opening chapters made it clear that an EMT-Basic can come in contact with an infectious disease, sustain injury, and get severely stressed out. How worried should I be about these hazards?**

A There certainly are a number of factors that should be taken very seriously. You will be doing a lot of lifting and moving, you will be working at hazardous accident scenes, you will be treating patients who may have infectious diseases, and your job may sometimes be quite stressful. However, by using appropriate protective clothing and equipment, exercising good health and hygiene practices, using the principles of body mechanics, and knowing how to manage stress, you can have a long, safe, and rewarding career in EMS.

Q **What about consent, abandonment, falsification — all those legal issues? Should I be afraid of getting sued?**

A You may be the subject of a lawsuit at some time during your career. However, you have some protection under the Good Samaritan laws, and you are not likely to be *successfully* sued if you do your job to the best of your ability according to the training you have received and if you carefully document every call.

(Module 1 Review continued)

Q **A lot of terminology was taught in Chapter 4. How much medical terminology do I have to know?**

A There is less and less emphasis on use of medical terminology by EMT-Bs. The terms you learned in Chapter 4 are enough to carry you through most situations. The object is to have enough understanding of the human body to be able to perform adequate assessment and emergency care and enough command of terminology to be able to communicate with other health care providers. If you forget a medical term, remember that others will understand you if you make clear use of plain English.

Q **It's hard to remember all those vital signs measurements and history-taking questions that were taught in Chapter 5. Are there any shortcuts?**

A Many EMTs carry basic vital signs ranges and the SAMPLE history questions on quick-reference cards. However, taking vital signs measurements and patient histories are among the most basic functions in of your profession as an EMT-B, and it is best to know this information "cold." Remembering them will get much easier as you practice your skills and gain experience.

AIRWAY MANAGEMENT, VENTILATION, AND OXYGEN THERAPY

COGNITIVE OBJECTIVES

Numbered objectives are from the United States Department of Transportation 1994 EMT-Basic National Standard Curriculum. Asterisked objectives, if any, pertain to material that is supplemental to the DOT curriculum.

2-1.1   Name and label the major structures of the respiratory system on a diagram.

2-1.2   List the signs of adequate breathing.

2-1.3   List the signs of inadequate breathing.

2-1.4   Describe the steps in performing the head-tilt, chin-lift.

2-1.5   Relate the mechanism of injury to opening the airway.

2-1.6   Describe the steps in performing the jaw thrust.

2-1.7   State the importance of having a suction unit ready for immediate use when providing emergency care.

2-1.8   Describe the techniques of suctioning.

2-1.9   Describe how to artificially ventilate a patient with a pocket mask.

2-1.10 Describe the steps in performing the skill of artificially ventilating a patient with a bag-valve mask while using the jaw thrust.

2-1.11 List the parts of the bag-valve mask system.

2-1.12 Describe the steps in performing the skill of artificially ventilating a patient with a bag-valve mask for one and two rescuers.

2-1.13 Describe the signs of adequate artificial ventilation using the bag-valve mask.

2-1.14 Describe the signs of inadequate artificial ventilation using the bag-valve mask.

2-1.15 Describe the steps in artificially ventilating a patient with a flow restricted, oxygen-powered ventilation device.

2-1.16 List the steps in performing the actions taken when providing mouth-to-mouth and mouth-to-stoma artificial ventilation.

2-1.17 Describe how to measure and insert an oropharyngeal (oral) airway.

2-1.18 Describe how to measure and insert a nasopharyngeal (nasal) airway.

2-1.19 Define the components of an oxygen delivery system.

2-1.20 Identify a nonrebreather face mask and state the oxygen flow requirements needed for its use.

2-1.21 Describe the indications for using a nasal cannula versus a nonrebreather face mask.

2-1.22 Identify a nasal cannula and state the flow requirements needed for its use.

KEY IDEAS

▼

In this chapter your knowledge of the respiratory system and airway management will be put to use. After completion of this chapter you should be able to establish and maintain an airway, as well as ensure effective ventilation and oxygen administration. It is important to . . .

▶ Review the anatomy and physiology of the respiratory system in both adults and infants/children.

▶ Understand the two manual methods of opening an airway and explain the circumstances in which each should be used.

▶ Understand that the EMT-B may insert an oropharyngeal or nasopharyngeal airway adjunct to assist in establishing and maintaining an open airway, and understand the circumstances in which they should be used.

▶ Understand how to assess for adequate or inadequate breathing.

▶ Know the methods that the EMT-B can use to artificially ventilate the patient, and understand the advantages and disadvantages of each.

▶ Know the techniques for ventilating patients with and without suspected spinal injury.

▶ Know the signs that indicate the patient is being ventilated adequately.

▶ Describe the appropriate procedure for initiating oxygen therapy, including preparing the equipment, and the steps for discontinuing oxygen administration.

TERMS AND CONCEPTS

▼

1. In each space, write the number of the term described by the statement. Not all terms will be used.

   1. agonal respirations
   2. alveoli
   3. bradypnea
   4. cricoid cartilage
   5. cyanosis
   6. epiglottis
   7. esophagus
   8. hemoglobin
   9. hypoxia
   10. mucous membrane
   11. nasal cannula

   12. nasopharynx
   13. nonrebreather mask
   14. oropharyngeal airway
   15. oropharynx
   16. oxygenated
   17. pleura
   18. retractions
   19. tachypnea
   20. tidal volume
   21. tracheostomy

_____ **a.** A breathing rate slower than the normal rate

_____ **b.** Gasping respirations that have no pattern and occur infrequently

_____ **c.** Two layers of connective tissue that surround the lungs

_____ **d.** Air sacs in the lungs, point of gas exchange with the pulmonary capillaries

_____ **e.** Bluish color of skin and mucous membranes that indicates poor oxygenation

_____ **f.** Depressions seen in the neck, above the clavicles, between the ribs, or below the rib cage from excessive muscle use during breathing

_____ **g.** A surgical procedure that creates a stoma in the neck for the patient to breathe through

_____ **h.** Volume of air inhaled and exhaled in one respiration

_____ **i.** A breathing rate faster than the normal rate

_____ **j.** Molecule that carries oxygen in the blood

_____ **k.** Portion of the pharynx that extends from the mouth to the base of the tongue

_____ **l.** A reduction of oxygen delivery to the tissues

_____ **m.** Portion of the pharynx that extends from the nostrils to the soft palate

_____ **n.** Passage for foods and liquids to enter the stomach

_____ **o.** Flap of tissue that closes over the trachea during swallowing

_____ **p.** Oxygen delivery device that includes a one-way valve and reservoir and can deliver up to 100% oxygen

_____ **q.** Semicircular hard plastic device that is inserted into the mouth and holds the tongue away from the back of the pharynx

CONTENT REVIEW

1. Which anatomical feature(s) may cause more frequent airway obstruction in infants and children than in adults?
   a. Nose and mouth are smaller.
   b. Cricoid cartilage is narrower and less rigid.
   c. Tongue takes up relatively more space.
   d. All of the above are correct.

2. Fill in each term naming a structure of the upper airway on the appropriate line.

cricoid cartilage   oropharynx
epiglottis   soft palate
esophagus   thyroid cartilage
larynx   tongue
mandible   trachea
nasal cavity   vocal cords
nasopharynx

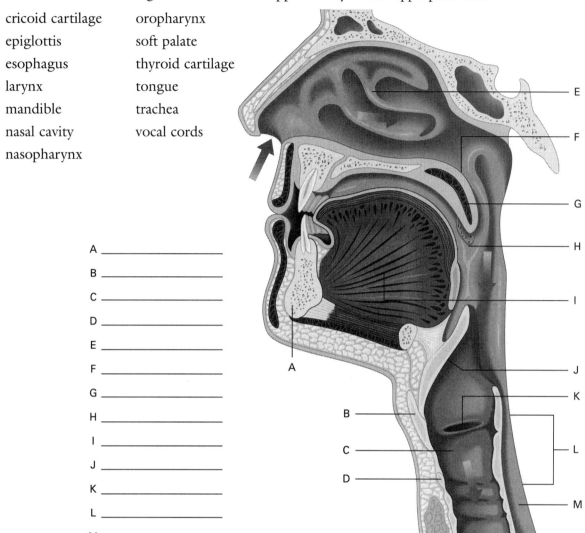

A _____
B _____
C _____
D _____
E _____
F _____
G _____
H _____
I _____
J _____
K _____
L _____
M _____

3. A major muscle of breathing that separates the chest cavity from the abdominal cavity is the
   a. Diaphragm
   b. Alveolus
   c. Visceral pleura
   d. Bronchiole

4. While inspecting a patient's mouth, you find broken teeth in the oropharynx, and suctioning equipment is not immediately available. You should
   a. Perform five quick abdominal thrusts
   b. Perform five back blows with your hand
   c. Sweep the mouth with your index finger
   d. Sit the patient up to help secure the airway

5. Describe the steps to perform the head-tilt, chin-lift maneuver.

6. When treating a patient with a suspected spinal injury, which method of opening the airway should be used?
   a. Jaw-thrust maneuver
   b. Head-tilt, chin-lift maneuver
   c. Lateral-flexion maneuver
   d. Hyperextension maneuver

7. To help prevent obstruction of the trachea when performing the head-tilt, chin-lift maneuver on infants or children, the head should be placed in which position?
   a. Flexed
   b. Tilted
   c. Extended
   d. Neutral

8. When suctioning, you should use what type of body substance isolation protection?
   a. Gloves
   b. Mask
   c. Protective eyewear
   d. All of these

9. Your patient is unresponsive and has a large amount of vomitus in the oropharynx. Which suction catheter should be used?
   a. English catheter
   b. French catheter
   c. Hard catheter
   d. Soft catheter

10. Suction should only be applied for _____ seconds in the adult patient and _____ seconds for infants and children.
    a. 20 seconds for the adult and 10 seconds for the infant or child
    b. 20 seconds for the adult and 5 seconds for the infant or child
    c. 15 seconds for the adult and 5 seconds for the infant or child
    d. None of the above

11. If the patient with inadequate breathing is producing large amounts of frothy secretions that are continuous and require constant suctioning, you should
    a. Suction for 15 seconds, provide oxygen by nonrebreather mask for 15 seconds, repeat
    b. Suction for 15 seconds, provide oxygen by nonrebreather mask for 5 minutes, repeat
    c. Suction for 15 seconds, provide positive pressure ventilation for 2 minutes, repeat
    d. Suction for 15 seconds, provide positive pressure ventilation for 10 minutes, repeat

12. You have decided to use an oropharyngeal airway on an unresponsive patient. How would you measure for the proper size?
    a. Measure the airway from the tip of the patient's nose to the tip of the earlobe.
    b. Measure the airway from the patient's earlobe to the bottom of the angle of the jaw.
    c. Measure the airway from the corner of the patient's mouth to the tip of the earlobe.
    d. Oropharyngeal airways should not be used if the patient is unresponsive.

13. After selecting the correct size nasopharyngeal airway and lubricating the airway with a water-soluble lubricant, the airway should be inserted into the larger nostril until
    a. The patient gags and then back out slightly
    b. Resistance is met or bleeding occurs
    c. The flange rests on the flare of the nostril
    d. The bevel comes in contact with the septum

14. You must assess your patient for adequate or inadequate breathing. Briefly describe what you would observe about the following four factors in a patient who is breathing adequately.

    a. Rate

    b. Rhythm

    c. Quality

    d. Depth

15. What are the normal respiratory rate limits for the following patients?

    Adult: _____ to _____ respirations a minute

    Child: _____ to _____ respirations a minute

    Infant: _____ to _____ respirations a minute

16. All of the following indicate inadequate breathing EXCEPT
    a. Bilateral chest rise
    b. Tachypnea
    c. Bradypnea
    d. Agonal breathing

17. After auscultating the chest of a elderly patient who has fallen out of bed, you note that the breath sounds on both sides are dramatically decreased. You should
    a. Place the patient back into bed
    b. Administer oxygen by nonrebreather mask
    c. Provide positive pressure ventilation
    d. Help the patient to a sitting position

18. From the selection below, choose the order of preferred methods to ventilate patients, from most to least desirable.

   1. Flow restricted, oxygen-powered ventilation device
   2. Bag-valve mask (one person)
   3. Bag-valve mask (two person)
   4. Mouth-to-mask

   a. 4, 2, 3, 1
   b. 3, 4, 2, 1
   c. 4, 3, 1, 2
   d. 3, 1, 4, 2

19. Exhaled breath contains about 16 percent oxygen. If you are the rescuer, how can you improve the amount of oxygen you deliver when performing mouth-to-mask ventilation?
   a. Raise one edge of the pocket mask to release the exhaled air more rapidly.
   b. Inhale oxygen from a cannula or oxygen mask between ventilations.
   c. Place the patient on a nonrebreather mask at a liter flow of 10 per minute.
   d. None of the above is correct.

20. All of the following are advantages of performing mouth-to-mask ventilations with a pocket mask EXCEPT
   a. The mask eliminates direct contact with the patient.
   b. Ventilations can be delivered automatically.
   c. A one-way valve prevents exposure to the patient's exhaled air.
   d. This method of ventilating can provide adequate tidal volumes.

21. When artificially ventilating, the adult patient should be ventilated every _____ seconds, and infants and children should be ventilated every _____ seconds.
   a. Adults every 5 seconds, infants and children every 3 seconds
   b. Adults every 3 seconds, infants and children every 5 seconds
   c. Adults every 10 seconds, infants and children every 5 seconds
   d. Adults every 15 seconds, infants and children every 10 seconds

22. Fill in the parts of the bag-valve mask unit on the appropriate lines.

A _____   bag   nonrebreathing patient valve

B _____   face mask   oxygen reservoir

C _____   intake valve/oxygen reservoir valve   oxygen supply connecting tube

D _____

E _____

F _____

23. The bag-valve mask with a reservoir, when attached to an oxygen source, can deliver nearly 100% oxygen. What percentage of oxygen is delivered to the patient by bag-valve mask without an oxygen source?
    a. 61%
    b. 41%
    c. 21%
    d. 11%

24. The following are desirable features of the bag-valve mask EXCEPT
    a. It allows a single operator to easily maintain a tight mask seal.
    b. It allows delivery of ventilations enriched from an oxygen source.
    c. Self-refilling bag is easy to clean and sterilize.
    d. Transparent mask allows for the detection of vomitus.

25. Your patient is experiencing agonal breathing, and you suspect a spinal injury. You should
    a. Perform a head-tilt, chin-lift to open the airway, then ventilate
    b. Pull on the head to align the airway, then ventilate
    c. Establish in-line stabilization and perform a jaw-thrust maneuver, then ventilate
    d. Establish in-line stabilization, but do not ventilate because the patient is breathing

26. All of the following are true of the flow-restricted, oxygen-powered ventilation device EXCEPT
    a. It is also known as a demand-valve device.
    b. It is recommended for children and infants.
    c. Gastric distention often occurs.
    d. Improper use may rupture the lungs.

27. When ventilating with the flow-restricted, oxygen-powered ventilation device, the trigger or button on the valve should be released
    a. As soon as the chest begins to rise
    b. After the chest has risen fully
    c. After the audible alarm sounds
    d. After 5 to 7 seconds of activation

28. While ventilating a patient with the flow-restricted, oxygen-powered ventilation device, the chest does not rise adequately. You should FIRST
    a. Depress the trigger or button up to twice as long
    b. Follow foreign body airway obstruction maneuvers
    c. Reevaluate the position of the head, chin, and mask seal
    d. Use an alternative means to ventilate the patient

29. To determine the correct tidal volume and rate for the automatic transport ventilator (ATV), you should
    a. Watch the stomach rise and fall
    b. Consult with medical direction
    c. Set the inspiration time for 10 seconds
    d. None of the above is correct

30. Although there are different sizes of oxygen tanks, when full all contain the same pressure:
    a. Approximately 1,000 pounds per square inch
    b. Approximately 2,000 pounds per square inch
    c. Approximately 3,000 pounds per square inch
    d. Approximately 4,000 pounds per square inch

31. When _____ comes into contact with oxygen under pressure, an explosion may occur.
    a. Oil
    b. Petroleum jelly
    c. Some adhesive tapes
    d. All of the above

32. Which type of pressure regulator has only one gauge, which registers the content of the oxygen tank?
    a. Therapy regulator
    b. Treatment regulator
    c. High pressure regulator
    d. Continuous flow regulator

33. To remove any debris, before placing the yoke of the pressure regulator onto the oxygen cylinder you should
    a. Tap the valve with the yolk of the regulator
    b. Wipe the valve stem with a clean, damp cloth
    c. Quickly open and shut the valve on the cylinder
    d. Gently rinse the valve under running water

34. When discontinuing oxygen administration, to help prevent a decreased tidal volume and blood oxygen content, you should
    a. Remove the tubing from the nipple, then remove the mask from the patient's face
    b. Remove the mask from the patient's face, then disconnect the tubing from the nipple
    c. Hyperventilate the patient for 5 minutes prior to disconnecting the tubing
    d. Ask the patient to breathe more rapidly before removing the tubing from the nipple

35. What liter flow is typically needed to keep the reservoir bag filled on the nonrebreather mask?
    a. 2 liters per minute
    b. 5 liters per minute
    c. 10 liters per minute
    d. 15 liters per minute

36. You are attempting to treat a child with a nonrebreather mask, but the child will not tolerate the mask. What is the recommended way to continue the treatment?
    a. Hold the mask on the face, while diverting the child's attention.
    b. Ask the parent to hold the mask on the face until the child accepts the mask.
    c. Have someone familiar with the child hold the mask close to the patient's face.
    d. Put the child on a flow restricted, oxygen-powered ventilation device.

37. The nasal cannula is not a preferred method of administering oxygen in the prehospital setting and is mainly indicated
    a. When the patient will not tolerate a nonrebreather mask
    b. As an adjunct to the nonrebreather mask
    c. When the patient requests its use
    d. For transports lasting longer than 30 minutes

38. The proper liter flow range for the nasal cannula is commonly set at
    a. 1–6 liters per minute
    b. 8–10 liters per minute
    c. 15 liters per minute
    d. 22–44 liters per minute

39. The only mask recommended for oxygen delivery in the prehospital setting is the
    a. Simple face mask
    b. Partial rebreather mask
    c. Nonrebreather mask
    d. Venturi mask

40. If your patient's dentures are securely in place, before ventilating you should
    a. Remove them to achieve a better mask seal
    b. Remove them to avoid the danger of breaking them in the mouth
    c. Leave them in the mouth so they will not be misplaced
    d. Leave them in the mouth to achieve a better mask seal

CASE STUDY 1

You and your partner, Ashley, are dispatched to a local church for an elderly woman suffering from shortness of breath. As you walk in, a clergyman directs you to the back of the church where you find a woman sitting bolt upright in a chair in a tripod position, obviously very anxious. You introduce yourselves to the patient, and she replies with gasping breaths, "I'm Mary. Help me. I can't breathe." You reassure her and, anticipating possible respiratory arrest, call for paramedic backup from another station.

1. From your brief interaction with Mary, what indications lead you to believe she is experiencing serious respiratory distress? (Name at least three.)

2. At this time, which of the following would be the most appropriate for Mary?
    a. Nasal cannula at 6 liters per minute
    b. Venturi mask at 10 liters per minute
    c. Simple face mask at 10 liters per minute
    d. Nonrebreather mask at 15 liters per minute

A friend of Mary's tells you that Mary has emphysema (chronic obstructive pulmonary disease) and sometimes has to be on oxygen at home. As you assess Mary's breathing sounds, you detect a gurgling noise and then notice a pink frothy secretion coming from her mouth. Ashley advises you that Mary's respiratory rate is 36 per minute.

3. Which suction catheter and technique would be most appropriate for Mary in this situation?
   a. Use a rigid catheter, insert the catheter without suction, apply suction for 15 seconds.
   b. Use a rigid catheter, insert the catheter with suction, suction for 20 seconds.
   c. Use a French catheter, insert into the mouth without suction, apply for 15 seconds.
   d. Use a soft catheter, insert into the mouth without suction, apply for 20 seconds.

   It becomes apparent that Mary's breathing is inadequate and that positive pressure ventilation is needed. You decide to use the bag-valve mask with you and Ashley delivering the ventilations. Before using the mask and the associated airway adjuncts, Ashley explains the procedure to Mary.

4. Keeping in mind that Mary is still slightly responsive, which of the following adjuncts and techniques is most appropriate for Mary at this time?
   a. Oropharyngeal airway inserted by using the 180-degree-turn advancing technique
   b. Oropharyngeal airway inserted by using a tongue-depressor technique
   c. Nasopharyngeal airway inserted bevel first until the flange rests on the nostril
   d. Nasopharyngeal airway inserted flange first until the bevel rests on the nostril

   Despite your best team efforts, Mary becomes unresponsive and is no longer breathing on her own. Her pulse can be felt and is bounding. Dispatch advises you that the estimated time of arrival for the paramedic backup unit is less than 1 minute.

5. What should you and Ashley do, now that Mary is not breathing on her own?
   a. Start cardiopulmonary resuscitation (CPR) until the paramedic unit arrives.
   b. Continue to ventilate and suction the patient as you did when she was responsive.
   c. Continue to ventilate the patient but, because she is unresponsive, suction is not needed.
   d. Roll the patient to clear the airway, and start CPR immediately.

CASE STUDY 2

You and your partner, Joshua, are dispatched to a construction site where there is a report of a young female worker who fell from the third floor. Dispatch advises you that Engine Company 4 and a paramedic backup unit from your system are both responding. Your unit arrives on scene. As you approach the patient, a co-worker states that the patient fell head-first from the third floor onto the dirt where she lies now. Another worker tells you the patient was unconscious when they rolled her from her stomach to her back. As you visually examine the patient, you notice that she is breathing with agonal respirations and is bleeding freely from the mouth.

1. In the above situation, how would you open the mouth and airway?
   a. Jaw pull with the head-tilt, chin-lift maneuver
   b. In-line stabilization with head-tilt, chin-lift
   c. In-line stabilization with jaw-thrust maneuver
   d. In-line stabilization with crossed-finger technique

2. After opening the mouth and airway, you find an abundant amount of blood with teeth in the oropharynx. How should you remove the foreign material?
   a. Turn the patient's head to the side to permit drainage.
   b. Roll the patient to a prone position and perform back blows.
   c. Suction, using the soft or French catheter.
   d. Suction, using the rigid or hard catheter.

   The patient's agonal respirations are clearly inadequate. With the oral airway in place, Joshua will stabilize the patient's head and hold the bag-valve mask in place while you squeeze the bag to ventilate the patient. You squeeze the bag, but the patient's chest does not rise.

3. Which of the following may cause the chest not to rise with ventilations?
   a. Incorrect position of the head and chin
   b. Air escaping from around the mask
   c. Airway obstruction
   d. Any or all of the above may cause a failure

   After reevaluating and adjusting your patient and airway technique, the patient's chest is rising and falling normally with every squeeze of the bag. The backup paramedic unit arrives with the engine company following. The paramedic lieutenant states, "This type of airway problem can be very difficult to control. You did a good job." You and Joshua assist the paramedics with spinal immobilization and give them your report. Joshua assists the paramedics further on the way to the hospital.

MODULE 2 REVIEW
AIRWAY: CHAPTER 7

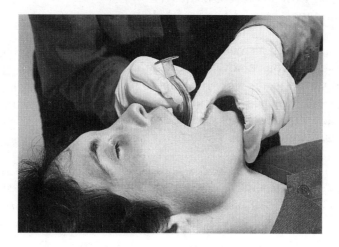

The module on airway management concerns basic techniques for establishing and maintaining an open airway and providing artificial ventilation and oxygen therapy.

Q **Why is Chapter 7 an entire module all by itself?**

A Because of the critical importance of airway care. Without a patent airway, no patient will survive, no matter what else is done for him.

Q **How important is it to learn the head-tilt, chin-lift, and jaw thrust maneuvers; suctioning procedures; and how to insert an airway adjunct?**

A These are essential. When a patient's mental status declines, perhaps to the point of unresponsiveness (unconsciousness), the muscles of the airway relax and the tongue may fall back into the airway. The patient's head may flex forward or extend backward, causing poor alignment or closing-off of airway passages. The patient may lose the gag reflex or the ability to cough and clear his own airway, so that fluids and foreign particles must be suctioned to keep the airway clear. An airway adjunct may be required to help keep the airway open once you have opened it. These are the basic airway management techniques every EMT-B must master and be ready to use.

Q **Why is it important to know both child and adult airway anatomy?**

A The airway anatomy of infants and children differs from that of adults in several significant ways. The head is larger and thus more likely to tip forward when the child is supine. The mouth and nose are smaller, but the tongue is relatively larger in the mouth. The trachea is narrower and thus more likely to become blocked. The chest wall is softer and should respond more obviously to artificial ventilations. These differences must be kept in mind when performing airway and ventilation procedures, and appropriate sizes of equipment such as airway adjuncts must be chosen.

Q   **Why does breathing have to be assessed? Isn't it easy to tell if a person is breathing or not breathing? What does "inadequate breathing" mean?**

A   It's easy to tell if a person is breathing or not breathing. It is not so easy to tell if a person is breathing inadequately — that is, not taking in enough oxygen to sustain life. A person is breathing inadequately when the rate is outside of normal ranges, either too fast or too slow; when the breathing pattern is irregular; or when there is a poor quality of breathing (breath sounds are decreased or absent when you listen to the chest with a stethoscope; the chest wall is not rising and falling adequately with each breath or the two sides of the chest rise and fall unequally; the breathing is shallow and you cannot feel an adequate amount of air coming from the person's mouth or nose with exhalation). When a person is breathing inadequately (or not breathing at all), positive pressure ventilation with supplemental oxygen must be provided.

Q   **What is "positive pressure ventilation?"**

A   "Positive pressure ventilation" is another term for artificial ventilation or artificial respiration. It is any of several means of forcing air into a patient's lungs (by exerting positive pressure) when the patient cannot breathe or breathe adequately on his own. Mouth-to-mask ventilation is preferred because it protects the rescuer from the patient's secretions, delivers a greater tidal volume of air than the bag-valve mask, and requires only a single rescuer. Bag-valve-mask ventilation performed by two rescuers is the next preferred method, followed by the flow-restricted, oxygen-powered ventilation device. One-rescuer bag-valve-mask ventilation is the least preferred method because of the difficulties of one person holding a mask seal and providing adequate tidal volumes of air.

Q   **What about providing oxygen by nonrebreather mask? Is this another form of positive pressure ventilation?**

A   When a patient is one who can benefit from additional oxygen and the patient is able to breathe adequately on his own, oxygen may be provided (at a flow rate of 15 liters per minute) by nonrebreather mask. This is not the same as positive pressure ventilation because no pressure is exerted to force the oxygen into the lungs. The oxygen supplied through the nonrebreather mask is breathed in by the patient. Oxygen may be supplied by nasal cannula, which provides oxygen at a maximum flow rate of 6 lpm, only if the patient will not tolerate a nonrebreather mask.

CHAPTER

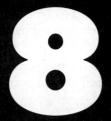

8

SCENE SIZE-UP

COGNITIVE OBJECTIVES

Numbered objectives are from the United States Department of Transportation 1994 EMT-Basic National Standard Curriculum. Asterisked objectives, if any, pertain to material that is supplemental to the DOT curriculum.

3-1.1 Recognize hazards/potential hazards.

3-1.2 Describe common hazards found at the scene of a trauma and medical patient.

3-1.3 Determine if the scene is safe to enter.

3-1.4 Discuss common mechanisms of injury/nature of illness.

3-1.5 Discuss the reason for identifying the total number of patients at the scene.

3-1.6 Explain the reason for identifying the need for additional help or assistance.

KEY IDEAS

This chapter covers the importance of proper scene size-up. Because the prehospital environment can be hostile and uncontrolled, it is extremely important to follow basic guidelines and use good sense when working as an EMT-Basic. It is imperative that the EMT-B pay close attention to the scene size-up on every call. By doing so you may save your life as well as that of your partner and patient.

▶ The EMT-B must ensure the safety of the EMS crew first, then that of the patient and bystanders.

▶ Note scene characteristics such as blood and other hazards that may require the use of protective clothing and body substance isolation (BSI) measures.

▶ Survey the total scene before entering, looking for hazards that make the scene unstable, and do not enter if you are not trained to stabilize them.

▶ Beware of low-oxygen and toxic-substance areas, such as sewers and caverns.

▶ Never enter a known crime scene unless it has been secured by the police. Be cautious and ready to retreat.

▶ At a crime scene take steps to help preserve evidence. However, remember that your primary concern is treating the patient.

▶ Alter the environment around the patients to help protect them.

▶ Protect bystanders by controlling the scene.

▶ Note whether the patient's problem is traumatic or medical in nature.

▶ The trauma scene size-up includes determining the mechanism of injury.

▶ The medical scene size-up requires collecting evidence that may help identify the nature of the illness.

▶ Determine the number of patients and call for additional resources, if needed, prior to making contact with the patient.

TERMS AND CONCEPTS

1. **The EMT-B may encounter patients who suffer from medical conditions and/or from trauma. Define, and explain the difference between, medical and trauma emergencies:**

    a. Medical emergency

    b. Trauma emergency

2. **Write the number of the correct term next to each definition. Not every term will be used.**

    1. index of suspicion
    2. mechanism of injury (MOI)
    3. nature of illness (NOI)
    4. scene safety
    5. scene size-up

    _____ **a.** An overall assessment of the scene to which an EMT-B has been called

    _____ **b.** An anticipation that certain types of accidents and mechanisms will produce specific types of injuries

    _____ **c.** Factor involved in producing an injury to a patient, including the strength, direction, and nature of the force that caused the injury

    _____ **d.** Steps taken to ensure the safety and well-being of the EMT-B, coworkers, patients, and bystanders

    _____ **e.** The type of medical condition or complaint a patient is suffering from

CONTENT REVIEW

1. One of the first goals of an EMT-B responding to a scene is scene safety. With this goal in mind, the EMT-B is concerned with the well-being of
   a. The EMT-Bs, patients, and bystanders
   b. The EMT-Bs and patients only
   c. The EMT-Bs only
   d. The patients only

2. Ensuring scene safety begins
   a. After patient contact is made
   b. After arrival at the scene
   c. While approaching the scene
   d. While receiving dispatch information

3. The EMT-B must use different levels of body substance isolation protection. Which BSI protection device should be used with every patient contact?
   a. Protective gown
   b. Eye protection
   c. Protective gloves
   d. HEPA respirator

4. To help protect the patient's privacy from onlookers, it is most effective to
   a. Ask some of the bystanders to turn their backs to the patient while holding an unfolded bed sheet at shoulder height
   b. Advise the bystanders to immediately leave the scene or you will be forced to notify the police
   c. Request that the police immediately remove the bystanders from the scene
   d. Request the police to arrest curious bystanders for interfering with the patient's confidentiality

5. As you arrive on the perimeter of a motor vehicle accident scene, you notice that there appear to be more patients than your unit can effectively handle. You should FIRST
   a. Proceed to the scene and evaluate the patient's needs
   b. Proceed to the patients and begin treatment
   c. Stage off the scene until law enforcement arrives
   d. Call for additional resources

6. You are on a motor vehicle accident scene where power lines are lying across the vehicle. Which statement is correct?
   a. Consider all power lines to be energized until a power company representative advises you they are not.
   b. If the power lines are not arcing or smoking, you may assume the lines are safe and not energized.
   c. You should approach the vehicle and remove the wires by using a wooden or fiberglass pole.
   d. If a local firefighter states, "The power was cut by the fire department," you can presume that it is safe.

7. If you are called to a vehicle crash involving a steep grade, and you are not trained to deal with this situation, you should
   a. Improvise and use whatever means are immediately available to reach the vehicle
   b. Notify your dispatcher of the situation and wait for a properly trained rescue crew
   c. Call out to the victims in the vehicle and ask them to try to exit the vehicle
   d. Notify your dispatcher of the situation, then proceed to try to reach the vehicle

8. Upon arrival at a known crime scene, you should
   a. Advise dispatch that you are entering the scene
   b. Enter the scene to reach the patient, exercising extreme caution
   c. Wait for police and enter the scene as the police arrive
   d. Enter the scene only after it has been secured by police

9. When approaching a residence, what is the correct way to knock on the door?
   a. Knock while standing in front of the door.
   b. Knock while standing off to the hinged side.
   c. Knock while standing off to the knob side.
   d. None of the above

10. Which of the following is NOT considered a mechanism of injury?
    a. A large-caliber gunshot
    b. A large laceration to the head
    c. A vehicle crash with heavy damage
    d. A fall from a great height

CASE STUDY 1

▼

You are dispatched to a possible shooting at Unit 101 of the Cheap-O Motel, a local hostelry known for its violent clientele. As you are en route, dispatch advises you that the police are on the scene and that the scene is secure. The police are requesting EMS to expedite; the patient is critical. ALS back-up has been dispatched, but is delayed.

1. As you approach the scene, you should
   a. Advise dispatch and respond to the scene with the lights and siren on
   b. Advise dispatch and respond to the scene with only the lights on
   c. Respond to the scene and park just outside the door of Unit 101 until police confirm that the scene is safe
   d. Stage your vehicle outside the scene, no lights and siren, until scene safety is confirmed

2. As you arrive on scene, a police officer advises you that they have just located a second victim who has also been shot. You should
   a. Treat and transport both victims to the best of your abilities
   b. Immediately call for additional transporting units
   c. Treat and transport the most critical patient, then return for the other
   d. Treat both patients, then call for an additional unit to transport

You start to treat one of the shooting victims, an unresponsive 32-year-old male with multiple large-caliber gunshot wounds to the chest. As you cut the clothes off the patient, being careful not to cut through the bullet holes (evidence), a small-caliber hand gun falls from his pants pocket.

3. You should
    a. Immediately pick up the gun by the barrel so you don't disturb fingerprints on the grip and take it to the nearest police officer
    b. Pick up the gun by putting a pencil through the trigger guard and place it in your ambulance until the police are available
    c. Not touch the gun but immediately advise the police of the situation
    d. Any of the above is acceptable in this situation.

While you are treating your patient, a crowd has begun to form and is becoming agitated and hostile.

4. You should
    a. Ask the crowd to "please stand back or I will have you arrested"
    b. Not let the crowd divert your attention, and keep on working
    c. Retreat temporarily until the police can give you support
    d. Leave the scene and request that police transport the patient

CASE STUDY 2

You are dispatched to 100 Cherry Lane for an elderly woman not feeling well. You immediately get under way and, en route, you ask the dispatcher to call the residence back to gain more information. The dispatcher states that the original caller was an elderly male, and the only information he gave was that his "wife has had a cough for months and is not feeling well." The dispatcher advises that there is no further information available because no one is now answering the phone.

1. List at least three details dispatch relayed and explain what each detail may tell you about the scene or the patient.

An elderly man answers the door and thanks you for being so prompt. You ask the man, "What seems to be the problem this evening?" He replies, "My wife hasn't felt well for months and she is always coughing." You ask, "Has your wife been diagnosed as having tuberculosis?" The gentleman replies, " I'm not sure, but she has been sick for some time."

2. What type of body substance isolation precautions should you take?
    a. After entering the house, both EMT-Bs should put on gloves and protective eye wear.
    b. After entering the house, only the EMT-B who is treating should put on gloves and protective eyewear.
    c. Before entering the house, both EMT-Bs should put on gloves and a HEPA respirator.
    d. Before entering the house, both EMT-Bs should put on gloves, eye protection, and a HEPA respirator.

You introduce your partner and yourself to the patient, and your partner radios dispatch to inform them that patient contact has been made and that you are okay. You explain to the patient that the mask you are wearing is a precaution you take when a patient is coughing a lot. When you ask the patient to tell you why she had her husband call the ambulance, the patient replies, "I've been coughing uncontrollably for the past week. I need relief." The patient says she has not seen a doctor about her condition and doesn't know what may be causing it. She denies having any other symptoms, but you make a note of some clues in the environment that you will report to the hospital staff: a thermometer on the night stand and pink-tinged tissues in a wastebasket by the bed, indications that the patient may be running a fever and spitting up blood. You gather up a couple of bottles of over-the-counter cough medications the patient has been taking in an effort to control her cough, to bring along to the hospital.

3. While you are transporting this patient to the hospital, which of the following would be appropriate?
    a. Because the patient and the scene present signs of TB, you continue to wear the respirator and advise the hospital of the precaution.
    b. The patient and the scene present signs of TB, but because TB is not contagious you take off the HEPA respirator.
    c. Because the patient has not received a doctor's diagnosis of TB, you take off the HEPA respirator.
    d. Because you are in the ambulance and not in the patient's house, the HEPA respirator is not needed and you take it off.

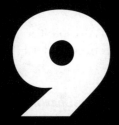
COGNITIVE OBJECTIVES

Numbered objectives are from the United States Department of Transportation 1994 EMT-Basic National Standard Curriculum. Asterisked objectives, if any, pertain to material that is supplemental to the DOT curriculum.

Part 1: Scene Size-up

3-1.4   Discuss common mechanisms of injury/nature of illness.

3-1.5   Discuss the reason for identifying the total number of patients at the scene.

3-1.6   Explain the reason for identifying the need for additional help or assistance.

*   Explain how to gain scene control.

*   Explain how to establish rapport with the patient.

Part 2: Initial Assessment

3-2.1   Summarize the reasons for forming a general impression of the patient.

3-2.2   Discuss methods of assessing altered mental status.

3-2.3   Differentiate between assessing the altered mental status in the adult, child, and infant patient.

3-2.4   Discuss methods of assessing the airway in the adult, child, and infant patient.

3-2.5   State reasons for management of the cervical spine once the patient has been determined to be a trauma patient.

3-2.6   Describe the methods used for assessing if a patient is breathing.

3-2.7   State what care should be provided to the adult, child, and infant patient with adequate breathing.

3-2.8   State what care should be provided to the adult, child, and infant patient without adequate breathing.

3-2.9   Differentiate between a patient with adequate and inadequate breathing.

3-2.10 Distinguish between methods of assessing breathing in the adult, child, and infant patient.

3-2.11 Compare the methods of providing airway care to the adult, child, and infant patient.

3-2.12 Describe the methods used to obtain a pulse.

3-2.13 Differentiate between obtaining a pulse in an adult, child, and infant patient.

3-2.14 Discuss the need for assessing the patient for external bleeding.

3-2.15 Describe normal and abnormal findings when assessing skin color.

3-2.16 Describe normal and abnormal findings when assessing skin temperature.

3-2.17 Describe normal and abnormal findings when assessing skin condition.

3-2.18 Describe normal and abnormal findings when assessing capillary refill in the infant and child patient.

3-2.19 Explain the reason for prioritizing a patient for care and transport.

Part 3: Focused History and Physical Exam

For a Trauma Patient

3-3.1 Discuss the reasons for reconsideration concerning the mechanism of injury.

3-3.2 State the reasons for performing a rapid trauma assessment.

3-3.3 Recite examples and explain why patients should receive a rapid trauma assessment.

3-3.4 Describe the areas included in the rapid trauma assessment and discuss what areas should be evaluated.

3-3.5 Differentiate when the rapid assessment may be altered in order to provide patient care.

3-3.6 Discuss the reason for performing a focused history and physical exam.

For a Medical Patient

3-4.1 Describe the unique needs for assessing an individual with a specific chief complaint with no known prior history.

3-4.2 Differentiate between the history and physical exam that are performed for responsive patients with no known prior history and responsive patients with a known prior history.

3-4.3 Describe the needs for assessing an individual who is unresponsive.

3-4.4 Differentiate between the assessment that is performed on a patient who is unresponsive or has an altered mental status and other medical patients requiring assessment.

Part 4: Detailed Physical Exam

3-5.1 Discuss the components of the detailed physical exam.

3-5.2 State the areas of the body that are evaluated during the detailed physical exam.

3-5.3 Explain what additional care should be provided while performing the detailed physical exam.

3-5.4 Distinguish between the detailed physical exam that is performed on a trauma patient and that of the medical patient.

Part 5: Ongoing Assessment

3-6.1 Discuss the reasons for repeating the initial assessment as part of the ongoing assessment.

3-6.2 Describe the components of the ongoing assessment.

3-6.3 Describe trending of assessment components.

KEY IDEAS

Performing an accurate and reliable assessment is your most important function as an EMT-Basic. All treatment and transport decisions will be based upon the information gathered during the assessment. It is important to develop a consistent routine for assessing all patients. This chapter introduces basic assessment skills.

▶ The purposes of assessing patients include: to determine the nature of the illness/mechanism of injury; to identify and manage life threats; to determine transport requirements; to examine the patient; to provide care based upon the findings; to monitor the patient; to assess and adjust the care provided; to communicate information to the medical staff; and to document the call.

▶ The key steps of patient assessment are scene size-up, initial assessment, focused history and physical exam (conducted somewhat differently for a trauma patient and a medical patient), detailed physical exam, and ongoing assessment. Communication and documentation are also key elements of patient assessment.

▶ The scene size-up comprises three phases: (1) determining scene safety, (2) determining the mechanism of injury or the nature of the illness, and (3) determining the number of patients. The latter two phases are actually the beginning of patient assessment.

▶ The initial assessment includes six steps conducted in this sequence: (1) forming a general impression of the patient, (2) assessing mental status, (3) assessing the airway, (4) assessing breathing, (5) assessing circulation, and (6) establishing patient priorities for transport and further assessment and care.

▶ The focused history and physical exam has three parts. For a trauma patient or unresponsive medical patient, they are conducted in this sequence: (1) physical exam, (2) baseline vital sign assessment, (3) history taking (using the acronym SAMPLE to represent categories of information to obtain during the history). For a responsive medical patient, the steps of the focused history and physical exam are generally conducted in this sequence: (1) SAMPLE history, (2) physical exam, (3) baseline vital sign assessment. For a patient who is unresponsive or with a significant mechanism of injury, the physical exam is a rapid head-to-toe trauma or medical assessment. For a responsive patient who has a specific, localized injury or medical complaint and no significant mechanism of injury, the physical exam will focus on the area of the injury or complaint.

▶ The detailed physical exam is a more thorough version of the rapid trauma or rapid medical assessment. It is a detailed head-to-toe examination typically conducted in the ambulance en route to the hospital, if time and the patient's condition permit, to discover any additional injuries or conditions that may previously have been overlooked.

▶ The ongoing assessment is conducted at frequent intervals, beginning immediately after the focused history and physical exam, or immediately after the detailed physical exam if one is conducted. The purposes of the ongoing assessment are to determine any changes in the patient's condition, to assess the effectiveness of your emergency care, and to intervene as necessary.

TERMS AND CONCEPTS

▼

1. **Write the number of the correct term next to each definition.**

1. apnea
2. aspiration
3. AVPU
4. Battle's sign
5. cerebrospinal fluid
6. chief complaint
7. decerebrate posturing
8. decorticate posturing

9. flail segment
10. focused medical assessment
11. focused trauma assessment
12. initial assessment
13. paradoxical motion
14. rapid medical assessment
15. rapid trauma assessment

_____ a. Head-to-toe physical exam that is swiftly conducted on a patient with a significant mechanism of injury

_____ b. Breathing a substance into the lungs

_____ c. Two or more adjacent ribs that are fractured in two or more places

_____ d. The patient's answer to the question "Why did you call the ambulance?"

_____ e. The patient arches the back and flexes the arms inward toward the chest

_____ f. Black-and-blue discoloration to the mastoid area behind the ear, a late sign of skull or head injury

_____ g. The movement of a section of the chest in the opposite direction to the rest of the chest during respiration

_____ h. A head-to-toe physical exam that is swiftly conducted on an unresponsive medical patient or a medical patient who is suspected to also have injuries

_____ i. The patient arches the back and extends the arms straight out parallel to the body

_____ j. Exam that is focused on a specific injury site, performed on a patient with no significant mechanism of injury

_____ k. The portion of the assessment conducted immediately following scene size-up for the purpose of discovering immediately life-threatening conditions

_____ l. Exam that is focused on the parts of the body indicated by the ill patient's chief complaint, signs, or symptoms

_____ m. The absence of breathing

_____ n. Fluid that surrounds and cushions the brain and spinal cord

_____ o. A mnemonic for alert, responds to verbal stimulus, responds to painful stimulus, unresponsive—to characterize levels of responsiveness

CONTENT REVIEW

1. Select the item that best describes the purpose(s) for performing a patient assessment.
   a. To identify and manage immediately life-threatening conditions
   b. To determine priorities for further assessment and care
   c. To monitor the patient's condition and assess the effectiveness of care provided
   d. The purposes for patient assessment include all of these.

Scene Size-up

2. Which of the following items is NOT a component of the scene size-up?
   a. Determining scene safety
   b. Determining the mechanism of injury or nature of illness
   c. Determining a detailed patient history
   d. Determining the total number of patients

3. Which statement best describes how to achieve a smooth transition of care when treating a critically injured unresponsive patient?
   a Gain patient care information from any bystanders who may be on scene.
   b. Proceed directly to the patient and obtain information as you begin your assessment.
   c. Gain patient care information from law enforcement officers who may be on scene.
   d. Announce your arrival: "I'm _____ and this is _____. We're EMT's. Can you tell us what happened and what care has been given?"

4. You have been dispatched to a scene where the patient's family is extremely hostile. A family member has made physical threats to you and your partner. Select the best action to take in this situation.
   a. Use scene control techniques to regain control.
   b. Move as rapidly as possible to leave the scene.
   c. Request immediate law enforcement back-up.
   d. Work back-to-back with your partner for protection.

Initial Assessment

5. Whenever there is a significant mechanism of injury, you must immediately
   a. Notify the police
   b. Establish in-line stabilization of the head and neck
   c. Call for paramedic back-up
   d. Begin the detailed physical exam

6. Once in-line stabilization of the head and neck is established, it must be maintained until
   a. A cervical spine immobilization device is applied
   b. The rapid trauma assessment has been completed
   c. The patient is fully immobilized to a backboard with straps and head immobilization device
   d. The patient is transferred to the care of hospital personnel

7. An initial assessment
   a. Must be completed prior to treatment of any life threats that may be discovered
   b. Does not necessarily need to be completed in a specific sequence to be effective
   c. Must be performed on all patients, regardless of the mechanism of injury or nature of illness
   d. Must only be performed on those patients who are critically injured or are critically ill

8. Select the correct sequence for performing the initial assessment.

   1. Form a general impression
   2. Assess circulation
   3. Assess mental status
   4. Assess airway
   5. Assess breathing
   6. Establish patient priorities

   a. 6, 4, 5, 2, 3, 1
   b. 1, 4, 5, 2, 3, 6
   c. 1, 3, 4, 5, 2, 6
   d. 3, 4, 5, 2, 2, 6

9. The patient's general age, sex, whether the patient seems well or injured, and items you notice in the patient's immediate environment can be obtained during which of the following steps of the initial assessment?
   a. General impression
   b. Assessment of breathing
   c. Assessment of mental status
   d. Establishment of patient priorities

10. Which question will best help you to establish a patient's chief complaint?
   a. "Where do you hurt?"
   b. "Can you take one finger and point to the pain?"
   c. "Does anything make the pain worse?"
   d. "Why did you call the ambulance?"

11. On approach to a patient, you note that his eyes are closed. The sound of your voice causes the patient to open his eyes. This patient would be considered
   a. Alert and oriented
   b. Alert and disoriented
   c. Alert and responds to verbal stimuli
   d. Responsive to verbal stimuli

12. Which patient has the "highest" or best level of consciousness?
   a. A patient who grabs your hand when you do a sternal rub
   b. A patient who displays decorticate posturing when you do a sternal rub
   c. A patient who mumbles incoherent words when you speak to him
   d. A patient who displays no response to a sternal rub

13. Assessment of the airway in the responsive patient
   a. Is accomplished by talking with the patient
   b. Is performed prior to the evaluation of mental status
   c. Is not necessary if the patient is looking at you
   d. Is performed as part of the scene size-up

14. Unresponsive patients have a high incidence of airway occlusion due to
   a. Uncontrolled coughing
   b. Relaxation of the muscles in the upper airway
   c. Spasm of the muscles in the upper airway
   d. Brain damage

15. Which management technique is INCORRECT for a partial airway obstruction based upon airway sounds?
   a. Gurgling: Suction out the contents immediately.
   b. Snoring: Use a head-tilt, chin-lift or jaw thrust maneuver.
   c. Crowing: Insert an oropharyngeal airway.
   d. Stridor: Be prepared to provide positive pressure ventilation with oxygen if required.

16. Which item is NOT considered a life-threatening breathing problem in an adult patient?
   a. A respiratory rate of 26 in a responsive patient
   b. A respiratory rate of 26 in an unresponsive patient
   c. Poor chest wall movement and nasal flaring
   d. Signs such as cyanosis or decreased mental status

17. Positive pressure ventilation can be delivered by all of the following means EXCEPT
   a. Mouth-to-mask
   b. Bag-valve mask
   c. Nonrebreather mask
   d. Flow-restricted, oxygen-powered ventilation device

18. Assessment of the circulation includes all of the following items EXCEPT
   a. Skin temperature, color, and condition
   b. Capillary refill in adults
   c. Pulse
   d. Possible major bleeding

19. When assessing the pulse in the initial assessment, the EMT-B should assess all of the following EXCEPT
   a. The exact heart rate
   b. The approximate heart rate
   c. If the pulse is present or not
   d. The regularity and strength

20. When assessing the circulation in the initial assessment, the EMT-B should perform all of the following EXCEPT
   a. Cut away areas of clothing that are completely blood soaked.
   b. Scan the body looking for major bleeding.
   c. Control arterial or venous bleeding.
   d. Control oozing capillary bleeding.

21. The least reliable place to check for skin color is the
   a. Mucous membranes of the mouth
   b. Nail beds
   c. Mucous membranes that line the eyelids
   d. Under the tongue

22. Select the skin color that is INCORRECTLY paired with a potential cause.
    a. Cyanotic: Reduced oxygenation
    b. Red: Blood loss either external or internal
    c. Yellow: Liver dysfunction
    d. Pale or mottled: Decrease in perfusion and the onset of shock

23. Which of the following skin temperature and skin condition combinations is most commonly a sign of shock?
    a. Hot, dry skin
    b. Cool, dry skin
    c. Cold, dry skin
    d. Cool, clammy skin

24. If capillary refill is _____ in the child or infant, tissue perfusion is inadequate. (Select the shortest time period that indicates inadequate perfusion.)
    a. Greater than 1 second
    b. Greater than 2 seconds
    c. Greater than 3 seconds
    d. Greater than 4 seconds

25. Your supervisor has asked you to assist with quality improvement (QI) by reviewing records of patient care. The supervisor wants you to determine if the following patients required rapid transport. Next to each patient description write Y (yes) if rapid transport is required or N (no) if rapid transport is not required.

    _____ 1. An unresponsive diabetic who does not respond to verbal or painful stimuli
    _____ 2. A patient complaining of severe right lower abdominal pain
    _____ 3. A responsive patient complaining of minor chest discomfort with a BP of 120/80
    _____ 4. A responsive patient who collapsed at work with cool, clammy skin
    _____ 5. A responsive patient with a minor cut on his leg
    _____ 6. A patient who was stung by a bee and looks ill
    _____ 7. A patient who is complaining of a headache and is unable to obey commands
    _____ 8. A patient complaining of shortness of breath

Focused History and Physical Exam—Trauma Patient

26. You have determined that a trauma patient requires rapid transport after completion of the initial assessment. You should next
    a. Move the patient to the stretcher, then perform a rapid trauma assessment
    b. Perform a rapid trauma assessment, then move the patient to the stretcher
    c. Perform a focused trauma assessment (focused on specific injuries), then move the patient to the stretcher
    d. Move the patient to the stretcher, then perform a focused trauma assessment

27. You performed such a good job reviewing patient care reports for your supervisor that she has returned and asked you to perform additional quality improvement reviews. The supervisor asks you to review reports to see if significant mechanisms of injury are present to justify a rapid trauma assessment. Next to each description write Y (yes) if there is significant mechanism of injury present or N (no) if there is not.

_____ 1. A patient involved in a roll-over collision

_____ 2. A patient who fell from 6 feet

_____ 3. A patient who was struck by a car

_____ 4. A patient with a gunshot wound to the hand

_____ 5. A patient whose impact causes deformity to a steering wheel

_____ 6. A patient who was in the passenger seat of vehicle in which the driver died

28. Select the mechanism of injury for infants and children that is NOT NECESSARILY considered significant.
    a. Fall greater than 10 feet
    b. Fall while running
    c. Bicycle collision
    d. Vehicle collision in which infant or child is unrestrained

29. Select the proper order for performing the focused history and physical exam in the trauma patient with a significant mechanism of injury.

    1. Rapid trauma assessment

    2. Focused trauma assessment

    3. Baseline vital signs

    4. SAMPLE history

    a. 2, 3, 4
    b. 1, 3, 4
    c. 3, 4, 1
    d. 3, 4, 2

30. Select the proper order for performing the focused history and physical exam in the trauma patient with no significant mechanism of injury.

    1. Rapid trauma assessment

    2. Focused trauma assessment

    3. Baseline vital signs

    4. SAMPLE history

    a. 3, 2, 4
    b. 4, 2, 3
    c. 1, 3, 4
    d. 2, 3, 4

31. You have responded to a traffic accident in which the patient sustained an injury to his head. He was unresponsive just after the accident. When you first arrived he was alert and oriented. When you reassess his mental status, he responds to your verbal stimuli with inappropriate words. What is the appropriate management for this patient?
  a. Rapid transport and if possible hyperventilate at 12–20 per minute with a bag-valve mask.
  b. Rapid transport and if possible hyperventilate at 24–30 per minute with a bag-valve mask.
  c. Administer oxygen by nonrebreather mask, then transport.
  d. Complete the focused history and physical exam, then administer oxygen by nonrebreather mask.

32. Of the following, which are necessary during the rapid trauma assessment?

  1. Inspect

  2. Palpate

  3. Auscultate

  4. Use the sense of smell

  a. 1 and 2

  b. 1, 2, and 3

  c. 2 and 3

  d. 1, 2, 3, and 4

33. During the rapid trauma assessment, it is necessary to examine the patient for DCAP-BTLS. Write what each letter in DCAP-BTLS stands for.

  D _____

  C _____

  A _____

  P _____

  B _____

  T _____

  L _____

  S _____

34. When assessing the head during the rapid trauma assessment, the EMT-B is PRIMARILY concerned with
  a. Identifying cerebrospinal fluid in the nose or ears
  b. Determining any possible head injury
  c. Identifying fractured facial bones
  d. All of these

35. When assessing the neck during the rapid trauma assessment, the EMT-B should inspect for
  a. Tracheal deviation or tracheal tugging
  b. Jugular vein distention and subcutaneous emphysema
  c. Large lacerations or punctures
  d. All of these

36. Regarding assessing the chest for breath sounds during the rapid trauma assessment, which is the MOST CORRECT statement?
    a. The EMT-B should determine the presence of the breath sounds bilaterally.
    b. The EMT-B should determine the equality of the breath sounds bilaterally.
    c. The EMT-B should do both a and b.
    d. It is not necessary to listen to the breath sounds during the rapid trauma assessment.

37. When assessing the abdomen during the rapid trauma assessment, the EMT-B should palpate for all of the following EXCEPT
    a. Crepitus
    b. Tenderness
    c. Distention
    d. Rigidity

38. For the rapid trauma assessment, which is the BEST statement about when the EMT-B should NOT palpate the pelvis?
    a. When the patient complains of pain in the pelvic area
    b. When there is deformity to the pelvic area
    c. Both a and b are reasons not to palpate the pelvis
    d. Neither a nor b (Always palpate the pelvis.)

39. Following inspection and palpation of the extremities in the rapid trauma assessment, the EMT-B should check for PMS. "PMS" refers to
    a. Pulses, motor function, and sensation
    b. Pulses, motor function, and severity
    c. Pain, motor function, and sensation
    d. Pain, motor function, and severity

40. In order to inspect the posterior body during the rapid trauma assessment, the EMT-B should
    a. Log-roll the patient while maintaining in-line stabilization
    b. Reach under the patient's body to palpate the spine
    c. Have the patient sit up so the back can be examined
    d. Not attempt to examine the posterior body

41. When spinal injury is suspected, the cervical spine immobilization device (CSID) should be applied
    a. Before the rapid trauma assessment is begun
    b. After the head is assessed
    c. After the neck is assessed
    d. After the rapid trauma assessment is completed

42. The vital signs should be reassessed and recorded every _____ minutes in the unstable trauma or medical patient.
    a. 15
    b. 10
    c. 8
    d. 5

43. During the focused history and physical exam, the EMT-B should obtain a SAMPLE history. Write the type of information that each of the letters in SAMPLE stands for.

S _____

A _____

M _____

P _____

L _____

E _____

44. You are treating a responsive trauma patient who complains of a minor injury. There is no significant mechanism of injury or critical finding. During the focused history and physical exam, however, you develop a suspicion that more injuries may exist. Your next action should be to
a. Secure the patient to the stretcher and transport immediately
b. Secure the patient to the stretcher and perform a rapid trauma assessment en route to the hospital
c. Immediately perform a rapid trauma assessment
d. Immediately perform a detailed physical exam

Focused History and Physical Exam—Medical Patient

45. Select the proper order for performing the focused history and physical exam in the responsive medical patient.

1. Perform a focused medical assessment

2. Obtain baseline vital signs

3. Perform a rapid medical assessment

4. Obtain the SAMPLE history

a. 2, 3, 4

b. 2, 4, 1

c. 4, 2, 1

d. 4, 1, 2

46. Select the proper order for performing the focused history and physical exam in the unresponsive medical patient.

1. Perform a focused medical assessment

2. Obtain baseline vital signs

3. Perform a rapid medical assessment

4. Obtain the SAMPLE history

a. 2, 1, 4

b. 3, 2, 4

c. 1, 2, 4

d. 4, 3, 2

47. During the rapid medical assessment, the abdomen should be inspected for scars, discoloration, or distention. Palpate for
    a. Tenderness, bowel obstruction, distention, and rigidity
    b. Deformity, tenderness, penetrations, and pulsating masses
    c. Rigidity, abdominal pain, distention, and lacerations
    d. Tenderness, rigidity, distention, and pulsating masses

48. When assessing the extremities during the rapid medical assessment, be sure to check around the hands, feet, and ankles for all of the following EXCEPT
    a. Swelling
    b. Rigidity
    c. Pulses, motor function, and sensation
    d. Medical identification device

49. Which baseline vital sign is missing from the list below?

    Respiration   Pulse   Skin   Blood pressure

    a. Pupils
    b. Capillary refill
    c. Patent airway
    d. Chest auscultation

50. During the SAMPLE history for a responsive medical patient, the OPQRST questions are asked to elicit more information about the patient's symptoms, especially pain. Write the type of information that each of the letters OPQRST stands for.

    O _____

    P _____

    Q _____

    R _____

    S _____

    T _____

51. The unresponsive medical patient should be transported in which position?
    a. Supine
    b. Prone
    c. Lateral recumbent
    d. Fowler's

52. Which statement is most correct regarding patient medications?
    a. Gather prescription medications only.
    b. Gather prescription and over-the-counter medications.
    c. Gather over-the-counter medications only.
    d. It is not important to gather medications.

53. You have responded to a call for a medical patient who just "doesn't feel well." You should
    a. Perform a focused medical assessment of the head and neck
    b. Perform a detailed physical exam
    c. Perform a rapid medical assessment
    d. Transport rapidly without additional interventions

Detailed Physical Exam and Ongoing Assessment

54. A complete detailed physical exam most often is performed
   a. Just prior to transport in all patients
   b. On a patient who required a head-to-toe rapid medical or trauma assessment
   c. When requested by medical direction
   d. On all patients who request EMS services

56. The basic reason(s) for performing an ongoing assessment are
   a. To detect any change in the patient's condition
   b. To identify any missed injuries or conditions
   c. To adjust the emergency care as needed
   d. All of these

CASE STUDY 1

▼

You have responded to a motor vehicle accident. You determine that the scene is safe. You observe a car that has rolled over and has significant damage. The only patient was ejected from the vehicle. As you approach, you can see that the patient is about 45 years old and looks severely injured. His eyes are closed and he looks pale. You direct your partner to provide in-line stabilization of the head and neck. The patient does not respond to your voice. He responds to a painful stimulus by arching his back and extending his arms and legs. His airway is open and clear; his breathing is shallow at 6 per minute. Your partner slides his finger up to palpate the carotid pulse and tells you it is strong and regular.

1. What are the most appropriate actions to take, given the above description?
   a. Provide oxygen via nonrebreather mask at 15 lpm, then check for pulses.
   b. Place a cervical spine immobilization collar and complete the initial assessment.
   c. Provide positive pressure ventilation at 24-to-30 per minute while maintaining in-line stabilization.
   d. Complete the initial assessment and then provide oxygen via nonrebreather mask at 15 lpm.

2. This patient will require
   a. A rapid trauma assessment on scene and a detailed physical exam—if time and the patient's condition permit—while en route to the hospital
   b. A rapid trauma assessment and components of the detailed physical exam while en route to the hospital
   c. A focused trauma assessment and a detailed physical exam—if time and the patient's condition permit—while en route to the hospital
   d. A focused trauma assessment and components of the detailed physical exam while en route to the hospital

3. You know that the patient's blood pressure is at least
   a. 80 mmHg
   b. 70 mmHg
   c. 60 mmHg
   d. 50 mmHg

CASE STUDY 2

You have responded to a house call for an unknown medical emergency. You have your disposable gloves and eye protection on. The scene appears safe as you approach an older home. An elderly woman meets you at the door and says, frantically, "George won't wake up! He takes a nap every afternoon, and I can't wake him up." In response to additional questioning she tells you there is no trauma involved, and her husband is the only patient. As you enter the room, you observe the patient (an approximately 70-year-old male) lying face up on his bed. You hear a snoring sound on inhalation and exhalation of each breath. He has a pillow behind his head and his skin looks blue. There are no signs of trauma. His eyes remain closed in spite of your attempts to arouse him with your voice. The patient also fails to respond to a painful stimulus. You tell your partner to remove the pillow from behind the patient's head and open the airway. Your partner opens the airway and assesses the patient's breathing. You assess the patient's circulatory status.

1. List at least three clues that this patient may have an airway problem.

2. What is the preferred method your partner should use to open the airway?
   a. Jaw-thrust maneuver
   b. Head-tilt, neck-lift maneuver
   c. Head-tilt, chin-lift maneuver
   d. Head-tilt maneuver

3. In this patient, a respiratory rate less than _____ and greater than _____ would require positive pressure ventilation.
   a. 10/23
   b. 9/22
   c. 8/24
   d. 11/21

4. Management of this patient should include
   a. A focused medical assessment
   b. A focused trauma assessment
   c. A rapid medical assessment
   d. A rapid trauma assessment

CASE STUDY 3

You have responded to a call for a patient who cut his hand. You have your disposable gloves and eye protection on as you leave the vehicle. Two young men greet you on the street before you can exit the vehicle. They yell, "Hurry up, man! Fred is gonna die!" The scene appears safe as you approach the residence located in a run-down neighborhood. As you are walking to the back of the house, you ask, "Why did you call the ambulance?" One of the two replies, "Fred got mad at his girlfriend and put his fist through the window." You ask him if Fred is the only patient injured. He nods.

As you enter the backyard, you see the patient sitting on the back steps holding his arm. His girlfriend is yelling at him, then starts yelling at you: "He's not hurt! He doesn't need an ambulance!" "Knock it off!" the patient snaps at her. The patient, who appears to be about 25 years old, has a towel wrapped around his lower arm. He looks up in disgust as you approach. Obviously, his girlfriend is upsetting him, and he is upsetting her. His color is pink. He appears to be in minor distress. His shirt is covered with blood. He responds to your questions appropriately and relates the same story his friend told you. You ask your partner to get the baseline vitals. The patient's respirations are adequate and you place him on oxygen by nonrebreather mask. You check the patient's radial pulse and it feels strong and regular at about 90 per minute. His skin is warm and dry. On examination, you discover a large laceration on the anterior surface of the patient's wrist that is bleeding moderately.

1. To maintain scene control you should
   a. Transport the patient rapidly from the scene
   b. Suggest a task for the girlfriend that will remove her from the area
   c. Actively listen to the patient's description of the injury that occurred
   d. Order the girlfriend to leave the area at once

2. Explain the best method to control this patient's bleeding.

3. This patient would most likely require a
   a Rapid trauma assessment followed by SAMPLE history, then vitals
   b. Rapid trauma assessment followed by vitals, then SAMPLE history
   c. Focused trauma assessment followed by vitals, then SAMPLE history
   d. Focused trauma assessment followed by SAMPLE history, then vitals

CASE STUDY 4

You have responded to a downtown office for a patient complaining of chest pain. You have disposable gloves and eye protection on. The scene appears safe as you arrive in front of a local insurance company. Several employees are awaiting your arrival. You ask them, "Why did you call the ambulance?" A young worker replies, "It's my boss. He says he is OK, but he doesn't look well at all. He told me his chest hurts." The worker tells you there is no trauma involved in this incident and the boss is the only patient.

As you enter a plush office, you observe the patient, who appears to be approximately 55 years old, leaning back in a large desk chair. He is pale, and your general impression is that he looks ill. There is no sign of trauma. You introduce yourself and ask the patient, "What seems to be the problem?" The patient replies, "Nothing, really. A little indigestion, maybe. I don't know why they called you, but I guess as long as you're here you may as well check me out. My chest hurts. But I'm sure it must be something I ate." His breathing appears adequate. His radial pulse is weak and slow. His skin is cool and clammy. While you are obtaining a history, your partner obtains the baseline vital signs. He reports the following: respirations normal at 20 per minute; pulse weak and regular at 50 per minute; skin pale, cool, and moist; pupils equal and reactive; blood pressure 90/60.

1. What history-taking method should you use on this patient?
    a. OPQRST questions only
    b. SAMPLE history including OPQRST questions
    c. SAMPLE history only
    d. DCAP-BTLS and SAMPLE history

2. The best way to evaluate the quality of this patient's pain is to ask
    a. Is the pain dull and squeezing?
    b. Where do you feel the pain?
    c. Can you take one finger and point to where the pain is located?
    d. How would you describe the pain?

3. The physical exam on this patient should be
    a. A medical assessment focused on the neck, chest, abdomen, and extremities
    b   A head-to-toe rapid medical assessment
    c. A head-to-toe rapid trauma assessment
    d. A detailed physical exam

4. Appropriate management for this patient should include
    a. Cardiopulmonary resuscitation
    b. Oxygen by nonrebreather mask and immediate transport
    c. Positive pressure ventilation and immediate transport
    d. Departing the scene, as the patient has refused treatment

CASE STUDY 5

You have responded to a house call for a "sick child." You are wearing disposable gloves and eye protection. The scene appears safe as you arrive in front of a neatly kept home in a working-class neighborhood. As you enter the home you observe the patient on a couch. The patient's mother tells you the patient is 5 years old. He is lying on his back. He does not look at you as you enter the room. He looks pale, and your general impression is that he looks ill. His eyes appear to be sunken into the sockets. There is no sign of trauma, and the mother reports no traumatic event. You introduce yourself, gain consent, and ask the mother, "Why did you call the ambulance?" The mother replies, "Ryan has been sick for the last week. He's been throwing up constantly." The patient does not respond to your voice, but he responds appropriately to pain. His breathing appears adequate at 20 per minute. His radial pulse is weak and rapid. His skin is cool and clammy.

1. You should next
   a Check for bleeding only
   b. Check the capillary refill and check for bleeding
   c. Check for pulse, motor, and sensory function in the extremities
   d. Check for a carotid pulse

2. This patient should be given
   a. A medical assessment focused on his abdomen
   b. A head-to-toe rapid medical assessment
   c. A trauma assessment focused on his chest and abdomen
   d. A head-to-toe rapid trauma assessment

3. Regarding a transport decision, this patient should be considered
   a. A medium priority patient
   b. A high priority patient
   c. Stable and would not be assigned to a category
   d. A low priority patient

4. Your treatment for this patient should include
   a. Oxygen by nasal cannula
   b. Oxygen by nonrebreather mask
   c. Insertion of an oropharyngeal airway
   d. Positive pressure ventilation by bag-valve mask

CHAPTER

10

ASSESSMENT OF THE GERIATRIC PATIENT

Numbered objectives are from the United States Department of Transportation 1994 EMT-Basic National Standard Curriculum. Asterisked objectives, if any, pertain to material that is supplemental to the DOT curriculum.

*   Discuss at least four factors that contribute to the geriatric patient being at a higher risk for medical emergencies.

*   Discuss the general physiological changes in the body systems of the geriatric patient that are due to the normal aging process.

*   Discuss special considerations for assessing the geriatric patient suffering from a medical or traumatic emergency.

*   Outline the special considerations for obtaining an accurate medical history from a geriatric patient.

*   List the emergency care steps and considerations for the geriatric patient suffering either a medical or a traumatic emergency.

*   Discuss positioning, immobilization, and packaging of the elderly trauma patient with consideration of physical deformity.

*   Recite and explain common disease processes in the geriatric patient that cause generalized complaints in the elderly.

KEY IDEAS

This chapter focuses on the assessment of the geriatric patient, one who is over the age of 65. Since this is the fastest growing segment of the population in the United States, and because the majority of EMS calls involve geriatric patients, it is important to understand the characteristics of this age group and how to tailor your assessment to their special needs. Key concepts include:

▶ The elderly are at greater risk for nearly all types of injuries and illness.

▶ Due to physiologic changes caused by aging, the geriatric patient will present problems with different signs and symptoms than you would expect to find if your patient were younger.

▶ Geriatric patients often have one or more coexisting long-term conditions or health problems which can mask or change the presentation of their current emergency problem.

TERMS AND CONCEPTS

▼

1. Write the number of the correct term next to each definition.

1. arteriosclerosis
2. cardiac hypertrophy
3. chronic
4. dementia
5. kyphosis
6. osteoporosis
7. silent heart attack
8. syncope

_____ a. Heart attack that does not cause chest pain

_____ b. Condition resulting in the malfunctioning of normal cerebral processes

_____ c. Long term, progressing gradually

_____ d. Abnormal curvature of the spine

_____ e. Disease process that causes the loss of elasticity in the vascular walls

_____ f. Disease characterized by an abnormal loss of bone minerals

_____ g. A brief period of unconsciousness due to lack of blood flow to the brain

_____ h. Thickening of the cardiac walls without an increase in the size of the chamber

CONTENT REVIEW

▼

1. Illness is an inevitable part of aging.
   a. True
   b. False

2. Cardiovascular system changes associated with aging include all of the following EXCEPT
   a. Degeneration of the conduction system that causes changes in rate or rhythm
   b. Increased arterial elasticity that speeds reaction to stimulation
   c. Decreased cardiac output due to cardiac hypertrophy
   d. Increased blood pressure due to increased vascular resistance

3. Aging causes a generalized deterioration of the respiratory system. This is characterized by decreased flexibility of the rib cage, alveolar degeneration, decreased elasticity of the lung tissue, and
   a. Increased resistance to infection
   b. Blunted sensitivity to hypoxia
   c. Increased gas exchange through diffusion
   d. Enhanced cough and gag reflex

4. _____ is the most significant musculoskeletal change associated with aging.
   a. Arthritis
   b. Kyphosis
   c. Fibrosis
   d. Osteoporosis

5. Slowing of reflexes commonly seen in the elderly is due to
   a. Degeneration of nerve cells
   b. Increased muscle elasticity
   c. Increased impulse transmission
   d. Increased brain mass and weight

6. Aging of the gastrointestinal system contributes to a variety of medical conditions as well as
   a. Enhanced drug absorption
   b. Increased peristalsis
   c. Malnutrition
   d. Obesity

7. Changes in the renal system (kidneys) due to aging increase the potential for the geriatric patient to develop
   a. Fluid and electrolyte imbalance
   b. Drug toxicity
   c. Renal failure
   d. All of these

8. Your scene size-up at an emergency call involving an elderly patient should include
   a. Body substance isolation (BSI) precautions
   b. Environmental concerns (fumes and temperature)
   c. Determining the number of patients
   d. All of these

9. Signs of dehydration in the elderly would include all of the following EXCEPT
   a. Eyes appear "sunken" in the orbits.
   b. Membranes of the eyes appear dry.
   c. Tongue appears furrowed.
   d. Lips appear swollen.

10. The elderly patient has a depressed perception of pain. Therefore the severity of pain is an unreliable indicator of the seriousness of an injury.
    a. True
    b. False

11. When completing a physical exam on a geriatric medical patient, you should remember that your patient may
    a. Have multiple complaints
    b. Minimize or deny symptoms out of fear of losing their independence
    c. Wear multiple layers of clothing that interfere with your exam
    d. All of these

12. Miss Spencer is a 75-year-old woman with an altered mental status and no history of trauma. She should be transported
    a. In a Fowler's position (sitting up)
    b. Lying on her side to protect her airway
    c. Immobilized on a long spine board after applying a cervical collar
    d. Wearing a cervical collar but placed in a position of comfort

13. Mr. Fitzgerald, a 78-year-old, fell from a ladder onto his concrete patio and is complaining of back and neck pain. Because of his severe kyphosis, he should be transported
    a. In whatever position is most comfortable
    b. Fully immobilized on a long spine board wearing a rigid cervical collar
    c. On a long spine board after immobilizing his cervical spine with blankets
    d. Lying on his left side to prevent aspiration

14. Due to depressed pain perception, geriatric patients may have a "silent heart attack" and instead of chest discomfort will complain of
    a. Fatigue
    b. Weakness
    c. Difficulty breathing
    d. Any of these

15. Congestive heart failure commonly occurs in older patients because the heart no longer pumps effectively and blood begins to "back up" into the lungs or peripheral vessels. Results may include fatigue and difficulty breathing. Treatment includes administering oxygen and expediting transport
    a. Immobilized to a long spine board
    b. In a Fowler's position (sitting up)
    c. Lying on the side to prevent aspiration
    d. Supine on the stretcher

16. Your 80-year-old patient, Mrs. Williams, suffers from chronic obstructive pulmonary disease. She is alert and complains of increasing difficulty breathing over the past couple of days. She denies having any pain. Emergency care for Mrs. Williams would include administering oxygen by nonrebreather mask and
    a. Assisting her in taking nitroglycerin
    b. Assisting her ventilations with positive pressure
    c. Transporting her in a Fowler's position if tolerated
    d. Assisting her in using a metered dose inhaler

17. Mr. Herbert, a 77-year-old patient, is complaining of a sudden onset of difficulty breathing and chest pain which is localized and does not radiate. He is slightly cyanotic. His breathing is labored at 15 per minute. He has a history of heart problems and recently had surgery. Your first priority in emergency treatment is
    a. Administering oxygen by nonrebreather mask
    b. Administering positive pressure ventilation
    c. Having him sit up with pillows behind his back
    d. Placing him in a lateral recumbent position

18. After you perform the emergency treatment in item 17, Mr. Herbert's respiratory rate decreases to 8 per minute. Your most accurate conclusion would be that
    a. Your treatment has caused his condition to improve, and no further treatment is required
    b. Your treatment has caused his condition to deteriorate, and you will contact medical direction for advice
    c. His condition is deteriorating because he is unable to sustain the labor of breathing, and you need to provide positive pressure ventilation
    d. His condition is improving because these spells come and go spontaneously, and you encourage him to contact EMS if he begins to feel ill again

19. Since senility is common in the elderly, an altered mental status is rarely an emergency.
    a. True
    b. False

20. List at least five causes for altered mental status in the geriatric patient.

21. Key treatment of a cerebrovascular accident (CVA, or stroke) includes
    a. Aggressive oxygenation and ventilation
    b. Complete immobilization of the head and neck
    c. Rapid transport to the hospital with delayed assessment en route
    d. Administering fluids to maintain hydration and perfusion

22. Your first priority when caring for an elderly patient who is suffering from drug toxicity is to determine what drug is causing the problems.
    a. True
    b. False

23. Your patient is an 82-year-old man who fell while getting off an escalator. He is awake but somewhat confused. His airway is patent and his breathing is rapid and very shallow. His pulse is strong, but rapid and irregular. His skin is pale and cool. What type of injuries might you expect to find during your physical exam?
    a. Head injury
    b. Hip fracture
    c. Fractures of the wrist or forearm
    d. Any of these

24. In obtaining the history for the patient described above, you should be sure to determine
    a. If the patient has medical insurance
    b. If the patient is able to walk
    c. If the fall was preceded by dizziness
    d. How severe the patient's pain is

25. Factors that contribute to the development of environmental emergencies among the elderly include all of the following EXCEPT
    a. Situational factors, such as inability to afford adequate heat
    b. Aging enhances the body's ability to control temperature.
    c. Physical impairments may limit mobility so they cool down more quickly.
    d. Medications may limit the body's ability to control temperature.

26. Number the list below in the proper order from 1 to 5 to provide emergency care to an elderly patient who is suffering from hypothermia.

_____ Remove wet clothing.

_____ Remove the patient from the environment.

_____ Protect the airway.

_____ Wrap the patient in a dry blanket.

_____ Maintain normal breathing and circulation.

27. You have been called to see an elderly male for an "unknown medical problem" after his granddaughter arrived unexpectedly for a visit and found him tied to his bed. He is disoriented, has wet clothing, and has defecated in his bed. His care has recently been provided by someone who responded to an ad placed in the local paper. Your immediate impression is that he may have been abused. When completing your physical exam, you should be alert for
    a. Bruises and bite marks
    b. Broken bones and deformities of the chest
    c. Cigarette burns and trauma to the ears
    d. All of these

28. In the situation above, your FIRST priority is to
    a. Contact the police and request assistance
    b. Confront the caretaker with your suspicions
    c. Provide appropriate medical treatment
    d. Contact your local adult protective services

CASE STUDY

You have been dispatched to an 88-year-old woman, Mrs. Walter, who has suffered a fall. As you enter the house, Mrs. Walter's daughter tells you that her mother had pneumonia three months ago but has been doing well since then. You note no hazards nor find any obstacles to extrication. You find your patient seated on the couch holding her right arm very carefully across her chest. When you introduce yourself and your partner, Mrs. Walter apologizes for bothering you on a Sunday afternoon. She goes on to say that she lost her balance and fell while coming down a flight of stairs. You find Mrs. Walter to be alert and oriented. Her airway is patent and her breathing is regular at 16 breaths per minute with good air exchange. Core and peripheral pulses are strong and regular at 78 per minute. Her skin is slightly pale and moist but warm to the touch. Your partner auscultates her blood pressure at 168/103 in her left arm. Mrs. Walter complains that her right shoulder is very painful where she hit the wall as she fell. You note that there is an obvious deformity near her shoulder and that her right arm seems to droop at an unnatural angle, even though she is supporting it with her left hand.

1. How should you proceed to further assess and care for Mrs. Walter?

2. Should you consider Mrs. Walter's apparent injury a critical finding? Why or why not?

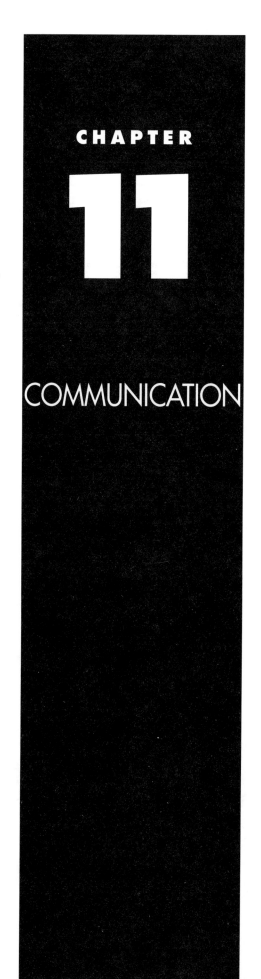

CHAPTER

11

COMMUNICATION

Numbered objectives are from the United States Department of Transportation 1994 EMT-Basic National Standard Curriculum. Asterisked objectives, if any, pertain to material that is supplemental to the DOT curriculum.

3-7.1   List the proper methods of initiating and terminating a radio call.

3-7.2   State the proper sequence for delivery of patient information.

3-7.3   Explain the importance of effective communication of patient information in the verbal report.

3-7.4   Identify the essential components of the verbal report.

3-7.5   Describe the attributes for increasing effectiveness and efficiency of verbal communications.

3-7.6   State legal aspects to consider in verbal communication.

3-7.7   Discuss the communication skills that should be used to interact with the patient.

3-7.8   Discuss the communication skills that should be used to interact with the family, bystanders, and individuals from other agencies while providing patient care and the difference between skills used to interact with the patient and those used to interact with others.

3-7.9 List the correct radio procedures in the following phases of a typical call:

To the scene
At the scene
To the facility
At the facility
To the station
At the station

KEY IDEAS

This chapter focuses on the role of communications in the delivery of emergency medical services. A good understanding of EMS communications skills and equipment is essential to your success as an EMT-Basic. Reliable communications systems are critical to all aspects of an EMS call. Key concepts include:

▶ Standard components of an emergency communications system include a base station and mobile or portable transmitters/receivers. Additional components, such as repeaters and digitalized encoders and decoders, are used to enhance communication capabilities within an EMS system.

▶ The Federal Communications Commission (FCC) has jurisdiction over all radio operations in the country, including those used by EMS systems.

▶ Communications within an EMS system are dependent on adhering to basic rules of radio communication at all times.

▶ Effective interpersonal communications depend on the three "Cs": competence, confidence, and compassion.

▶ Patients with special needs, such as the hearing impaired, children, and the elderly, require special consideration to ensure effective communication at the scene of an emergency.

TERMS AND CONCEPTS

1. **Write the number of the correct term next to each definition.**

    1. base station
    2. decoder
    3. encoder
    4. repeater

____ **a.** Device that converts sound waves into digital codes for transmission
____ **b.** The central dispatch and coordination area of an EMS communications system
____ **c.** Devices that receive transmissions from one source and rebroadcast them at a higher power on another frequency
____ **d.** Device that recognizes and responds to only certain codes imposed on a radio broadcast

CONTENT REVIEW

1. Which of the following are characteristics of a base station?
    a. High power output equipped with a suitable antenna
    b. Located in proximity to the hospital which serves as the medical command center
    c. Has communications contact with all other elements of the system
    d. All of these

2. Repeaters are used within an EMS communications system to
   a. Allow communications over a wide geographic area
   b. Allow all personnel the opportunity to monitor all statewide radio transmissions
   c. Allow communications between EMS agencies in adjoining jurisdictions
   d. Allow communications to be transmitted through the air via cells

3. List three benefits associated with the use of cellular telephones within EMS system.

4. One role of the Federal Communications Commission (FCC) in EMS communication systems is to
   a. Purchase all radio equipment
   b. License base stations
   c. Serve as a repeater for base station operations
   d. Conduct radio operations training for EMS personnel

5. All of the following are ground rules for radio operations EXCEPT
   a. Use the radio just as if you were talking on a telephone.
   b. Keep transmissions brief, organized, and to the point.
   c. Always listen before transmitting.
   d. Use the "echo method" when receiving orders or information.

6. The role of dispatch in an EMS communication system is to obtain information about the nature of the emergency, direct the appropriate emergency service(s) to the scene, and
   a. Notify the medical command center of the request for service
   b. Alert the local news media of the emergency situation
   c. Provide the caller with instructions about what to do until help arrives
   d. Contact the medical director to provide a link for medical direction

7. In addition to communicating with dispatch to acknowledge the dispatch information and again while en route to report your estimated time of arrival at the scene, arrange in order (1 to 5) the other times you should communicate with dispatch.

   _____ To announce your arrival back at base

   _____ To announce your arrival on scene and request further assistance

   _____ To announce you are "clear" and available for another call

   _____ To announce your arrival at the hospital

   _____ To announce your departure from the scene and your estimated hospital arrival time

8. When communicating with medical direction you should use a standard format which includes your unit identification and service level; the patient's age, sex, and chief complaint; a brief, pertinent history of the present illness, including scene assessment and mechanism of injury; past major illnesses; and
   a. The patient's mental status and baseline vital signs
   b. Pertinent physical examination findings
   c. Description of care given and the patient's response
   d. All of these

9. After receiving an order or instructions from medical direction you should
   a. Always say thank you before you "sign off"
   b. Repeat the instructions word for word
   c. Click your "press to talk" button twice to signal your understanding
   d. Acknowledge the instructions by saying "10-4"

10. If you receive orders from medical direction which do not appear to be appropriate, you should always
    a. Question the order to clarify if there has been a misunderstanding
    b. Do what you're told by medical direction
    c. Double check with your partner before following the orders
    d. Request to speak with someone else

11. All of the following describe how you should interact with bystanders or other first responders when you arrive on the scene EXCEPT
    a. Obtain permission from police and fire personnel before beginning patient care.
    b. Identify yourself as an emergency medical technician.
    c. Ask for information about what happened and what care has been given.
    d. Comment positively on the care that has already been provided.

12. Your patient is a non-English-speaking foreign traveler in your community. Which of the following would be the LEAST appropriate action in this situation?
    a. See if one of his companions or a bystander can interpret.
    b. Talk loudly and slowly to make yourself understood.
    c. Contact dispatch to see if they have an interpreter available.
    d. Check with medical direction to see if someone could interpret via radio.

CASE STUDY

You were dispatched to the carousel on the playground at 1031 Bruce Road for an injured child. Your partner notifies dispatch of your arrival. You note no signs of danger as you park the ambulance and then put on your gloves and protective eyewear. As you approach the group gathered near a picnic table, you can hear the sound of a crying child. You introduce yourself to the woman holding the crying child on her lap and ask what happened and what you can to do to help. The mother of your patient, Mrs. Smith, thanks you for coming so quickly and tells you that her son, Mikey, tripped while running and cut his chin. She says he did not lose consciousness. Mikey's crying has quieted and he's watching you closely. You ask him if you can look at his chin. He nods his okay. His mother removes the washcloth which she had been using to control the bleeding. You observe an approximately 1-inch cut. You explain what you're going to do and then, as you gently apply a sterile dressing and bandage to Mikey's injury, you talk to him quietly. He tells you that he is three years old, has a dog and three big sisters. He also says he never rode in an "ambliance." You see no other signs of injury.

Your partner obtains a set of baseline vitals. Mikey's blood pressure is 80/68 mmHg. His heart rate is strong at 80 beats per minute. His respirations are 28 per minute, full and adequate. His skin is slightly flushed, warm, and moist. His capillary refill is less than 2 seconds. His pupils are normal and equal in size and reactivity. You obtain a SAMPLE history. When asked, Mikey says his chin "hurts bad." His mother reports that he is a healthy child who takes no medications and has no known allergies. Mikey tells you that he had a popsicle in the car on his way to the park. Mrs. Smith says that they arrived about an hour ago. Mrs. Smith says that Mikey was fine before he fell as he ran to get on the carousel. You secure Mikey in the child restraint seat on the stretcher in the back of the ambulance and then help Mrs. Smith get settled and secured to the jump seat. You perform the ongoing assessment on Mikey, finding him still completely alert and oriented. His dressing remains dry. His vital signs are essentially unchanged. You radio the hospital with your report.

1., 2., 3. In the space below, write the report you would give orally at the following times: (1) arrival on scene, (2) en route to the hospital, and (3) at the hospital when you transfer care.

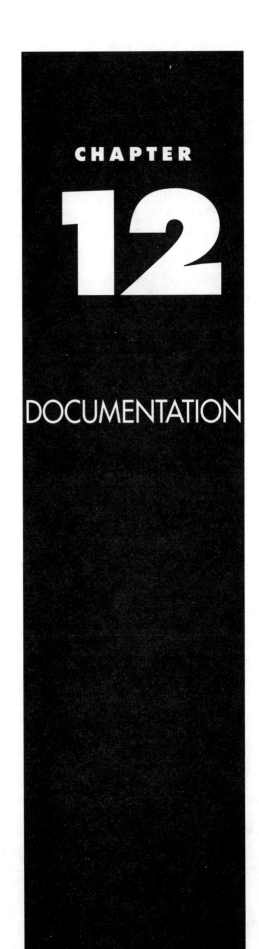

CHAPTER

12

DOCUMENTATION

Numbered objectives are from the United States Department of Transportation 1994 EMT-Basic National Standard Curriculum. Asterisked objectives, if any, pertain to material that is supplemental to the DOT curriculum.

3-8.1 Explain the components of the written report and list the information that should be included in the written report.

3-8.2 Identify the various sections of the written report.

3-8.3 Describe what information is required in each section of the prehospital care report and how it should be entered.

3-8.4 Define the special considerations concerning patient refusal.

3-8.5 Describe the legal implications associated with the written report.

3-8.6 Discuss all state and/or local record and reporting requirements.

KEY IDEAS

The focus of this chapter is the written documentation of patient care. As an EMT-Basic, the documentation of all of your encounters with patients is an essential part of doing your job. Key ideas and concepts include:

▶ Documentation serves many functions. Among them are medical uses, such as ensuring continuity of care and establishing a baseline of patient status; administrative uses, such as billing and insurance information; and as a legal record of assessment, care given, and patient response. Documentation may also be used for educational, research, and quality improvement purposes.

▶ The traditional format for the patient care report is the written prehospital care report (PCR), which is designed to provide a complete and accurate picture of your contact with the patient.

▶ Documentation is governed by two basic rules: "If it wasn't written down, it wasn't done," and "If it wasn't done, don't write it down."

TERMS AND CONCEPTS

1.   Write the number of the correct term next to each definition.

    1.   minimum data set
    2.   pertinent negatives
    3.   prehospital care report (PCR)
    4.   triage tag

_____   **a.**   Tag containing key patient information used during a multiple casualty incident

_____   **b.**   Signs/symptoms that might be expected in certain situations but the patient denies

_____   **c.**   Information that the U. S. Department of Transportation recommends all patient care reports include

_____   **d.**   Documentation of an EMT-Basic's contact with a patient

CONTENT REVIEW

1.   The PRIMARY purpose of high-quality documentation is
    a. As a resource for quality improvement review
    b. To assist in the preparation of patient bills
    c. To ensure the continuity of patient care
    d. As a resource in malpractice suits

2.   State and explain the two basic rules of documentation.

3.   An important element of documentation is the use of accurate and synchronous clocks.
    a. True
    b. False

4.   The narrative section of the patient care report should include the patient's chief complaint, the SAMPLE history, and
    a. Your diagnosis of the patient's problem
    b. Pertinent information about the scene
    c. All remarks made by bystanders
    d. Your conclusions about the incident

5. Which of the following would be considered a pertinent negative for a patient who was the unrestrained driver of a car involved in a serious motor vehicle accident?
   a. The patient complains of abdominal pain.
   b. The patient reports that it hurts to take a deep breath.
   c. The patient denies back and neck pain.
   d. The patient denies any allergies to food or drugs.

6. To ensure that patient care reports are as brief and concise as possible, you should use radio codes, medical terminology, and abbreviations.
   a. True
   b. False

7. Under most state laws, you may provide confidential information about a patient in all of the following situations EXCEPT
   a. Reporting to another health-care provider when transferring care
   b. In response to questions from friends of the patient
   c. When providing information to the police as part of a criminal investigation
   d. If you are subpoenaed to appear in court and provide information in a legal case

8. Although any competent adult has the right to refuse treatment, which of the following would be an appropriate action for you to take before leaving the scene?
   a. Document your explanation of possible consequences of failing to accept care, and have the patient sign the form acknowledging his refusal of treatment.
   b. Discuss the situation with medical direction as required by local protocol.
   c. Complete as much of the assessment as the patient will permit, and ensure that the patient is not under the influence of drugs or alcohol.
   d. All of these

9. Falsification of patient data on a patient care report is punishable by a $1000 fine and imprisonment.
   a. True
   b. False

10. Which of the following best describes the appropriate way to correct an error on the patient care report?
    a. Use correction fluid to cover the incorrect entry.
    b. Use multiple heavy lines to block out the incorrect entry.
    c. Draw a single line through the incorrect entry and initial it.
    d. Report the error verbally but do not alter the report.

11. _____ are commonly used for patient care reports in a multiple casualty incident.
    a. Triage tags
    b. Casualty codes
    c. Regularly used patient care reports
    d. Multiple casualty forms

12. All of the following situations may require additional special documentation by the EMT-Basic EXCEPT
a. Suspected abuse of a child or elderly patient
b. Possible exposures to communicable diseases
c. Patient care given to victims of motor vehicle accidents
d. Injury to a member of the EMS crew

CASE STUDY

You get dispatched to the local high school on a report of a fall. On arrival at the school, you report to the office where you find that your patient slipped on a wet floor and "twisted his ankle." Your 50-year-old patient is Mr. Henderson, the school principal. He says, "I'm sorry you were sent out for nothing. I'm more embarrassed than hurt." You introduce yourself and ask if you can check him over anyway, as long as you're here. He agrees.

On your initial assessment, you find him to be alert and oriented, having no apparent difficulty breathing and in no apparent distress. You see no signs of bleeding. Mr. Henderson lets your partner check his pulse, which is strong and regular. His skin is pink, warm, and dry.

During your focused physical exam, you find that Mr. Henderson's right ankle, which he reports is "a little sore," is markedly swollen, discolored, and very tender to gentle palpation. His foot is slightly pale but warm to the touch. His pedal pulse is present and he has good sensation and motion. Vital signs: blood pressure 138/78 mmHg, pulse 68 beats per minute, and respirations 18 per minute and adequate. Skin is still normal, as are pupils. You complete your SAMPLE history and find that Mr. Henderson has no allergies and takes no medications. He denies any medical problems or any other injuries. He had soup and a sandwich for lunch about a half hour ago. He says that he has felt fine all day, but slipped on some water on the floor as he was leaving the cafeteria.

You urge Mr. Henderson to allow you to splint his ankle and transport him to the hospital so that he can get x-rays to see if his ankle is broken. He refuses, saying, "Thanks for checking me out, but you guys have to be available for real emergencies. I've already called my wife and she's on her way to take me to the doctor. She ought to be here in 10 minutes or so. Bad enough that I fell down in front of half of the school. There's no way I'm going out of here on that stretcher." You agree that he's stable enough to be transported by car, but remind him that he shouldn't bear any weight on his ankle until he's been seen by the doctor. You also remind him that if any problems arise or he changes his mind that he should call 9-1-1.

1. In the space below, write the narrative section of the patient care report for this call.

_____
_____
_____
_____
_____
_____
_____
_____
_____
_____
_____
_____
_____
_____
_____
_____
_____
_____
_____

2. What else should be done before you leave the scene from this call?

MODULE 3 REVIEW
PATIENT ASSESSMENT: CHAPTERS 8-12

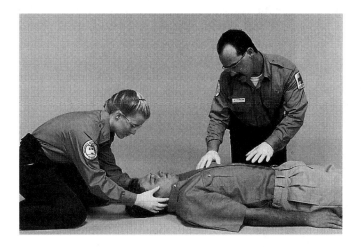

As an EMT-B, your most important functions will be assessing the patient plus providing emergency care and transport to the hospital. Of these, performing an accurate and reliable patient assessment will be the most important, because all of your decisions about care and transport will be based on it.

Q Why is the patient assessment procedure broken down into separate steps?

A Because it is very important to follow an assessment routine that is systematic. This will ensure that you assess every patient consistently and appropriately, based on that patient's illness or injury, and that you will not overlook any important parts of the assessment.

Q Why is scene size-up considered part of patient assessment?

A Because, in addition to the scene safety considerations involved in sizing up the scene, important clues to the patient's condition can also be observed. The most important of these observations is whether or not there is a mechanism of injury that would indicate that this is a trauma patient, as well as clues to the nature of a medical patient's illness, such as medications or an unusually warm or cold environmental temperature.

Q Why is the initial assessment so important?

A The purpose of the initial assessment is to identify any immediate life threats and treat them at once, as they are found. Once life threats have been controlled, a more thorough assessment and additional care can be provided.

Q Why is there a different sequence to the focused history and physical exam for a trauma patient and for a medical patient?

A For a trauma patient, the physical exam and baseline vital signs measurements are performed first and the SAMPLE history last. This is because the greatest amount of information about a traumatic injury can be gathered from physical assessments and because life-threatening injuries not discovered during the initial assessment must be quickly found and managed. For a medical patient, on the other hand, the greatest amount of information is usually gained from the SAMPLE history — the patient's symptoms, for example, what medical conditions has he been suffering from, what medications has he been taking, and what brought on the current emergency. Because the patient who is responsive and able to provide this information may become unresponsive or have a deteriorating mental status, it is important to gain this information first for a medical patient.

Q **For whom, and when, should the detailed physical exam be performed?**

A If a patient required a head-to-toe physical exam (rapid trauma assessment or rapid medical assessment) during the focused history and physical exam, that patient is a candidate for a detailed physical exam en route to the hospital. The purpose of the detailed physical exam is to discover any conditions previously overlooked. However, if the patient is critical or unstable, there may not be time to perform a detailed exam. Perform a detailed physical exam only when time and the patient's condition permit.

Q **Why must an ongoing assessment be performed on every patient?**

A A patient's condition may change, and treatments or interventions may become ineffective. To monitor the patient's condition and interventions, an ongoing assessment must be performed at least every 5 minutes on an unstable patient, and every 15 minutes on a stable patient.

COGNITIVE OBJECTIVES

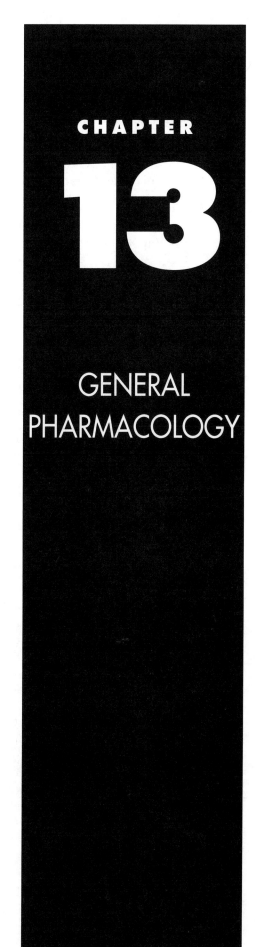

CHAPTER

13

GENERAL PHARMACOLOGY

Numbered objectives are from the United States Department of Transportation 1994 EMT-Basic National Standard Curriculum. Asterisked objectives, if any, pertain to material that is supplemental to the DOT curriculum.

4-1.1   Identify which medications will be carried on the unit.

4-1.2   State the medications carried on the EMS unit by the generic name.

4-1.3   Identify the medications the EMT-Basic may assist the patient with administering.

4-1.4   State the medications the EMT-Basic can assist the patient with by the generic name.

4-1.5   Discuss the forms in which the medications may be found.

*   List and explain the various routes of drug administration used by the EMT-Basic.

*   List and describe the essential medication information that should be understood by the EMT-Basic.

*   Describe the reassessment strategies used following medication administration.

*   List sources that can be used to gather medication information.

KEY IDEAS

As an EMT-Basic, you will have the responsibility of administering certain medications carried on the EMS unit. You also may assist with the administration of certain prescribed medications that may be taken by the patient. Improper administration of these medications can result in dangerous or fatal consequences. It is vital that you be completely familiar with the medications and the proper procedures for administration. This chapter reviews these important concepts.

▶ You may NOT administer or assist with administration of any medication other than the six medications covered in this chapter and that are also identified in local protocol.

▶ The three medications carried on the EMS unit that may be administered under the approval of medical direction are oxygen, oral glucose, and activated charcoal.

▶ The three medications prescribed for the patient that may be administered under the approval of medical direction are prescribed metered-dose inhaler, nitroglycerin, and epinephrine.

▶ Medications can have up to four different names: chemical, generic, trade, and official. The EMT-Basic must be familiar with the generic and trade names.

▶ Drugs can be administered by the following common routes: sublingual, oral, inhalation, and injection (intramuscular).

▶ There are six essential terms associated with medication administration: indications, contraindications, dose, administration, actions, and side effects.

▶ There are seven key steps to administering medications: Obtain an order from medical direction; select the proper medication; verify the patient's prescription; check the expiration date; check for discoloration or impurities; verify the form, route, and dose; and provide documentation.

TERMS AND CONCEPTS

1. Write the number of the correct term next to each definition.

    1. medication

    2. drug

    3. pharmacology

_____ **a.** A chemical substance that creates a change in one or more body functions
_____ **b.** Treatment with a substance that is used as a remedy for illness
_____ **c.** The study of drugs

CONTENT REVIEW

1. The EMT-Basic may not administer or assist in the administration of any medication other than the six medications listed in this chapter. In addition, these drugs must be
   a. Clearly identified by the official name on all prescriptions
   b. Clearly identified by the official or chemical name on all prescriptions
   c. Identified in local protocols as acceptable for the EMT-Basic to administer
   d. Only administered by oral or sublingual route

2. Medications administered by the EMT-Basic are
   a. Administered without medical direction
   b. Carried on the unit or prescribed for the patient
   c. Only given by the oral or sublingual route
   d. Only those medications that are prescribed for the patient

3. Which of the following is a medication that can be administered by the EMT-Basic?
   a. Epinephrine
   b. Diazepam
   c. Lasix
   d. Lidocaine

4. You have responded to a patient complaining of chest pain. The patient states that his medication is upstairs on his dresser. Select the best response to this situation.
   a. Leave the patient momentarily to retrieve the patient's medication.
   b. Ask the patient to walk upstairs and retrieve the medication.
   c. Ask a family member to retrieve the medication.
   d. Help the patient up the stairs to retrieve the medication.

5. Which of the following is also known as the brand name of a drug?
   a. Trade name
   b. Generic name
   c. Chemical name
   d. Official name

6. Which of the following generic and trade names are INCORRECTLY paired?
   a. Metaproterenol–Alupent, Metaprel
   b. Isoetharine–Serevent
   c. Epinephrine–Adrenalin
   d. Albuterol–Proventil, Ventolin

7. Which of the following generic and trade names are INCORRECTLY paired?
   a. Nitroglycerin–Nitrostat
   b. Glucose–OralSuctrose
   c. Oxygen–oxygen
   d. Nitroglycerin spray–Nitrolingual Spray

8. Medication that is placed under the tongue is an example of medication given by
   a. The inhalation route
   b. The intramuscular route
   c. The oral route
   d. The sublingual route

9. A suspension must be
   a. Shaken before it is administered
   b. Given sublingually
   c. Inhaled
   d. Injected

10. Situations when a drug should not be given are known as
    a. Actions
    b. Contraindications
    c. Side effects
    d. Negative markers

11. What are the six essential items of medication information that the EMT-Basic should understand to ensure safe, proper, and effective medication administration?
    a. Indications, contraindications, dose, administration, actions, and side effects
    b. Indications, negative markers, dose, administration, actions, and side effects
    c. Indications, negative markers, dose, forms, prescriptions, and side effects
    d. Indications, negative markers, dose, administration, actions, and adverse actions

12. An example of a drug given by the injection or intramuscular route is
    a. Alupent
    b. Epinephrine
    c. Glutose
    d. Isoetharine

13. All of the following are key steps for medication administration EXCEPT
    a. Obtain an order from medical direction.
    b. Select the proper medication.
    c. Verify that the medication is prescribed to the patient.
    d. Verify the expiration date.
    e. Check for discoloration or impurities (if in liquid form).
    f. Verify the form, route, and dose.
    g. Contact the patient's physician for permission to administer the medication.
    h. Document the administration and the patient's response.

14. Which of the following is NOT a source of information for a patient's prescription medication
    a. AMA Drug Evaluation
    b. Physicians Desk Reference
    c. Wilson's Formulary Service
    d. Package inserts

Complete the following chart:

Generic Name	Trade Name	Used for
Oxygen	15.	wide range of emergencies
16.	Glutose, Insta-glucose	17.
Activated charcoal	SuperChar, InstaChar, Actidose, LiquiChar	18.
Nitroglycerin	Nitrostat	19.
20.	Nitrolingual Spray	21.
Epinephrine	22.	allergic reactions
Albuterol	23.	breathing difficulty associated with respiratory conditions
Metaproterenol	24.	25.
26.	Bronkosol, Bronkometer	27.
Salmeterol Xinafoate	28.	breathing difficulty associated with respiratory conditions

CASE STUDY

▼

You have responded to a call for a patient complaining of chest pain. You've completed the scene size-up and the initial assessment. The patient is a 56-year-old male who responds to painful stimuli only. The patient's wife tells you that he has been complaining of chest pain for the past 2 hours. A neighbor of the patient suggests that you give the patient her nitroglycerin. She takes it for a heart problem.

1. What is your best reaction to the neighbor's suggestion?
   a. Give the patient the neighbor's nitroglycerin.
   b. Contact the patient's personal physician for orders to administer the medication to the patient.
   c. Never administer medication to a patient unless it is prescribed and/or you are ordered to do so by medical direction.
   d. Take the medication with you and administer en route after checking the patient's vital signs.

2. Suppose that nitroglycerin prescribed to this patient is discovered on his person. *The nitroglycerin can and should be placed into the mouth of this patient.* Select the best response to this statement.
   a. The statement is true; you should administer the medication while holding the mouth closed with one hand.
   b. The statement is false; the medication should not be administered to a patient with an altered level of consciousness.
   c. The statement is true if the medication is administered by the oral route instead of the sublingual route.
   d. The statement is false; the patient must be unresponsive to pain before the medication can be administered.

3. Nitroglycerin is used for
   a. Altered mental status
   b. Poisoning and overdose
   c. Chest pain
   d. Difficulty breathing

Note: Medication Reference Cards appear at the back of this workbook. There is a card for each of the following medications EMT-Bs are permitted to administer or assist with administering, with approval from medical direction: **activated charcoal, epinephrine auto-injector, metered dose inhaler, nitroglycerin,** and **oral glucose.** Each card includes information on medication names, indications, contraindications, form, dosage, administration, actions, side effects, and reassessment. You will be able to carry these cards with you for ready reference.

CHAPTER

14

RESPIRATORY EMERGENCIES

COGNITIVE OBJECTIVES

Numbered objectives are from the United States Department of Transportation 1994 EMT-Basic National Standard Curriculum. Asterisked objectives, if any, pertain to material that is supplemental to the DOT curriculum.

4-2.1   List the structure and function of the respiratory system.

4-2.2   State the signs and symptoms of a patient with breathing difficulty.

4-2.3   Describe the emergency medical care of the patient with breathing difficulty.

4-2.4   Recognize the need for medical direction to assist in the emergency medical care of the patient with breathing difficulty.

4-2.5   Describe the emergency medical care of the patient with breathing distress.

4-2.6   Establish the relationship between airway management and the patient with breathing difficulty.

4-2.7   List signs of adequate air exchange.

4-2.8   State the generic name, medication forms, dose, administration, action, indications, and contraindications for the prescribed inhaler.

4-2.9   Distinguish between the emergency medical care of the infant, child, and adult patient with breathing difficulty.

4-2.10 Differentiate between upper airway obstruction and lower airway disease in the infant and child.

KEY IDEAS

This chapter describes respiratory distress and respiratory failure. Emphasis is placed on ensuring an open airway and providing high-flow oxygen or positive pressure ventilation, as needed, and not on trying to diagnose a specific underlying disease.

▶ There is a wide variety of signs and symptoms of breathing difficulty. They may include any of these: shortness of breath; restlessness; increased pulse rate or breathing rate; decreased breathing rate; skin color changes; noisy breathing; inability to speak; retractions; shallow, slow, or irregular breathing; abdominal breathing, coughing; patient in a tripod position; unusual anatomy (barrel chest); altered mental status; nasal flaring; tracheal tugging or deviations; paradoxical motion; and/or pursed-lip breathing.

▶ Time is critical to the patient who is breathing inadequately. If signs of inadequate breathing are exhibited by the patient, you should immediately begin positive pressure ventilation with supplemental oxygen. If the breathing is adequate, but the patient is complaining of breathing difficulty or showing signs of respiratory distress, oxygen must be administered by a nonrebreather mask at 15 lpm.

▶ Metered dose inhalers (MDI) are used by some patients with chronic or recurring breathing problems. If the patient has a prescribed MDI, contact medical direction for an order to assist the patient with administering the medication. It may be necessary to coach the patient during the procedure to be sure the medication is taken in by the patient in an effective manner.

▶ An increased work of breathing in the infant and child is an indication that he is compensating for inadequate oxygen and carbon dioxide exchange and may deteriorate into respiratory failure. You must recognize the wide range of symptoms and immediately provide oxygen if the infant or child is breathing adequately or provide positive pressure ventilation with supplemental oxygen if there are signs of inadequate breathing.

TERMS AND CONCEPTS

1. **Write the number of the correct term next to each definition.**

   1. apnea
   2. bronchodilator
   3. bronchospasm
   4. dyspnea
   5. grunting

   6. metered dose inhaler (MDI)
   7. respiratory arrest
   8. respiratory failure
   9. spacer
   10. tripod position

   _____ a. A drug that relaxes the smooth muscle of the bronchi and bronchioles

   _____ b. When breathing stops completely

   _____ c. Constriction of the smooth muscle of the bronchi and bronchioles

   _____ d. Device consisting of a plastic container and a canister used to inhale an aerosolized medication

   _____ e. A chamber that is connected to MDI to collect medication until it is inhaled

   _____ f. A period with absence of breathing

   _____ g. A sound heard during exhalation in infants suffering from severe respiratory distress

   _____ h. Inadequate oxygenation of the blood and elimination of carbon dioxide

   _____ i. Shortness of breath or difficulty in breathing

   _____ j. Patient sits upright, leans slightly forward, and supports the body with arms in front and elbows locked

2. **Which two of the terms listed in item 1 above have essentially the same meaning?**

   _____ and _____

CONTENT REVIEW

1. Which of the following may produce difficulty in breathing?
   a. Cardiac compromise
   b. Emotional anxiety
   c. Face and neck trauma
   d. All of the above

2. Which condition causes a drastic increase in resistance to air flow in the bronchioles?
   a. Dyspnea
   b. Bronchodilation
   c. Bronchoconstriction
   d. Respiratory arrest

3. The respiratory patient who is found in a reclining or supine position could indicate
   a. The patient is in mild distress
   b. The patient is in severe distress
   c. Either of the above
   d. Neither of the above

4. The tripod position is commonly indicative of
   a. Severe respiratory distress
   b. Moderate respiratory distress
   c. Mild respiratory distress
   d. None of the above

5. All of the following are signs of severe respiratory distress EXCEPT
   a. Speaks a couple of words between breaths
   b. Bluish-gray skin
   c. Cyanosis under the tongue
   d. Respiratory rate of 50 in infants

6. List four abnormal upper airway sounds that are common signs of breathing difficulty.

7. You are treating an unresponsive 3-year-old child who is exhibiting signs of breathing difficulty. The respiratory rate is 14 breaths per minute. Which of the following is correct?
   a. Immediately begin positive pressure ventilation.
   b. Begin positive pressure ventilation after the physical exam.
   c. Immediately apply oxygen by nonrebreather mask at 15 lpm.
   d. Apply oxygen by nasal cannula at 6 lpm after the physical exam.

8. You are treating an elderly man with a complaint of difficulty in breathing. He is breathing 18 times a minute with good chest rise and fall, and you feel a good volume of air at his nose and mouth upon exhalation. Which of the following is correct?
   a Begin positive pressure ventilation.
   b. Apply oxygen by nasal cannula at 6 lpm.
   c. Apply oxygen by nonrebreather mask at 15 lpm.
   d. No ventilation or oxygen therapy is required.

9. The adult with breathing difficulty and increased pulse rate and the infant or child with breathing difficulty and slow pulse rate should both be transported immediately
   a. Following the initial assessment
   b. Following the focused history
   c. Following the physical exam
   d. Following the ongoing assessment

10. Suprasternal notch retractions indicate that the patient
    a. Has a history of heart surgery
    b. Is experiencing substernal chest pain
    c. Is making an extreme effort to breathe
    d. Has a history that includes asthma

11. Bradycardia in the adult, infant, or child is a sign of
    a. Extremely poor oxygenation
    b. Impending respiratory failure
    c. Possible cardiac arrest
    d. All of the above

12. When an area of the chest moves inward during inhalation and outward during exhalation, it is a common sign of chest injury leading to breathing difficulty known as
    a. Diaphragm breathing
    b. Accessory muscle use
    c. Paradoxical motion
    d. Intercostal retractions

13. If you are in doubt whether to ventilate with positive pressure or not, you should
    a. Use a nonrebreather mask
    b. Contact medical direction for orders
    c. Provide the positive pressure ventilation
    d. All of the above

14. For the patient with adequate breathing who is complaining of difficulty in breathing, number the emergency care steps in the correct sequence (1–5).
    _____ Complete the focused history and physical exam.
    _____ Place the patient in a position of comfort and transport.
    _____ Assess the vital signs.
    _____ Administer oxygen at 15 lpm by nonrebreather mask.
    _____ Determine if the patient has a prescribed MDI and contact medical direction for permission to administer it.

15. To determine if your emergency medical care has decreased the patient's breathing difficulty or if further intervention is necessary, you should
    a. Perform an ongoing assessment prior to transporting the patient
    b. Perform an ongoing assessment while en route to the hospital
    c. Perform the focused history and physical exam while transporting
    d. Perform the focused history and physical exam before transporting

16. For administering an MDI, all of the following procedures are correct EXCEPT
    a. Coach the patient to breathe through the nose.
    b. Coach the patient to hold his breath as long as possible after inhalation of the medication.
    c. Depress the canister as the patient begins to inhale.
    d. Shake the canister for 30 seconds before removing the cap.

17. It is imperative that you recognize the early signs of respiratory difficulty in infants and children and treat aggressively. List at least five early signs.

18. All of the following are signs of respiratory failure in infants and children EXCEPT
    a. See-saw or rocky breathing
    b. Increased muscle tone
    c. Diminished breath sounds
    d. Bradycardia or hypotension

19. Your 4-year-old patient displays head bobbing with irregular breathing. You should
    a. Administer oxygen; transport after completing the assessment
    b. Hold the nonrebreather mask next to the child's face; transport at once
    c. Immediately begin positive pressure ventilation; transport at once
    d. Immediately administer oxygen by nonrebreather mask; transport after completing the assessment

20. A child experiencing respiratory difficulty should be placed in which position?
    a. Supine position
    b. Prone position
    c. Position of comfort
    d. Tripod position

21. Regarding epiglottitis in the infant or child, all of the following are true EXCEPT
    a. It can completely block the opening to the trachea.
    b. The child usually sits straight up, juts the neck out, and drools.
    c. You should not inspect or insert anything inside the mouth.
    d. You should perform foreign body airway obstruction maneuvers if respiratory distress is evident.

22. A cough that produces a sound like a barking seal is the hallmark sign of
    a. Complete airway obstruction
    b. Partial airway obstruction
    c. Epiglottitis, swollen epiglottis
    d. Croup, swelling of the larynx

CASE STUDY

▼

It's 8:15 in the morning. You and your partner, Angie, have just received the report from the previous shift. With a cup of coffee in hand, you walk to the ambulance to inventory the supplies and equipment. The alerting system sounds: "Unit 105 respond to 155 Wick Avenue for an elderly patient complaining of difficulty breathing. Alert time 0816 hours." You and Angie get underway at once. En route, dispatch advises that they are on the phone with the son of the patient and that he is very apprehensive. You arrive at the scene and are met at the ambulance by the son. "Hurry! My mother is having trouble breathing." You quickly reassure him as he leads you to the patient. You find an elderly woman, Mrs. Frederick, sitting on the side of the bed with slight use of accessory muscles. A quick survey of the house and room doesn't reveal indications of trauma. The patient's chest is rising and falling adequately. There is good air volume exchange. Auscultation of the lungs reveals breath sounds bilateral with a slight wheezy sound. The respiratory rate is 20 per minute. The patient responds appropriately, and states "I've been—short of breath—over an hour—Hope—you can—help me."

1. From the information provided, what should your assessment and first emergency care step be?
   a. The patient is critical. Immediately begin positive pressure ventilation.
   b. Breathing is adequate. Apply oxygen via nonrebreather mask at 15 lpm.
   c. Patient is hyperventilating. Apply a nasal cannula at 6 lpm.
   d. Patient is hyperventilating. Place a paper bag over the nose and mouth.

2. Using the OPQRST questions to evaluate the history of the present illness, the question *Does lying flat make the breathing difficulty worse?* relates to
   a. Provocation
   b. Quality
   c. Radiation
   d. Severity

   During the focused history and physical exam, you learn that Mrs. Frederick has a history of asthma, and has no known allergies. She does take Albuterol when her breathing is difficult, but she has not taken any today. You inspect around the lips and mouth for cyanosis; none is found. Angie advises that the vitals are blood pressure 160/76, breathing rate 22 per minute, pulse of 100 and regular.

3. Which of the following might cause the rapid breathing in this patient?
   a. Most asthmatics have rapid breathing continuously.
   b. The body attempts to make up for inadequate oxygenation.
   c. The patient's age (the elderly have higher respiratory rates).
   d. This is a common side effect to Albuterol.

4. Which of the following is correct regarding the drug Albuterol?
   a. Alpha agonist bronchoconstrictor, constricts the smooth muscles, dilates the airway
   b. Alpha agonist bronchodilator, relaxes the smooth muscles and dilates the airway
   c. Beta agonist bronchodilator, relaxes the smooth muscles and dilates the airway
   d. Beta pacifist bronchoconstrictor, contracts the smooth muscles, constricts the airway

5. Before you and Angie assist in the administration of the patient's MDI, what three criteria must first be met (indications)?

6. After you administer an MDI, if there is little or no effect you should
   a. Check the expiration date, then re-administer the dose
   b. Consult medical direction to consider re-administering
   c. Shake the MDI for 15 seconds, then re-administer the dose
   d. Have the patient begin deep breathing to increase the effect of the medication

   After administering the MDI you perform an ongoing assessment. Mrs. Frederick advises that her breathing difficulty has decreased dramatically. The vitals are blood pressure 140/62, respiratory rate 14 per minute, and pulse 74 and regular. After auscultating the lungs you hear bilateral breath sounds without wheezes. Angie records and documents all the findings and readies the patient for transport.

7. In what position should you place this patient on the stretcher?
   a. Trendelenburg
   b. Lateral recumbent
   c. Supine
   d. Fowlers or semi-Fowlers

COGNITIVE OBJECTIVES

Numbered objectives are from the United States Department of Transportation 1994 EMT-Basic National Standard Curriculum. Asterisked objectives, if any, pertain to material that is supplemental to the DOT curriculum.

4-3.1 Describe the structure and function of the cardiovascular system.

4-3.2 Describe the emergency medical care of the patient experiencing chest pain/discomfort.

4-3.5 Define the role of the EMT-Basic in the emergency cardiac care system.

4-3.7 Discuss the position of comfort for patients with various cardiac emergencies.

4-3.8 Establish the relationship between airway management and the patient with cardiovascular compromise.

4-3.9 Predict the relationship between the patient experiencing cardiovascular compromise and basic cardiac life support.

4-3.40 Recognize the need for medical direction of protocols to assist in the emergency medical care of the patient with chest pain.

4-3.41 List the indications for the use of nitroglycerin.

4-3.42 State the contraindications and side effects for the use of nitroglycerin.

KEY IDEAS

In this chapter the cardiac system and cardiac emergencies involving chest pain are discussed. Key ideas include the following:

▶ Signs and symptoms of cardiac compromise may vary widely from patient to patient.

▶ All adult patients complaining of chest pain should be treated as cardiac patients until proven otherwise.

▶ Prehospital treatment by the EMT-B of the responsive patient suffering chest pain should focus on assessment, early interventions such as administration of high-flow oxygen, and transport —not on diagnosing the specific type of cardiac emergency the patient is experiencing.

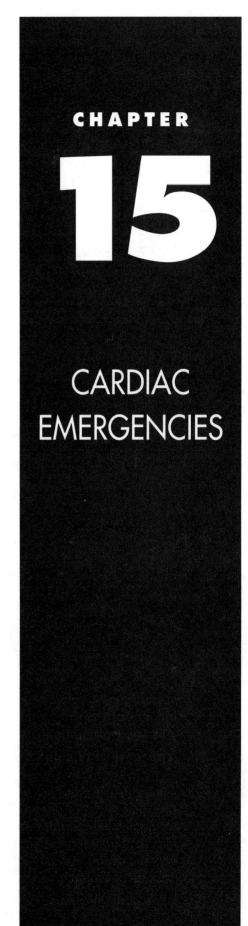

CHAPTER

15

CARDIAC EMERGENCIES

► Not all patients experiencing chest pain will go into cardiac arrest. If the patient does go into cardiac arrest, the EMT-B must be prepared to perform CPR and to apply the AED (automated external defibrillator) as detailed in Chapter 16.

TERMS AND CONCEPTS

▼

1. **Write the number of the correct term next to each definition. Not all terms will be used.**

   1. aorta
   2. atrium
   3. cardiac conduction system
   4. carotid artery
   5. coronary arteries
   6. diastolic pressure

   7. pulmonary vein
   8. radial artery
   9. systolic pressure
   10. valves
   11. venae cavae
   12. ventricle

_____ **a.** One of the two upper chambers of the heart

_____ **b.** Membranes located within the heart to prevent backflow of blood

_____ **c.** One of two lower chambers of the heart

_____ **d.** Vessel carrying oxygen-rich blood from the lungs to the left atrium of the heart

_____ **e.** Major artery in the neck

_____ **f.** The pressure exerted against the arterial wall during contraction of the ventricles of the heart

_____ **g.** The two major veins that carry oxygen-depleted blood back to the heart

_____ **h.** Major artery that starts at the left ventricle and carries oxygen-rich blood to the body

_____ **i.** Pressure exerted against the arterial walls during relaxation of the ventricle of the heart

_____ **j.** Specialized contractile and conductive tissue of the heart that generates electrical impulses and causes the heart to beat

_____ **k.** Network of arteries that supply the heart with blood

CONTENT REVIEW

1. Fill in each term, naming a structure of the circulatory system, on the appropriate line.

alveoli
arteries
arterioles
body capillaries
bronchi
lung capillaries
pulmonary artery
pulmonary vein
veins
venules

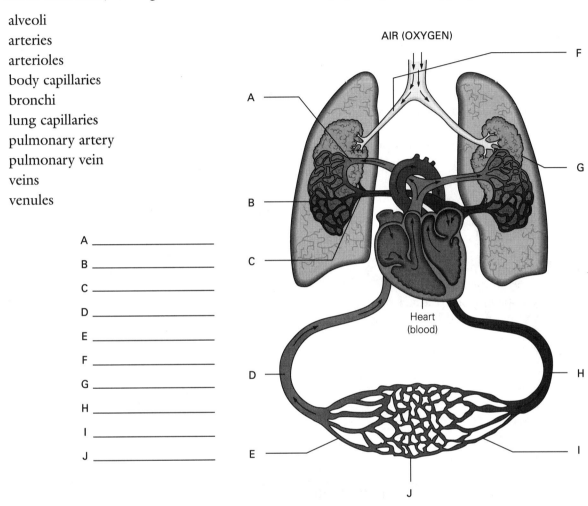

A _____

B _____

C _____

D _____

E _____

F _____

G _____

H _____

I _____

J _____

2. List and briefly explain the three major components of the circulatory system.

3. Hypoperfusion can occur as a result of
   a. Low blood volume
   b. Pump (heart) damage
   c. Nervous system interference
   d. Any of the above

4. Which is the proper sequence for the initial assessment of the responsive cardiac patient who is suffering chest pain?
   a. Assess circulation, breathing, airway, skin
   b. Assess airway, breathing, circulation, skin
   c. Assess breathing, circulation, airway, skin
   d. Assess skin, airway, breathing, circulation

5. Which is the FIRST emergency care step for the responsive patient who is suffering chest pain?
   a. Administer nitroglycerin.
   b. Perform positive pressure ventilation with supplemental oxygen.
   c. Administer oxygen at 15 lpm by nonrebreather mask.
   d. Perform cardiopulmonary resuscitation (CPR).

6. Using the OPQRST questions to evaluate the history of the present illness, the question, "On a scale of 1 to 10, how would you rate your pain?" is an example of
   a. Onset
   b. Quality
   c. Severity
   d. Provocation

7. Many cardiac patients will not experience pain during a cardiac emergency. This painless attack is widely known as
   a. A suspicious heart attack
   b. An unconfirmed heart attack
   c. A quiet heart attack
   d. A silent heart attack

8. Nitroglycerin spray or tablet form is administered by what route?
   a. Sublingual
   b. Topical
   c. Intravenous
   d. Intramuscular

9. Which of the following are contraindications for administering nitroglycerin?

   1. The patient has signs and symptoms of chest pain.

   2. The patient's systolic blood pressure is below 100.

   3. The patient has a suspected head injury.

   4. The patient has physician-prescribed nitroglycerin.

   5. Three doses have already been taken by the patient.

   6. Medical direction has given approval off-line but not on-line.

   a. 1, 2, and 4

   b. 2, 3, and 5

   c. 1, 4, and 6

   d. 1, 3, and 5

10. Which is the MOST CORRECT statement about the following possible causes of chest pain?

congestive heart failure   angina pectoris

coronary artery disease   indigestion

myocardial infarction (heart attack)   muscle spasm

    a. The EMT-B must be able to diagnose which of these conditions is the cause of the chest pain.
    b. The EMT-B's assessment and care will not change no matter what the cause of the patient's chest pain.
    c. The EMT-B will administer nitroglycerin only to the patient who is known to be suffering from angina pectoris.
    d. The EMT-B needs to know which of these conditions is likely to deteriorate into cardiac arrest.

CASE STUDY

You and your partner, Manny Rodriguez, are dispatched to a residence where there is a report of an elderly man having a heart attack. You are met at the door by the patient's wife, and she thanks you for your prompt response. She leads you to the back porch where you find her husband sitting clutching his chest. You introduce yourselves, and the patient says his name is Fred Hansen. A quick visual assessment reveals that the patient is pale, slightly short of breath, and seems very anxious.

1. You instruct Manny to place Mr. Hansen on oxygen. Which is the most appropriate means of delivering the oxygen?
    a. The patient's own home oxygen apparatus
    b. Nasal cannula at 6 lpm
    c. Nonrebreather mask at 15 lpm
    d. Positive pressure ventilation with supplemental oxygen

    As you perform the initial assessment, you note that Mr. Hansen's radial pulse is very weak and irregular. You compare his radial pulse with the carotid pulse and find that the carotid is strong and fast, but both are irregular.

2. On the basis of the information you gathered on arrival plus this additional information, you determine that
    a. Mr. Hansen is experiencing cardiac compromise; however, early transport is not necessary
    b. Mr. Hansen is experiencing cardiac compromise, and early transport is necessary
    c. Mr. Hansen is not experiencing cardiac compromise; however, early transport is necessary
    d. Mr. Hansen is not experiencing cardiac compromise, and early transport is not necessary

Mr. Hansen states the only medicine that his physician prescribes for him is an aspirin a day and nitroglycerin for chest pain. You ask Mr. Hansen if he took any nitroglycerin with this episode of chest pain. He states, "One about 5 minutes before you arrived, but the pain is getting worse." You reassure Mr. Hansen as you quickly obtain the vital signs: pulse 70 per minute, weak and irregular, respirations 24 per minute, BP 152/74. Skin is slightly pale and sweaty. Pupils are normal. Then you call medical direction for permission to administer additional nitroglycerin. Permission is granted by Dr. Smith for a total of three doses, including the dose Mr. Hansen has already taken, as long as the patient's blood pressure is stable.

3. Shortly after you administer a nitroglycerin tablet, Mr. Hansen complains of a headache. You should
   a. Reassure him that this is a common side effect and the pain should pass
   b. Immediately remove the tablet; the headache indicates an allergic response
   c. Have him swallow the tablet; this will speed its absorption
   d. Re-establish contact with medical direction to ask for advice

4. Mr. Hansen's chest pain has improved dramatically. You should
   a. Relax—the crisis is over
   b. Continue to evaluate him en route, and update the receiving emergency department of any changes
   c. Administer the third nitroglycerin tablet
   d. Contact medical direction for permission to administer an aspirin to reduce the chest pain

COGNITIVE OBJECTIVES

Numbered objectives are from the United States Department of Transportation 1994 EMT-Basic National Standard Curriculum. Asterisked objectives, if any, pertain to material that is supplemental to the DOT curriculum.

4-3.3   List the indications for automated external defibrillation (AED).

4-3.4   List the contraindications for automated external defibrillation.

4-3.6   Explain the impact of age and weight on defibrillation.

4-3.10   Discuss the fundamentals of early defibrillation.

4-3.11   Explain the rationale for early defibrillation.

4-3.12   Explain that not all chest pain patients result in cardiac arrest and do not need to be attached to an automated external defibrillator.

4-3.13   Explain the importance of prehospital ACLS intervention if it is available.

4-3.14   Explain the importance of urgent transport to a facility with Advanced Cardiac Life Support if it is not available in the prehospital setting.

4-3.15   Discuss the various types of automated external defibrillators.

4-3.16   Differentiate between the fully automated and the semi-automated defibrillator.

4-3.17   Discuss the procedures that must be taken into consideration for standard operations of the various types of automated external defibrillators.

4-3.18   State the reasons for assuring that the patient is pulseless and apneic when using the automated external defibrillator.

4-3.19   Discuss the circumstances which may result in inappropriate shocks.

4-3.20   Explain the considerations for interruption of CPR, when using the automated external defibrillator.

4-3.21   Discuss the advantages and disadvantages of automated external defibrillators.

4-3.22   Summarize the speed of operation of automated external defibrillation.

4-3.23   Discuss the use of remote defibrillation through adhesive pads.

4-3.24   Discuss the special considerations for rhythm monitoring.

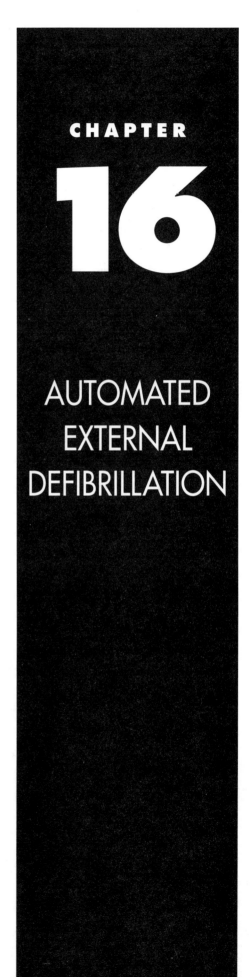

CHAPTER

16

AUTOMATED
EXTERNAL
DEFIBRILLATION

4-3.25 List the steps in the operation of the automated external defibrillator.

4-3.26 Discuss the standard of care that should be used to provide care to a patient with persistent ventricular fibrillation and no available ACLS.

4-3.27 Discuss the standard of care that should be used to provide care to a patient with recurrent ventricular fibrillation and no available ACLS.

4-3.28 Differentiate between the single rescuer and multi-rescuer care with an automated external defibrillator.

4-3.29 Explain the reasons for pulses not being checked between shocks with an automated external defibrillator.

4-3.30 Discuss the importance of coordinating ACLS-trained providers with personnel using automated external defibrillators.

4-3.31 Discuss the importance of post-resuscitation care.

4-3.32 List the components of post-resuscitation care.

4-3.33 Explain the importance of frequent practice with the automated external defibrillator.

4-3.34 Discuss the need to complete the Automated Defibrillator: Operator's Shift Checklist.

4-3.35 Discuss the role of the American Heart Association in the use of automated external defibrillation.

4-3.36 Explain the role medical direction plays in the use of automated external defibrillation.

4-3.37 State the reasons why a case review should be completed following the use of the automated external defibrillator.

4-3.38 Discuss the components that should be included in a case review.

4-3.39 Discuss the goal of quality improvement in automated external defibrillation.

4-3.43 Define the function of all controls on an automated external defibrillator, and describe event documentation and battery defibrillator maintenance.

KEY IDEAS

▼

One of the links in the American Heart Association's "chain of survival" for cardiac arrest patients is early defibrillation. Some believe it is the most important link—"the one thing in EMS that we know works." Therefore, an essential skill for EMT-Basics is correct application and operation of the automated external defibrillator, or AED.

▶ Successfully resuscitating a cardiac arrest patient is dependent upon the "Chain of Survival." This chain has four links: (1) early access, (2) early CPR, (3) early defibrillation, and (4) early advanced cardiac life support (ACLS).

▶ There are two basic types of external defibrillators, manual and automated. There are two types of automated external defibrillators (AEDs), fully automated and semi-automated.

▶ The rhythms for which automated external defibrillation is appropriate are ventricular fibrillation and ventricular tachycardia.

▶ The AED is indicated for use on the adult (over 12 and/or over 90 pounds) non-trauma patient who is unresponsive with no breathing and no pulse.

▶ The sequence for using the external semi-automated defibrillator is:

— Perform the initial assessment and verify absence of pulse and breathing.

— Begin CPR while your partner prepares the AED.

— Place the defibrillator electrodes on the patient's chest.

— Turn on the defibrillator and start your narrative.

— Stop CPR and get clear as the AED analyzes the rhythm.

— If a shock is advised, clear everyone from the patient and deliver the shock.

▶ Up to six total shocks may be delivered. Administer three shocks (analyze–shock, analyze–shock, analyze–shock), check pulse and resume CPR for 1 minute, and then deliver three more shocks. This six-shock rule starts over again if the patient's pulse returns and subsequently stops.

▶ The AED must be checked on a daily basis using the Automated Defibrillator: Operator's Shift Checklist to prevent device failure.

▶ AED operators should practice with the device every 90 days to refresh skills.

TERMS AND CONCEPTS

1. **The four terms below name heart rhythms and conditions that may be detected by an AED. Write the number of each term next to its definition.**

   1. asystole
   2. pulseless electrical activity (PEA)
   3. ventricular fibrillation (VF or V-Fib)
   4. ventricular tachycardia (V-Tach)

   _____ **a.** A condition in which the heart generates relatively normal electrical rhythms but there is decreased or absent cardiac output as a result of cardiac muscle failure or blood loss

   _____ **b** A very rapid heart rhythm that is generally too fast to perfuse the body's organs adequately

   _____ **c.** A continuous, uncoordinated trembling of the heart muscle which does not produce any cardiac output or perfusion of the body's organs

   _____ **d.** A heart rhythm indicating absence of electrical activity in the heart; also known as "flatline"

CONTENT REVIEW

1. Select the patient who is the BEST candidate for automated external defibrillation.
   a. An adult medical patient who is in cardiac arrest
   b. A child medical patient who is in cardiac arrest
   c. An adult trauma patient in cardiac arrest
   d. A responsive adult who is having chest pain

2. Which item is NOT a component of the "Chain of Survival?"
   a. Early assessment
   b. Early CPR
   c. Early defibrillation
   d. Early Advanced Cardiac Life Support (ACLS)

3. The application of an electric shock to help the heart reorganize its electrical activity and restore its normal rhythm is known as
   a. Vagal stimulation
   b. Shock therapy
   c. Defibrillation
   d. Cardiovascular therapy

4. Which of the following is NOT an advantage of using an automated external defibrillator (AED) instead of a manual defibrillator?
   a. AEDs can deliver a first shock quickly, usually within the first minute.
   b. AEDs allow for "hands-free" defibrillation by the use of adhesive pads.
   c. The operator analyzes the rhythm and make the decision to shock.
   d. Initial operational training is relatively short, and extensive training is not required.

5. Important factors in achieving successful resuscitation in a cardiac arrest patient include all of the following EXCEPT
   a. How rapidly CPR is established
   b. The speed with which defibrillation is accomplished
   c. The age of the patient
   d. How rapidly the incident is recognized and EMS is dispatched

6. Which of the following is NOT one of the indications for the use of the AED?
   a. Severe chest pain
   b. No breathing
   c. No pulse
   d. All of the above are indications for application of the AED.

7. Which of the following emergency care actions should take precedence over AED shock delivery?
   a. Inserting an airway device
   b. Setting up an oxygen delivery device
   c. Obtaining a detailed patient history
   d. No actions should take precedence over shock delivery.

8. Select the proper description for the anterior placement of the defibrillator electrodes.
   a. (-)(sternum) on left upper chest wall, (+)(apex) on right lower ribs at the anterior axillary line to the right of the nipple
   b. (+)(apex) on left upper chest wall, (-)(sternum) on right lower ribs at the anterior axillary line to the right of the nipple
   c. (-)(sternum) right upper border of the sternum, (+) (apex) on left anterior axillary line below and to the left of the nipple
   d. (-)(sternum) left upper border of the sternum, (+)(apex) on right anterior axillary line to the right of the nipple

9. Place the following steps for using a semi-automated AED in the proper sequence.
   1. Turn on power button.
   2. Attach pad to cables and apply pad to the patient's chest.
   3. Begin or resume CPR and prepare the AED.
   4. Stop CPR, say "Clear" and press the button to begin analysis.
   5. Begin narrative (if equipped with recorder).
   6. BSI and perform an initial assessment.
   7. Press button to deliver shock if "Deliver shock" message is given.

   a. 6, 3, 2, 1, 5, 4, 7
   b. 6, 3, 1, 4, 2, 5, 7
   c. 5, 6, 1, 3, 4, 7, 2
   d. 3, 6, 1, 5, 4, 2, 7

10. AED use is ideally performed by two EMT-Bs. Place the following steps for one-rescuer AED use in the proper sequence.
    1. Verify that the patient is unresponsive with no breathing and no pulse.
    2. Attach the AED's pads to the cable and attach the pads to the patient.
    3. Perform the initial assessment.
    4. Initiate the rhythm analysis.
    5. Turn on the AED and begin narrative (if equipped with recorder).
    6. Deliver shocks as the AED indicates.

    a. 1, 3, 5, 2, 4, 6
    b. 3, 1, 5, 2, 4, 6
    c. 3, 1, 2, 5, 4, 6
    d. 1, 3, 2, 5, 4, 6

11. You are transporting an unresponsive patient who has been defibrillated. The patient becomes pulseless and has no respiration. Select the best action to take.
    a. Stop the vehicle, deliver three stacked shocks, resume transport.
    b. Stop the vehicle, turn off the motor, deliver three stacked shocks, check pulse/resume CPR, deliver three stacked shocks (if indicated), resume transport.
    c. Stop the vehicle, deliver as many as 3 sets of 3 stacked shocks, recheck the pulse, if no pulse continue CPR until arrival at the hospital.
    d. Deliver 3 stacked shocks, recheck the pulse, if no pulse, continue CPR until arrival at the hospital.

12. ACLS care for a patient in cardiac arrest can be provided by all of the following means EXCEPT
    a. ACLS may be provided by EMT-Is or EMT-Ps.
    b. ACLS may be provided by the receiving hospital.
    c. ACLS may be provided by transporting the patient to a clinic with cardiac care capabilities.
    d. ACLS may be provided by the EMT-B following contact with medical direction.

13. AED failure is most commonly attributed to
    a. Operator error
    b. Cable failure
    c. Internal electronics failure
    d. Battery failure

14. It is recommended that every AED operator refresh or practice operational skills with the device every
    a. Month
    b. Three months
    c. Six months
    d. Year

15. Which of the following best describes an acceptable and safe use of an AED?
    a. Application of an AED on a patient who is lying in shallow water
    b. AED use on a patient who is on a metal catwalk
    c. Placement of an AED pad on top of a nitroglycerin patch
    d. AED use on a patient who is on the floor of his home

16. The Operator's Shift Checklist should be completed by the EMT-B at the beginning of
    a. Each EMS call
    b. Every third shift
    c. Every other shift
    d. Each shift

CASE STUDY 1

You have been dispatched to the scene of a cardiac arrest. Dispatch advises that an ALS vehicle is also responding to the incident. A family member is on scene providing CPR. You arrive and observe a male patient who appears to be in his mid-60s supine on the floor. The family member is performing adequate CPR on the patient. You hear the siren of the approaching ALS vehicle.

1. Your next best action is to
   a. Take over CPR, then stop and verify absence of pulse/breathing; do nothing further until ALS arrives
   b. Stop CPR, perform an initial assessment, and verify the absence of pulse/breathing
   c. Obtain a detailed history of the event as the family member continues CPR, then stop and verify the absence of pulse/breathing
   d. Have the family member continue CPR and radio dispatch to determine the exact ETA of the ALS vehicle, then verify the absence of pulse/breathing

2. The patient is pulseless and breathless. Your next best action is to
   a. Prepare the AED for operation by turning the power button on
   b. Resume CPR and prepare the AED for operation by turning the power button on
   c. Resume CPR and do nothing further until ALS arrival
   d. Place the adhesive monitoring-defibrillation pads on the patient's chest

3. The patient's rhythm is analyzed and the AED shows that applying a shock will not benefit the patient ("no shock"). What is your next best action?
   a. Resume CPR and transport the patient rapidly.
   b. Reanalyze the rhythm, wait 30 seconds, then reanalyze the rhythm again.
   c. Contact medical direction for additional orders.
   d. Recheck the pulse; if no pulse resume CPR for 1 minute, then reanalyze the rhythm.

CASE STUDY 2

You are working alone at a large public complex as an EMT-Basic providing emergency medical coverage. You have been assigned to cover a concert for the evening. At the completion of the concert you receive a call for a man down. You respond quickly to the site of the emergency. When you arrive you observe a 50-year-old male who is supine on the floor of the rest room. You perform an initial assessment on the patient and determine that he is unresponsive to pain and is breathless and pulseless.

1. What is your next best action?
   a. Turn on the AED and begin the narration (if equipped with recorder).
   b. Call EMS for assistance.
   c. Attach the AED's external adhesive pads.
   d. Use a pocket mask and attempt to give one ventilation to confirm an open airway.

2. You have delivered three shocks and rechecked the pulse. The patient is still pulseless. What is the next best action to take?
   a. Perform CPR for 1 minute, then call dispatch for EMS help.
   b. Reanalyze the rhythm and repeat three more shocks if indicated.
   c. Transport, performing CPR en route.
   d. Call for help from EMS dispatch, perform CPR for 1 minute, recheck pulse.

3. You recheck the pulse and find that the patient has a palpable radial and carotid pulse. What is your next best action?
   a. Check the blood pressure.
   b. Check the breathing.
   c. Check the pupils.
   d. Check skin color and temperature.

CASE STUDY 3

You are on scene treating a 70-year-old cardiac arrest patient. A neighbor tells you that he saw the patient collapse while mowing his yard. The neighbor's wife called EMS while the neighbor quickly started CPR. You have been working on the patient for what seems like a long time. The ALS unit has not yet arrived. You have administered a total of six shocks.

1. What is your next best action?
   a. Recheck the pulse, continue CPR (if required), and reanalyze for additional shocks.
   b. Recheck the pulse and continue CPR (if required) until the arrival of the ALS unit.
   c. Recheck the pulse, continue CPR (if required), and transport the patient.
   d. Continue CPR for 5 minutes and reanalyze for additional shocks.

2. You are now en route to the hospital with the patient. The patient's pulse has not returned. What of the following actions may be requested by medical direction?

   1. That you make further defibrillation attempts

   2. That you provide only CPR and rapid transport

   a. Only 1
   b. Only 2
   c. Either 1 or 2
   d. Neither 1 nor 2

3. The medical director stops by the hospital to visit you after the call has been completed. He asks for information on the call that may be used for quality improvement. This information may include which of the following items?
   a. Written reports
   b. Solid-state memory modules or magnetic tapes (if AED is so equipped)
   c. Voice or EKG tapes (if AED is so equipped)
   d. All of the above

COGNITIVE OBJECTIVES

Numbered objectives are from the United States Department of Transportation 1994 EMT-Basic National Standard Curriculum. Asterisked objectives, if any, pertain to material that is supplemental to the DOT curriculum.

4-4.1   Identify the patient taking diabetic medications with altered mental status and the implications of a diabetes history.

4-4.2   State the steps in the emergency medical care of the patient taking diabetic medicine with an altered mental status and a history of diabetes.

4-4.3   Establish the relationship between airway management and the patient with altered mental status.

4-4.4   State the generic and trade names, medication forms, dose, administration, action, and contraindications for oral glucose.

4-4.5   Evaluate the need for medical direction in the emergency medical care of the diabetic patient.

*   State the steps in the emergency care of the patient with an altered mental status and no known history.

KEY IDEAS

This chapter focuses on the patient with an altered mental status caused by a condition associated with diabetes. Emphasis is placed on assessing the patient's mental status, determining if the patient has a history of diabetes controlled by medication, and determining if the patient is alert enough to swallow before administering oral glucose with permission from medical direction.

▶ It is important to distinguish between the patient with an altered mental status who has a history of diabetes controlled by medication and the patient with an altered mental status who does not have a known history of diabetes.

▶ Airway management is a major concern in the patient with an altered mental status.

▶ With on-line or off-line approval from medical direction, oral glucose may be administered to the patient with an altered mental status and a history of diabetes controlled by medication who is alert enough to swallow.

CHAPTER

17

ALTERED MENTAL STATUS— DIABETIC EMERGENCIES

TERMS AND CONCEPTS

1. Write the number of the correct term next to each definition.

   1. altered mental status
   2. diabetes mellitus
   3. glucose
   4. hyperglycemia
   5. hypoglycemia
   6. insulin

   _____ **a.** High blood sugar

   _____ **b.** Hormone secreted by the pancreas that promotes the movement of glucose into the sugar-storing cells

   _____ **c.** Disease characterized by the body's inability to produce insulin

   _____ **d.** Condition in which the patient displays a change ranging from disorientation to complete unresponsiveness

   _____ **e.** Low blood sugar

   _____ **f.** Form of sugar that is the body's basic source of energy

CONTENT REVIEW

1. An altered mental status indicates that the central nervous system has been affected. Which of the following may affect the central nervous system, causing an altered mental status?
   a. A traumatic injury
   b. A change in blood sugar levels
   c. A change in blood oxygen levels
   d. Any of these

2. Which of the following can be considered a frequent medical cause of altered mental status?
   a. Poisoning
   b. Infection
   c. Stroke
   d. Any of these

3. Your altered mental status patient is lying in bed, and no mechanism of injury is evident. You would suspect that the altered mental status is a result of
   a. Head trauma
   b. Chest injury
   c. A medical illness
   d. Any of these

4. You are assessing a patient with an altered mental status. Which of the following signs would cause you to suspect that the decreased mental status is due to trauma rather than a medical illness?
   a. Pupils that are pinpoint, or dilated
   b. Decorticate or decerebrate posturing (arms flexed or extended, legs extended)
   c. Lacerations to the tongue indicating seizure
   d. Loss of bowel control

5. Your patient has had a rapid onset of altered mental status and has cool, moist skin, an elevated heart rate, and other signs that he is experiencing a diabetic emergency. He has no medical ID tag or medications on his person, and you are unable to confirm that he has a history of diabetes controlled by medication. However, he is clearly still able to swallow. Which of the following emergency care measures should you provide?

   1. Ensure an open airway.
   2. Provide oxygen by nonrebreather mask at 15 lpm.
   3. Administer oral glucose.
   4. Position the patient on his side and transport.

   a. 1, 3, and 4
   b. 1, 2, and 4
   c. 1 and 4
   d. 1, 2, 3, and 4

6. Briefly explain the two types of diabetes.
   Type I

   Type II

7. Which of the following may be true of the diabetic patient?

   1. A lack of insulin will prevent sugar from entering the cells.
   2. Too much insulin will cause too much sugar to enter the cells, leaving too little sugar in the blood.
   3. A lack of insulin will cause too much sugar to build up in the blood.
   4. An imbalance between the amount of insulin and the amount of sugar in the blood is likely to cause an altered mental status.

   a. 1, 3, and 4
   b. 1 and 3
   c. 2 and 3
   d. 1, 2, 3, and 4

8. Write the four questions that are particularly important when assessing the patient with a history of diabetes.

9. Signs and symptoms that mimic a stroke, such as weakness or paralysis on one side of the body, may occur more frequently in the diabetic patient who is
    a. Young
    b. Hyperglycemic
    c. Elderly
    d. On cardiac medications

10. List at least two possible indications that a patient has a history of diabetes that is controlled by medication.

11. You are treating a patient with an altered mental status who has diabetes that is controlled by medication. After establishing and maintaining the airway you should next
    a. Administer oral glucose per protocol
    b. Determine if the patient can swallow
    c. Reassess airway, breathing, and circulation
    d. Perform an ongoing assessment

12. Select the correct statement regarding reassessment following administration of oral glucose.
    a. Reassess the patient's mental status, expecting an improvement in 3 minutes or less.
    b. Reassess the patient's mental status, understanding that improvement may not be apparent for 20 minutes or more.
    c. Assume that the patient's mental status will not deteriorate once oral glucose has been administered.
    d. If the patient loses responsiveness or seizes, insert a tongue depressor to prevent the patient from biting his tongue.

CASE STUDY

You and your partner, Emil, are dispatched to a local park where there is a report of a young female acting strangely. You approach the scene and find an approximately 30-year-old female in a jogging outfit sitting on a bench. It appears that she is anxious and speaking with inappropriate words. You notice a medical identification bracelet that informs you she is an insulin-dependent diabetic. The patient's airway is patent and her breathing appears adequate. You place her on oxygen. The patient does not answer any of your questions appropriately, and none of the bystanders who have gathered know her. Her vital signs include heart rate 104 per minute, blood pressure 100/64, respirations 20 per minute. The skin is cool and moist. You and Emil both suspect a diabetic emergency and decide that she is alert enough to swallow. You ask Emil to prepare to administer oral glucose following the protocol established off line by your medical direction.

1. From the above information, list the signs that support your suspicion that the patient is suffering from a diabetic emergency.

2. You placed the patient on oxygen. Which of the following is most appropriate for this patient?
   a. Nasal cannula at 6 lpm
   b. Nonrebreather mask at 15 lpm
   c. Simple face mask at 15 lpm
   d. Positive pressure ventilation

3. You and your partner determined that the patient met the three criteria for administration of oral glucose. List the three criteria.

4. Approval to administer oral glucose was given off line in the above scenario. In some jurisdictions, approval to administer oral glucose must be given on line. Briefly explain the difference between off-line and on-line medical direction.

After you administered the oral glucose, the patient began feeling much better. En route to the hospital, she is able to converse normally. She informs you her name is Pat, that she lives on Third Avenue, and she knows it's Tuesday. She took her insulin this morning but went for a jog and forgot to eat lunch. You continue to assess her during the transport to the hospital.

CHAPTER 18

ALTERED MENTAL STATUS WITH LOSS OF FUNCTION

COGNITIVE OBJECTIVES

Numbered objectives are from the United States Department of Transportation 1994 EMT-Basic National Standard Curriculum. Asterisked objectives, if any, pertain to material that is supplemental to the DOT curriculum.

4-4.3 Establish the relationship between airway management and the patient with altered mental status.

* Describe the assessment of the patient with an altered mental status and a loss of speech, sensory, or motor function.

* List the common signs and symptoms of a nontraumatic brain injury.

* Describe the emergency care for a patient with an altered mental status and a loss of speech, sensory, or motor function.

* Describe the conditions most likely to cause altered mental status with a loss of speech, sensory, or motor function.

KEY IDEAS

An altered mental status may sometimes be accompanied by a loss of speech, sensory, or motor function. This chapter focuses on the assessment and management of patients with these signs.

▶ Altered mental status with loss of function may be caused by external trauma or by a nontraumatic brain injury, such as that caused by stroke.

▶ It is important to closely monitor and manage the airway and breathing of the patient who is suffering an altered mental status with loss of speech, sensory, and motor function.

TERMS AND CONCEPTS

1. **Write the number of the correct term next to each definition.**

    1. cerebrovascular accident (CVA)
    2. neurologic deficit
    3. nontraumatic brain injury
    4. transient ischemic attacks (TIAs)

_____ **a.** Brief, intermittent episodes with stroke-like symptoms that disappear within 24 hours

_____ **b.** A medical injury to the brain, such as a stroke, that is not caused by an external injury

_____ **c.** Any deficiency in the brain's functioning

_____ **d.** A sudden disruption in blood flow to the brain that results in brain cell damage; a stroke

CONTENT REVIEW

1. Which of the following is a sign or symptom of neurologic deficit?
   a. Slurred speech
   b. Paralysis
   c. Numbness
   d. Any of the above

2. One kind of nontraumatic (medical) brain injury is a stroke (cerebrovascular accident, or CVA). Using the illustrations as your guide, choose possible causes of a stroke from the list below.

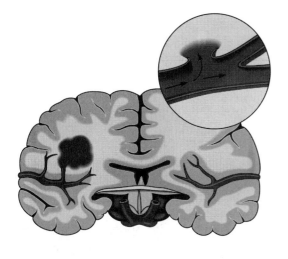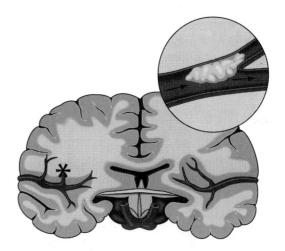

   1. Rupture of a blood vessel in the brain
   2. Blockage of a blood vessel in the brain
   3. Laceration of the carotid artery
   4. Dilation of the blood vessels in the brain

   a. 1 and 2
   b. 3 and 4
   c. 2 and 3
   d. 1 and 4

3. During scene size-up, you find a bucket next to the bed. Which of the following is most likely to be the reason for this?
   a. Frequent urination, which is a common sign of nontraumatic brain injury
   b. Nausea or vomiting, which is a common sign of nontraumatic brain injury
   c. Bloody sputum, which is a common sign of nontraumatic brain injury
   d. None of the above

4. Briefly explain why it is important to immediately assess the patient's airway when you suspect a nontraumatic brain injury.

5. Explain how you might interview the patient if your patient has lost the ability to communicate through speech.

6. All of the following are signs and symptoms of neurological deficit resulting from nontraumatic brain injury EXCEPT
   a. Hemiparesis of the right arm and foot
   b. Paralysis to both right and left legs
   c. Weak or absent vision in the right eye
   d. Garbled or incomprehensible speech

7. You are treating a patient with an altered mental status who has lost motor function. The patient's breathing has become inadequate. You should
   a. Administer positive pressure ventilation with supplemental oxgyen
   b. Administer oxygen via nonrebreather mask
   c. Administer oxygen via nasal cannula
   d. All of the above are appropriate treatments

8. You are treating a patient with signs and symptoms of a stroke who is unresponsive. Which position is most appropriate to place this patient in?
   a. Supine position, legs elevated
   b. Supine position, head and chest elevated
   c. Lateral recumbent position
   d. Prone position

9. Because the nontraumatic brain-injured patient may deteriorate rapidly, you should frequently perform
   a. A rapid trauma assessment
   b. A focused trauma assessment
   c. A detailed physical exam
   d. An ongoing assessment

10. Strokes most often affect elderly patients with any of the following kinds of medical history EXCEPT
    a. A history of heart disease
    b. A history of osteoporosis
    c. A history of hypertension
    d. A history of atherosclerosis

11. Your patient has experienced the signs and symptoms of a transient ischemic attack. However, he is feeling better and is refusing treatment. You must encourage the patient to be treated because
    a. Approximately one-third of the those who suffer a TIA will have a stroke
    b. Approximately one-half of the those who suffer a TIA will have a heart attack
    c. Nearly all of the patients who suffer a TIA sustain permanent neurologic deficit
    d. There is no need for treatment because there are no lasting effects to a TIA

12. You are assessing an elderly patient who appears to have suffered a stroke. Why is it important to determine if there is a history of diabetes?
    a. An elderly diabetic patient should not be given oxygen.
    b. An elderly stroke patient is likely to develop diabetes.
    c. Elderly hyperglycemic diabetics suffer more strokes than elderly non-diabetics.
    d. An elderly diabetic patient who is hypoglycemic may present with signs and symptoms similar to a stroke.

CASE STUDY

You and your partner, Lynn, are dispatched to an unknown medical problem in a high-rise apartment. You are met in the parking lot by a security guard who directs you to the elevator. He says, "Jose, the other guard, is with the patient, Mrs. Peters, and he will meet you up there." Jose directs you to the bedroom where you find an elderly female lying in bed. As you introduce yourself, the patient looks at you with a terrified glare. You reassure her and ask if she can understand you. She nods her head to indicate yes. The patient tries to communicate, but her speech is incomprehensible. Her feelings of frustration are obvious. You explain that you will ask yes-or-no questions, and she can reply by shaking or nodding her head.

1. Mrs. Peters's breathing appears to be adequate. Which is most appropriate?
    a. Place her on oxygen at 15 lpm via nonrebreather mask.
    b. Mrs. Peters's breathing is adequate, so there is no need for oxygen.
    c. Place her on oxygen at 6 lpm via nasal cannula.
    d. Administer positive pressure ventilation with supplemental oxygen.

    Further interviewing reveals that Mrs. Peters's only medical history is hypertension. You notice significant facial drooping and paralysis to the right side of her body. Lynn suggests that the portable suction unit be set up and ready for immediate use. You agree. You prepare Mrs. Peters for transport, carefully protecting her paralyzed extremities so as not to injure them.

2. Briefly explain why the suction unit may be needed although Mrs. Peters's airway is adequate.

As you and Lynn are transporting Mrs. Peters in the elevator, the patient grabs her head with her left hand. You ask her if she has a terrible headache. She nods yes, then becomes unresponsive, and her breathing becomes inadequate at 8 breaths per minute.

3. Recognizing that her breathing is inadequate, which of the following is now most appropriate for Mrs. Peters?
   a. Administer oxygen at 15 lpm via nonrebreather mask.
   b. Administer positive pressure ventilation at 12 ventilations per minute with supplemental oxygen.
   c. Administer positive pressure ventilation at 20 ventilations per minute with supplemental oxygen.
   d. Administer positive pressure ventilation at greater than 24 ventilations per minute with supplemental oxygen.

ALTERED MENTAL STATUS— SEIZURES AND SYNCOPE

COGNITIVE OBJECTIVES

Numbered objectives are from the United States Department of Transportation 1994 EMT-Basic National Standard Curriculum. Asterisked objectives, if any, pertain to material that is supplemental to the DOT curriculum.

*   Explain the assessment and emergency care for a seizing patient.

*   Recognize the common signs and symptoms of a generalized seizure.

*   Recognize signs and symptoms of status epilepticus.

*   Identify various conditions that cause seizures.

*   Recognize the common signs and symptoms of syncope.

*   Differentiate between syncope and seizures.

KEY IDEAS

This chapter focuses on seizures, their causes and characteristics, and their management in the prehospital setting. Syncope, or fainting, is also discussed.

▶ A common cause of seizures is epilepsy, but seizures are caused by a variety of conditions.

▶ The most common type of epileptic seizure is the generalized tonic-clonic seizure.

▶ It is important to protect the airway in the seizing and post-seizure patient.

▶ Oxygen should be administered to the seizure patient. If breathing is inadequate, it may be necessary to assist breathing.

▶ It is important to prevent injury to the seizing patient.

▶ Syncope (fainting) is a temporary loss of responsiveness and may be confused with a seizure. Among other distinctions between a seizure and syncope, the patient who has fainted usually becomes responsive and recovers almost immediately.

TERMS AND CONCEPTS

1. **Write the number of the correct term next to each definition.**

    1. aura
    2. epilepsy
    3. generalized tonic-clonic seizure
    4. postictal state
    5. seizure
    6. status epilepticus
    7. syncope

    _____ **a.** An unusual sensory sensation that may precede a seizure episode

    _____ **b.** A sudden and temporary alteration in the mental status caused by massive electrical discharge in a group of nerve cells in the brain

    _____ **c.** Recovery period that follows the clonic phase of a generalized seizure

    _____ **d.** A medical disorder characterized by recurrent seizures

    _____ **e.** A seizure lasting longer than 10 minutes or seizures that occur consecutively without a period of responsiveness between them

    _____ **f.** A brief period of unresponsiveness due to a lack of blood flow to the brain

    _____ **g.** A common type of seizure that produces unresponsiveness and a generalized jerking muscle activity; a grand mal seizure

CONTENT REVIEW

1. A seizure is a sign of an underlying defect. Which of the following may be a cause of seizures?
    a. Head injury
    b. Epilepsy
    c. High fever
    d. Any of these

2. Briefly list and describe in order the four stages of a typical generalized tonic-clonic seizure.

3. When you arrive on scene, in what state will you most often encounter the seizure patient?
   a. Aura phase
   b. Tonic phase
   c. Clonic phase
   d. Postictal phase

4. When you encounter a patient seizing with jerky body movements, to help prevent further injury you should
   a. Place a spoon in the mouth to stop the patient from swallowing his tongue
   b. Move objects away from the patient's area and guide his movements
   c. Physically restrain the patient's body movements until he is postictal
   d. Restrain the patient by securing him on a spine board

5. Which of the following patients is/are at risk of airway, breathing, or circulation compromise?
   a. The unresponsive seizure patient
   b. The patient who is actively seizing
   c. The patient seizing for more than 10 minutes
   d. All of the above are at risk.

6. Which of the following is the most appropriate treatment for a patient suffering status epilepticus?
   a. Positive pressure ventilation, transport after focused history and physical exam
   b. Positive pressure ventilation, immediate transport to a medical facility
   c. Oxygen at 15 lpm via nonrebreather mask, transport after focused history and physical exam
   d. Oxygen at 15 lpm via nonrebreather mask, immediate transport to a medical facility

7. Which of the following is a common cause of seizures in infants and young children?
   a. Head injury
   b. Diabetes
   c. High fever
   d. Epilepsy

8. All of the following patients are characterized as a priority for transport EXCEPT
   a. The seizing patient who is pregnant, has a history of diabetes, or is injured
   b. The patient whose seizure has occurred in the water, such as a swimming pool or lake
   c. The patient who has suffered a seizure, regained responsiveness, then suffered another seizure an hour later
   d. The patient who remains unresponsive following the seizure activity

9. Briefly explain why you should inspect and palpate for a painful, swollen, or deformed extremity in the seizure patient.

10. Briefly explain why the nasopharyngeal airway is preferred over the oropharyngeal airway in a patient who is seizing.

11. The postictal patient with no suspected spinal injury should be placed in which position?
a. Semi-Fowler's
b. Lateral recumbent
c. Trendelenburg
d. Prone

12. Briefly explain why the position you chose in Question 11 is preferred.

13. All of the following are true regarding syncope EXCEPT
a. The brain is briefly deprived of oxygen.
b. The skin is usually warm, pale, and dry.
c. The patient remembers feeling faint.
d. The event usually begins in a standing position.

CASE STUDY

▼

You and your partner, Sascha, are at a local grocery store picking up groceries for dinner when an elderly woman screams for help: "There's a man over here dying!" You ask Sascha to bring the ambulance closer to the building and bring the equipment and stretcher. You reach into your pocket for your extra pair of gloves and put them on as you hurry to the patient's side. You find an elderly man on the ground, shaking uncontrollably. A closer look reveals the identity of the patient. You recognize him as Karl Louis, a local homeless man with a history of epilepsy and chronic alcoholism. The bystander states, "I found him lying on the ground shaking. I don't know how long he was like that, but he's been shaking for 3 or 4 minutes just since I found him!"

1. While you are waiting for Sascha to bring the equipment, you should
a. Guide the body movements, move obstacles
b. Assess the airway and breathing
c. Look for signs of an injury to the head
d. All of the above are correct.

Sascha approaches with the stretcher and equipment. You advise him that it's Karl Louis and that you have never seen him this bad. The seizure stops and you try to arouse Karl, but he remains unresponsive. As you are assessing his breathing, he begins to seize again, violently. You notice blood flowing from his mouth.

2. Which of the following is the most appropriate emergency care?
   a. Administer oxygen via nonrebreather mask at 15 lpm, wait for the seizure to end, and suction.
   b. Suction, administer oxygen via nonrebreather mask at 15 lpm, and transport immediately.
   c. Suction, begin positive pressure ventilation with an oropharyngeal airway in place, and use rapid transport.
   d. Suction, begin positive pressure ventilation with a nasopharyngeal airway in place, and use rapid transport.

3. Briefly explain why you might see blood coming from the mouth of a seizure patient and how you would treat this problem.

En route to the medical facility, Karl stops seizing. While you are reassessing Karl's mental status, you ask Sascha to obtain baseline vital signs. Karl responds to a painful stimulus by pulling away. Then he opens his eyes sluggishly and asks you to stop. He looks exhausted. Your physical exam reveals no injuries. The vital signs include heart rate 118 beats per minute, blood pressure 164/68, breathing adequate at 20 per minute.

4. Now that Karl is responsive, you recognize that he is in which phase?
   a. Aura phase
   b. Clonic phase
   c. Postictal phase
   d. Tonic phase

5. What should you now do for Karl?
   a. Place Karl in a supine position, administer positive pressure ventilation with supplemental oxygen.
   b. Place Karl in a semi-sitting position, administer oxygen by bag-valve mask, and hyperventilate him at greater than 24 ventilations per minute.
   c. Place Karl in a full sitting position, administer oxygen by nonrebreather mask at 15 lpm.
   d. Place Karl in a lateral recumbent position and administer oxygen by nonrebreather mask at 15 lpm.

You arrive at the medical facility. Karl is feeling much better although still somewhat confused and disoriented. You reassure him and give your report to the emergency department nurse.

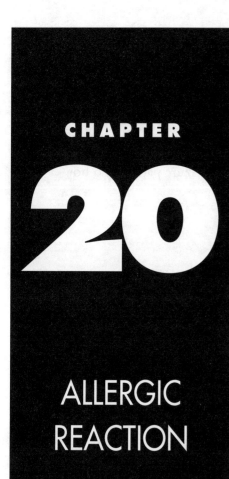

CHAPTER

20

ALLERGIC
REACTION

Numbered objectives are from the United States Department of Transportation 1994 EMT-Basic National Standard Curriculum. Asterisked objectives, if any, pertain to material that is supplemental to the DOT curriculum.

4-5.1   Recognize the patient experiencing an allergic reaction.

4-5.2   Describe the emergency medical care of the patient with an allergic reaction.

4-5.3   Establish the relationship between the patient with an allergic reaction and airway management.

4-5.4   Describe the mechanism of allergic response and implications for airway management.

4-5.5   State the generic and trade names, medication forms, dose, administration, action, and contraindications for the epinephrine auto-injector.

4-5.6   Evaluate the need for medical direction in the emergency medical care of the patient with an allergic reaction.

4-5.7   Differentiate between the general category of those patients having an allergic reaction and those patients having an allergic reaction and requiring immediate medical care, including immediate use of an epinephrine auto-injector.

KEY IDEAS

An allergic reaction can be quickly life threatening. It is important for the EMT-B to rapidly assess and manage patients suffering an allergic reaction. Appropriate assessment and management techniques for allergic reactions are the focus of this chapter.

▶ An allergic reaction is a misdirected or excessive response by the immune system to a foreign substance or allergen. An allergen can enter the body by injection, ingestion, inhalation, or contact.

▶ Common causes of allergic reactions include: venom from bites or stings, foods, pollen, and medications. Medications taken orally or injected are the most common cause.

▶ Hives and itching are the hallmark signs and symptoms of an allergic reaction.

▶ Most allergic reactions are mild. A severe form of allergic reaction is anaphylaxis, or anaphylactic shock.

▶ In anaphylactic shock, the entire body is affected by the release of chemical substances by the immune system. There is swelling in the upper airway, and bronchoconstriction and swelling in the lower airways. Blood vessels dilate and decrease the blood pressure. Anaphylaxis is a life-threatening condition that commonly leads to death without proper treatment.

▶ The two key categories of signs and symptoms that specifically indicate anaphylaxis are respiratory compromise and shock (hypoperfusion).

▶ Emergency medical care for the severe allergic reaction (anaphylaxis) includes maintaining a patent airway, oxygen therapy, administering epinephrine by prescribed auto-injector, considering calling for advanced life support, and early transport. It may be necessary to provide positive pressure ventilation to force air past the swollen upper airway.

TERMS AND CONCEPTS

1. **Write the number of the correct term next to each definition.**

    1. allergen
    2. allergic reaction
    3. anaphylactic shock
    4. antibodies
    5. hives
    6. immune system
    7. malaise
    8. sensitization

    _____ a. The process by which antibodies are produced after exposure to an antigen

    _____ b. Misdirected and excessive response by the immune system to a foreign substance or an allergen

    _____ c. Raised, red blotches associated with some allergic reactions

    _____ d. Special proteins produced by the immune system that search out antigens, combine with them, and destroy them

    _____ e. The body's defense mechanism against invasion by foreign substances

    _____ f. A state of hypoperfusion that results from dilated and leaking blood vessels related to severe allergic reaction

    _____ g. A substance that enters the body by ingestion, injection, inhalation, or contact and triggers an allergic reaction

    _____ h. A general feeling of weakness or discomfort

CONTENT REVIEW

1. Anaphylaxis is
   a. A life-threatening condition that commonly leads to death without proper treatment
   b. A condition that causes blood vessels to dilate and begin to leak, decreasing the blood pressure
   c. A condition that causes swelling in the upper airway that can cause obstruction and a reduction of air to the lungs
   d. All of these are true statements

2. The MOST common cause of allergic reactions and anaphylaxis is
   a. Glue
   b. Pollen from ragweed
   c. Medications
   d. Mosquito bites

3. Which of the following is NOT a route by which an allergen may enter the body?
   a. Injection
   b. Excretion
   c. Contact
   d. Ingestion

4. Which of the following are groups of items that commonly cause allergic reaction and anaphylaxis?
   1. venom
   2. foods
   3. metals
   4. pollen
   5. medications

   a. 1, 2, and 4
   b. 1, 2, and 3
   c. 1, 2, 4, and 5
   d. 1, 2, 3, 4, and 5

5. When assessing respiratory sounds, stridor or crowing indicates
   a. Significant swelling to the upper airway, requiring positive pressure ventilation
   b. Significant swelling to the upper airway, requiring insertion of an airway adjunct
   c. Significant swelling to the bronchioles, requiring oxygen at 15 lpm by nonrebreather mask
   d. Possible collapse of the alveoli of the lungs, requiring endotracheal intubation

6. You are providing positive pressure ventilation to an anaphylaxis patient who is breathing inadequately. The bag-valve mask device's pop-off valve releases air with each squeeze of the bag. What is the BEST action to take?
   a. Deactivate the valve or place your thumb over it and continue with ventilations.
   b. Continue ventilating the patient and increase the rate of ventilations.
   c. Continue until ALS arrives and report your finding to the crew.
   d. Reduce the pressure you are using to squeeze the bag to prevent the valve from opening.

7. Hives may be present all over the skin in a patient suffering an allergic reaction or anaphylaxis. Hives are usually accompanied by
   a. Severe coughing
   b. Severe stuffy nose
   c. Severe itching
   d. Severe headache

8. Most anaphylactic reactions are apparent within ____ minute(s) after exposure.
   a. 1
   b. 5
   c. 10
   d. 20

9. The two key categories of signs and symptoms that specifically indicate anaphylaxis are
   a. Gastrointestinal compromise and shock
   b. Respiratory compromise and shock
   c. Central nervous system compromise and shock
   d. Respiratory compromise and gastrointestinal complaints

10. Anaphylaxis can be mistaken for other conditions with similar signs and symptoms such as
    a. Anxiety attack
    b. Alcohol intoxication
    c. Hypoglycemia
    d. Any of the above

11. It is important to differentiate between a mild allergic reaction and a severe allergic reaction (anaphylaxis). For both, you will maintain an open airway, provide oxygen, and transport. Additionally, for a severe reaction you will
    a. Be prepared to suction and provide positive pressure ventilation
    b. Obtain an order from medical direction to administer the patient's prescribed epinephrine auto-injector
    c. Consider calling for advanced life support, and initiate early transport
    d. All of these

12. The bronchospasms associated with anaphylaxis
    a. May result in severe respiratory distress
    b. May be so severe that air movement is minimal through the bronchioles
    c. May prevent breath sounds or wheezing from being heard on auscultation
    d. All of these

13. The criteria that must be met before an EMT-B can administer epinephrine by auto-injector to a patient are (1) _____ , (2) the medication has been prescribed to the patient, and (3) the EMT-B has received an order from medical direction.
    a. Hives and itching
    b. Headache and low blood pressure
    c. Signs and symptoms of severe allergic reaction including respiratory distress and/or shock
    d. All of these

CASE STUDY

You have responded to a call for a child who has been stung by a bee. The scene appears safe as you arrive at a small frame home. A frantic-looking woman meets you at the front of the house and asks you to "Please hurry up!" As you follow her to the backyard you ask, "Why did you call the ambulance?" She replies, "My daughter was just stung by a bee!"

The patient looks to be about 10 years of age. She is sitting in a chair and looks up at you as you approach. Your general impression is that she looks well. Her skin color is red. She responds to your questions appropriately. She says her name is Caitlin. She tells you that she was stung by a bee about 5 minutes ago. She doesn't appear to have any difficulty breathing. She complains of a "lump" in her throat and her stomach feels "upset." Her pulse is strong and regular. There is no sign of trauma, and no bleeding is present.

You complete the OPQRST and SAMPLE history. You find out that she had an allergic reaction to a yellow jacket sting one year ago. She has a prescription for an EpiPen Jr. During the physical exam, you observe the small red sting site on her arm, but make no other findings.

1. The patient
   a. Is not showing signs of anaphylaxis or allergic reaction. Caitlin does not require transport or additional treatment.
   b. Is not showing signs of anaphylaxis or allergic reaction. Caitlin should be transported by her mother for additional evaluation at a local hospital.
   c. Is not showing signs of anaphylaxis or allergic reaction. Place Caitlin on oxygen and closely evaluate her during transport.
   d. Is showing early signs of anaphylaxis or allergic reaction. Place Caitlin on oxygen, call for ALS back-up, prepare for suction and to assist ventilations, and initiate early transport.

2. You should carefully monitor Caitlin for
   a. Signs of developing hives and itching
   b. Signs of abdominal cramping
   c. Loss of bowel control
   d. Airway and breathing compromise and poor perfusion

3. En route to the hospital, Caitlin develops breathing that sounds noisy, with a rattling sound on inspiration and exhalation. These sounds are probably caused by
   a. Swelling of the tongue
   b. Severe bronchoconstriction
   c. Excessive mucus in the upper airways
   d. Excessive mucus in the lower airways

4. What additional signs and symptoms may you expect Caitlin to develop?
   a. Severe headache
   b. Coughing and hoarseness
   c. Cyanotic skin
   d. All of the above

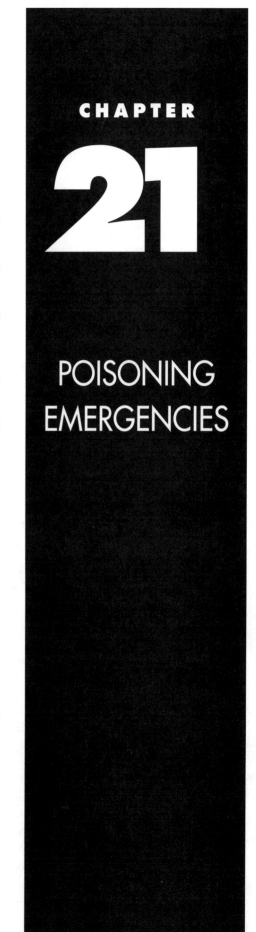

COGNITIVE OBJECTIVES

Numbered objectives are from the United States Department of Transportation 1994 EMT-Basic National Standard Curriculum. Asterisked objectives, if any, pertain to material that is supplemental to the DOT curriculum.

4-6.1   List various ways that poisons enter the body.

4-6.2   List signs/symptoms associated with poisoning.

4-6.3   Discuss the emergency medical care for the patient with possible overdose.

4-6.4   Describe the steps in the emergency medical care for the patient with suspected poisoning.

4-6.5   Establish the relationship between the patient suffering from poisoning or overdose, and airway management.

4-6.6   State the generic and trade names, indications, contraindications, medication form, dose, administration, actions, side effects, and reassessment strategies for activated charcoal.

4-6.7   Recognize the need for medical direction in caring for the patient with poisoning or overdose.

KEY CONCEPTS

This chapter focuses on the assessment and management of poisoning emergencies. Thousands of people become seriously ill or die each year due to accidental or suicidal poisonings. As an EMT-Basic, you may encounter these patients in homes, the workplace, or outdoors. It is important that you have a good understanding of the assessment and emergency care needed to effectively manage such patients. Key concepts include the following:

▶ A poison is any substance that impairs health or can cause death by its chemical effect when it enters the body or comes in contact with the skin.

▶ Poisons may enter the body via absorption, ingestion, inhalation, or injection.

▶ Children are the most frequent victims of accidental poisoning.

▶ Scene size-up is important when responding to a poisoning emergency to prevent the exposure of EMS personnel to the poison.

▶ The first priority of care in the management of poisoning emergencies is to maintain an airway and ensure oxygenation.

▶ The primary focus of your attention should be on managing the effects of the poisoning and not on the type of poisoning.

▶ Activated charcoal is an important adjunct to the emergency management of ingested poisoning since it inhibits the absorption of poisons.

▶ All poisoned patients need to be evaluated by a physician.

TERMS AND CONCEPTS

1. **Write the number of the correct term next to each definition.**

    1. absorption
    2. ingestion
    3. inhalation
    4. injection
    5. poison
    6. toxin

_____ **a.** Substance that can impair health or cause death
_____ **b.** Exposure that results from breathing a substance
_____ **c.** Passage of a substance through the skin surface upon contact
_____ **d.** Exposure that results from swallowing a substance
_____ **e.** A poison of animal, plant, or bacterial origin
_____ **f.** Forceful introduction of a substance through the penetration of the skin surface

CONTENT REVIEW

1. When performing the scene size-up at the site of a possible poisoning emergency, you should pay attention to
   a. Potential dangers to yourself or bystanders
   b. Evidence of a chemical or hazardous spill
   c. Possibility of trauma related to the poisoning
   d. All of these

2. On arrival at the scene of a poisoning emergency where you suspect an environmental exposure hazard, you should
   a. Contact your regional poison control center first
   b. Immediately rescue all patients from the scene
   c. Request assistance from a trained "hazmat" team
   d. Establish a command post for scene control

3. Which of the following indicators that you find at the scene would NOT suggest a poisoning emergency?
   a. Open chemical containers releasing noxious odors
   b. Hazardous material warning label on a locked cabinet door
   c. Chewed-up plants found near a child patient
   d. Empty pill bottles bearing the patient's name

4. At the scene of a poisoning emergency your medical priority is to
   a. Identify the poisonous substance
   b. Contact the regional poison center
   c. Maintain the patient's airway
   d. Verify the type of exposure

5. Poisons may affect your patient's airway by
   a. Alteration of his mental status
   b. Respiratory depression
   c. Direct damage to airway tissues
   d. Any of these

6. List five questions you should include in a SAMPLE history of a poisoning emergency.

7. The signs and symptoms of poisoning are specific to the substance (poison) and should rule out other possible causes of the emergency.
   a. True
   b. False

8. Possible indicators of ingested poisoning in children include
   a. Previous history of ingestion
   b. Burns or stains around mouth
   c. Altered mental status
   d. Any of these

9. Timmy is a 2-year-old who has ingested a corrosive acid. In addition to maintaining his airway and oxygenation, you should
   a. Dilute the substance by giving large amounts of milk or water
   b. Prevent further injury by rinsing the substance from his mouth and lips
   c. Administer activated charcoal per local protocol or medical direction
   d. Talk seriously with his mother about child safety issues

10. Activated charcoal is the medication of choice in the emergency medical care of poisonings because
    a. It is an antidote to most commonly ingested poisons
    b. It neutralizes caustic and corrosive poisonous substances
    c. It inhibits the absorption of poisons by the body
    d. It reverses the toxic effects of drugs and alcohol

11. When ordered by medical direction or the poison control center, activated charcoal is indicated for the patent who has
    a. Ingested poisons by mouth
    b. Inhaled toxic chemical substances
    c. Made skin contact with corrosive powders
    d. Been bitten by a poisonous snake

12. Activated charcoal is CONTRAINDICATED for all of following patients EXCEPT
    a. 16-year-old who is unresponsive from a drug ingestion
    b. 3-year-old who is responsive and crying after ingesting an unknown plant
    c. 58-year-old who is incoherent after ingesting multiple medications
    d. 30-year-old who is alert and has ingested bleach

13. The usual adult dosage of activated charcoal is
    a. 10 grams
    b. 12 to 20 grams
    c. 25 to 50 grams
    d. 100 grams

14. Activated charcoal is an effective binding agent against all poisons.
    a. True
    b. False

15. Allowing the patient to eat ice cream following a dose of activated charcoal will decrease its effectiveness.
    a. True
    b. False

16. A common side effect seen with administration of activated charcoal is
    a. Blackened stool
    b. Headache
    c. Rapid pulse
    d. All of these

17. The majority of toxic inhalations occur as a result of
    a. Recreational use of inhalants
    b. Industrial accidents
    c. Fire-related incidents
    d. Hazardous material incidents

18. The PRIMARY symptom associated with toxic inhalation is
    a. Altered mental status
    b. Difficulty breathing
    c. Increased tearing from the eyes
    d. Nausea

19. All of the following actions are appropriate in the emergency medical management of a toxic inhalation EXCEPT
    a. Remain outside the scene until your personal safety is assured.
    b. Remove the patient to fresh air as soon as possible.
    c. Administer activated charcoal to minimize absorption of substance.
    d. Administer positive pressure ventilation if breathing is inadequate.

20. When managing poisonings due to injection or absorption, you should pay attention to
    a. Preventing your own exposure to the poison
    b. Airway maintenance and supporting ventilation
    c. Identifying the poisonous agent if possible
    d. All of these

CASE STUDY

You have been dispatched to 1234 Early Lane for "one unconscious." You note no obvious hazards as you approach the house. Mrs. Johnson lets you in and reports she found her 50-year-old husband lying on the floor of his workshop in the basement when she returned from work. You are aware of a peculiar chemical odor as you begin to descend the stairs.

1. What should you do now?

2. After Mr. Johnson has been removed from his workshop, what should be done next?

You find Mr. Johnson to be unresponsive with rapid, shallow, labored breathing. His pulse is rapid. His skin is pale, cool, and sweaty. There are no signs of trauma.

3. What should you do now?

Mrs. Johnson reports that her husband has "never been sick a day in his life." He takes no medications and has no known allergies. She said that she left for work early and does not know when he last ate. Mrs. Johnson says that her husband enjoys refinishing furniture.

4. What special care does Mr. Johnson require en route to the hospital?

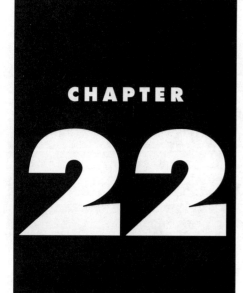

CHAPTER

22

DRUG AND ALCOHOL EMERGENCIES

COGNITIVE OBJECTIVES

4-6.3 Discuss the emergency medical care for the patient with possible overdose.

*   Describe the steps in the assessment of a drug or alcohol overdose patient.

*   Explain how to determine if an emergency is drug or alcohol related.

*   List six factors that may make a drug or alcohol emergency life-threatening.

*   Discuss the signs and symptoms that indicate a drug or alcohol emergency.

*   Discuss the techniques for managing a violent drug or alcohol patient.

KEY CONCEPTS

This chapter focuses on the assessment and management of emergencies related to drug and alcohol use and abuse. Since drugs and alcohol are abused by a number of people in a variety of ways, you may encounter such patients in virtually any setting. In addition to the medical emergency created by drug or alcohol ingestion or withdrawal, these patients are also often victims of trauma and may exhibit aggressive or violent behavior toward the EMS crew. Key concepts include the following:

▶ Safety must be a primary concern for the EMT-Basic at the scene of drug or alcohol emergencies, since these patients may exhibit aggressive or violent behavior and are also often infected with bloodborne or airborne diseases.

▶ Overdose and withdrawal are potentially life-threatening emergencies.

▶ Drug and alcohol emergency indicators include unresponsiveness or other altered mental status, respiratory difficulty, fever, abnormal pulse rates, vomiting, and seizures.

▶ Management of drug and alcohol emergencies requires careful attention to the maintenance of airway, breathing, and circulation status as well as to controlling potentially volatile situations with unpredictable patients.

TERMS AND CONCEPTS

1. Write the number of the correct term next to each definition.

    1. drug abuse
    2. overdose
    3. withdrawal

_____ **a.** Physical syndrome that occurs after a period of abstinence from a substance to which a person's body has become accustomed

_____ **b.** Self-administration of legal or illicit substances in a manner that is not in accord with approved medical or social patterns

_____ **c.** An emergency that involves poisoning or toxicity caused by drugs or alcohol

CONTENT REVIEW

1. What are the goals at the scene of a drug or alcohol emergency?
   a. Identify and reverse effects of the abused substance.
   b. Identify and treat potential life threats.
   c. Notify police of illegal drug use.
   d. Identify abused substance and control behavior of patient.

2. List three potential dangers at the scene of a drug or alcohol emergency.

3. Your patient is found unresponsive on the living room floor, surrounded by nearly a dozen empty and partially filled pill bottles. What should be done with those bottles?
   a. Do nothing with the pill bottles.
   b. Keep them with the patient as a source of information.
   c. Have your partner call Poison Control to verify they are dangerous.
   d. Contact the police; this may be evidence of a crime.

4. Drugs and alcohol produce signs and symptoms that mimic a number of systemic disorders and diseases.
   a. True
   b. False

5. Upon completion of your initial assessment, you suspect that your unresponsive patient's condition may be due to drugs or alcohol. What should you do?
   a. With a gloved hand, check the mouth for signs of pills or tablets.
   b. Smell the patient's breath for trace odors of alcohol.
   c. Ask bystanders for information about precipitating events.
   d. All of these

6. List the six signs and symptoms that indicate a life-threatening drug or alcohol emergency.

7. The most reliable indicators of a drug or alcohol emergency are likely to come from which two phases of the patient assessment?
a. Physical exam and vital signs
b. Vital signs and patient history
c. Scene size-up and patient history
d. Physical exam and ongoing assessment

8. You are on scene with a disoriented patient who reports taking an overdose of pain medication. Arrange in the proper order (1–5) the following emergency care steps for this patient.

_____ Administer oxygen at 15 lpm by nonrebreather mask or positive pressure ventilation with supplemental oxygen as necessary.

_____ Transport the patient to the hospital.

_____ Monitor vital signs and take measures to maintain body temperature and prevent shock.

_____ Establish and maintain a patent airway.

_____ Gather medications to bring to the hospital.

9. What type of response should you anticipate if your patient reports ingesting a hallucinogenic substance?

10. The EMT-B pictured here is talking with a patient suffering a behavioral emergency. Choose the most correct comment about the technique being demonstrated.
a. Touch can be comforting; always touch the behavioral emergency patient.
b. Touch can be comforting; however, never touch the patient without his permission.
c. Pat the patient on the back to help clear his airway.
d. Grasp the shoulder and forearm to initiate restraint.

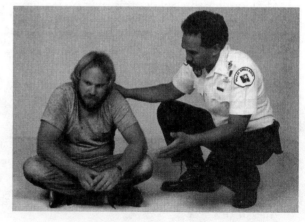

11. Briefly describe at least three elements of the "talk-down technique" for dealing with a drug-abuse patient who is experiencing a "bad trip."

12. Never use the talk-down technique for which kind of patient?
    a. A patient you know has used the drug PCP
    b. A patient you know is intoxicated on alcohol
    c. A patient you know has used LSD
    d. A patient you know has taken a depressant

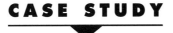

CASE STUDY

You are on scene with a 17-year-old female who was found unresponsive in her bedroom by her mother. She was last seen about 4 hours ago. Your initial assessment finds her unresponsive with snoring respirations at approximately 8 per minute. There is vomitus on the floor near her head. Her pulse is slow and irregular. Her skin is pale, cool, and dry.

1. What is your first priority?

The mother reports that her daughter has been depressed since the death of her boyfriend in a car crash last month, but she has no medical problems or allergies. Your partner finds four empty pill bottles and a partially full wine bottle in the adjacent bathroom.

2 Your local protocols allow you to administer activated charcoal for ingestions. Should this patient receive a dose? Why or why not?

3. What should be done now?

CHAPTER

23

ACUTE ABDOMINAL PAIN

COGNITIVE OBJECTIVES

Numbered objectives are from the United States Department of Transportation 1994 EMT-Basic National Standard Curriculum. Asterisked objectives, if any, pertain to material that is supplemental to the DOT curriculum.

* Describe the structure and function of the organs contained within the abdominal cavity.

* Define the term "acute abdomen."

* Describe the assessment of a patient with acute abdominal pain.

* Describe the signs and symptoms of acute abdominal pain.

* Discuss the appropriate emergency medical care for a patient with acute abdominal pain.

KEY IDEAS

Acute abdominal pain may indicate a serious condition. This chapter reviews assessment and emergency care for the patient suffering from acute abdominal pain.

▶ Acute abdominal pain, also called "acute abdomen" or "acute abdominal distress," is a common condition characterized by an acute onset of moderate to severe abdominal pain that may result from a variety of causes.

▶ All patients with acute abdominal pain should be considered to have a life-threatening condition until proven otherwise.

▶ Internal bleeding, peritonitis, and diarrhea are conditions that often involve considerable fluid loss, leading to shock (hypoperfusion). A top priority during the assessment of a patient with acute abdominal pain is to look for signs of shock.

▶ Rapid transport should be considered for the acute abdomen patient who meets any of the following criteria: poor general impression, unresponsive, responsive but not following commands, difficulty breathing, shock (hypoperfusion), uncontrolled bleeding, or severe pain.

▶ Perform the examination of the abdomen carefully and gently. If the patient is a priority for rapid transport, the focused history and physical exam should be conducted en route to the hospital.

▶ Emergency medical care for the patient with an acute abdomen includes maintaining a patent airway, placing the patient in a position of comfort, administering oxygen, not giving anything by mouth, calming and reassuring the patient, being alert for shock, and initiating a quick and efficient transport.

TERMS AND CONCEPTS

1. **Write the number of the correct term next to each definition.**

   1. abdominal aorta
   2. acute abdomen
   3. guarded position
   4. involuntary guarding

   5. peritoneum
   6. referred pain
   7. umbilicus
   8. voluntary guarding

   _____ a. The navel

   _____ b. Abdominal wall muscle contraction due to inflammation of the peritoneum that the patient cannot control

   _____ c. The lining of the abdominal cavity

   _____ d. Pain that is felt in a body part removed from its point of origin

   _____ e. Moderate to severe abdominal pain with an acute onset

   _____ f. A position generally adopted by patients with acute abdominal pain: knees drawn up and hands clenched over the abdomen

   _____ g. A major division of the heart's primary artery that runs through the abdomen

   _____ h. Abdominal wall muscle contraction that is controlled by the patient

CONTENT REVIEW

1. The abdomen is the area below the diaphragm to the top of the pelvis. It is helpful to reference the abdomen by dividing it into quarters, or quadrants. The central reference point is the umbilicus. Correctly place the following terms on the figure below.

   diaphragm

   left lower quadrant (LLQ)

   left upper quadrant (LUQ)

   right lower quadrant (RLQ)

   right upper quadrant (RUQ)

   umbilicus

   A _____

   B _____

   C _____

   D _____

   E _____

   F _____

2. Which of the following organs are found in the abdominal cavity?

1. appendix
2. female reproductive organs
3. gallbladder
4. heart
5. large intestine
6. liver
7. lungs
8. pancreas
9. small intestine
10. spleen
11. stomach
12. urinary bladder

a. All except 4 and 7
b. All except 8 and 10
c. All except 3, 4, 7, and 8
d. All except 3, 4, 8, and 10

3. A patient experiencing acute abdominal pain can also be reported as suffering from which of the following?

1. acute abdomen
2. acute abdominal distress
3. appendicitis
4. diarrhea
5. gastritis
6. heartburn

a. 2
b. 1 or 2
c. 1, 2, 3, or 5
e. Any of these

4. All patients with abdominal pain should be considered
a. To have a bowel obstruction until proven otherwise
b. To have a life-threatening condition until proven otherwise
c. To be stable until proven otherwise
d. To have a digestive system disorder until proven otherwise

5. A person with an acute abdomen generally appears very ill. The patient may
a. Adopt a position on his side with his legs straight
b. Adopt a position lying on his stomach with his legs flat
c. Adopt a position lying flat on his back with his legs flat
d. Adopt a position with his knees drawn up

6. The acute abdomen patient should be categorized as a priority for transport if he meets any of seven specific criteria. List the seven criteria.

7. Which statement is NOT true related to the scene size-up of the acute abdomen patient?
   a. Patients experiencing abdominal bleeding are likely to faint and usually do so in the bathroom.
   b. You should look for any mechanism of injury to rule out trauma as the cause of abdominal pain.
   c. Bloody vomitus is always present in the acute abdomen patient.
   d. Certain types of bleeding have a distinct smell and sometimes can be determined as you arrive on scene.

8. When palpating the abdomen of the acute abdomen patient, the EMT-B should
   a. Have the patient point to the site of the pain and palpate this quadrant last
   b. Have the patient point to the site of the pain and palpate this quadrant first
   c. Have the patient point to the site of the pain and do not palpate this quadrant
   d. Palpate all four quadrants, always with the upper quadrants first, then the lower quadrants

9. Which of the following is NOT a sign or symptom of an acute abdomen?
   a. Widespread or localized abdominal pain
   b. Bloody vomitus or blood in the stool
   c. Signs or symptoms associated with shock
   d. Soft abdomen that produces no pain on palpation

10. Which item is appropriate management for the patient with an acute abdomen?
    a. Give fluids when requested by the patient.
    b. Position the patient in a supine position with legs flat.
    c. Perform an ongoing assessment every 15 minutes for the unstable patient.
    d. Never give anything to the patient by mouth.

11. Which item is NOT appropriate management for the patient with an acute abdomen?
    a. Position the patient in a lateral recumbent position, if it does not increase discomfort, to protect against aspiration of vomitus.
    b. Administer oxygen at 15 lpm by nonrebreather mask.
    c. Provide care for shock.
    d. Do not transport until a detailed physical exam has been completed and findings reported to the receiving facility.

12. Which of the following is NOT a condition that can cause acute abdominal pain?
    a. Cholecystitis
    b. Transient ischemic attack
    c. Pancreatitis
    d. Abdominal aortic aneurysm

CASE STUDY

You have responded to a call for a patient complaining of abdominal pain. The scene appears safe as you arrive at a neat one-story home. A man meets you at the curb and escorts you to the front door. As you follow him you ask, "Why did you call the ambulance?" He replies, "My wife's stomach hurts really bad!" As you enter the house you see the patient. She looks to be about 25 years of age. She is lying on her side on the floor with her knees drawn up to her chest. She is holding her lower abdominal area. She doesn't look at you as you enter. Your general impression is that she looks ill. Her skin color is pale. She responds to your questions slowly but appropriately. She tells you, "My stomach started hurting about an hour ago. I think I'm going to throw up!" Her respirations are rapid and shallow. Her radial pulse is weak and rapid, and her skin is cool and moist. There is no sign of trauma and no obvious bleeding is observed.

1. This patient
   a. Is not showing serious signs. The patient does not require transport or additional treatment.
   b. Is showing serious signs. However, the patient should be allowed to be transported by her husband to the hospital for additional evaluation.
   c. Is not showing serious signs. However, the patient should be placed on oxygen and transported in a sitting-up position.
   d. Is showing early signs of shock. The patient should be placed on oxygen, positioned with feet up, and provided quick transport with suction unit ready.

2. When beginning the exam of the patient's abdomen you should
   a. Ask her to quickly drink a glass of water
   b. Ask her to straighten her legs
   c. Ask her to point to the area that is most painful
   d. Reassure the patient that palpation of her abdomen will not hurt

   En route to the hospital, the patient vomits several times.

3. The patient's emesis (vomitus)
   a. Should be saved for possible testing at the hospital
   b. Should be saved, but only if it looks bloody or dark in color
   c. Should be disposed of immediately in an infectious waste container
   d. Should not be considered a serious sign of acute abdomen

4. An ongoing assessment of this patient should be performed every
   a. 1 minute
   b. 3 minutes
   c. 5 minutes
   d. 15 minutes

COGNITIVE OBJECTIVES

Numbered objectives are from the United States Department of Transportation 1994 EMT-Basic National Standard Curriculum. Asterisked objectives, if any, pertain to material that is supplemental to the DOT curriculum.

4-7.1 Describe the various ways that the body loses heat.

4-7.2 List the signs and symptoms of exposure to cold.

4-7.3 Explain the steps in providing emergency medical care to a patient exposed to cold.

4-7.4 List the signs and symptoms of exposure to heat.

4-7.5 Explain the steps in providing emergency medical care to a patient exposed to heat.

4-7.8 Discuss the emergency medical care of bites and stings.

KEY IDEAS

Conditions brought on by interactions between people and the environment are reviewed in this chapter. The signs, symptoms, and expected emergency management of extremes of hot and cold, bites and stings are addressed.

▶ Hypothermia occurs when the body loses more heat than it gains or produces. Heat loss occurs through five mechanisms: radiation, convection, conduction, evaporation, and respiration.

▶ Exposure to cold can cause two kinds of emergencies. The first is generalized cold emergency (generalized hypothermia), which is an overall reduction in body temperature affecting the entire body. The second is local cold injury (commonly called "frost-bite") that results in damage to body tissues in a specific part or parts of the body.

▶ Signs and symptoms of generalized hypothermia include decreasing mental status, decreasing motor and sensory function, and changing vital signs.

▶ Emergency medical care for generalized hypothermia includes preventing further heat loss, rewarming the patient as quickly and safely as possible, and staying alert for complications. It is important to remove the patient from the cold environment, handle the patient gently, administer oxygen, and be prepared to resuscitate the patient if he goes into cardiac arrest.

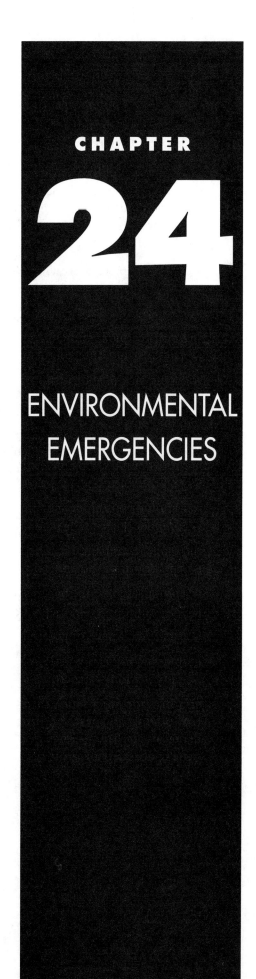

CHAPTER

24

ENVIRONMENTAL EMERGENCIES

▶ Local cold injury results from the freezing of body tissue. Local cold injury falls into two categories: early (superficial) or late (deep) injury.

▶ Signs and symptoms of early (superficial) cold injury include blanching of the skin and loss of feeling. The skin and tissue beneath it remain soft. There may be a tingling sensation during rewarming.

▶ Signs and symptoms of late (deep) cold injury include white, waxy skin, swelling, and blisters. The skin and tissues beneath the skin feel firm-to-frozen. If thawed, the skin may appear flushed or mottled.

▶ Emergency medical care for local cold injury includes removing the patient from the cold environment, avoiding thawing if there is danger of refreezing, administering oxygen, removing jewelry or wet or restrictive clothing if not frozen to the skin, covering the skin with dressings or dry clothing, avoiding rubbing, and not permitting the patient to walk on an injured extremity.

▶ Hyperthermia occurs when the amount of heat the body produces or gains exceeds the amount the body loses.

▶ Signs and symptoms of a heat emergency may include muscle cramps, weakness, dizziness, heartbeat becoming progressively weak and rapid, deep breathing that becomes progressively shallow and weak, headache, seizures, loss of appetite, nausea or vomiting, altered mental status, and possible unresponsiveness. The skin may be moist and pale with a normal-to-cool temperature, or the skin may be hot and either dry or moist.

▶ Emergency medical care for the patient with a heat emergency includes moving the patient to a cool place, administering oxygen, removing as much clothing as possible, and cooling the patient. The patient should be placed supine with elevated feet. If the patient is fully responsive and not nauseated, he may drink cool water. (If the patient has an altered mental status or is nauseated or vomiting, do **NOT** give fluids.)

▶ Hot skin (which may be either dry or moist, depending on how the sweat mechanisms are operating) represents a dire medical emergency. The patient requires rapid cooling and immediate transport.

▶ Emergency care for bites and stings includes removing the stinger by scraping, washing the area, removing jewelry or other constricting objects, lowering the injection site slightly below the heart, and applying cold packs (except for marine stings and snakebite). It is important to be alert for and prepared to treat anaphylaxis. Keep the patient calm and transport.

TERMS AND CONCEPTS

▼

1. **Write the number of the correct term next to each definition.**

   1. active rewarming
   2. conduction
   3. convection
   4. evaporation
   5. generalized cold emergency
   6. hyperthermia

   7. hypothermia
   8. local cold injury
   9. passive rewarming
   10. radiation
   11. water chill
   12. wind chill

   _____ **a.** Technique of aggressively applying heat to a patient to rewarm his body

   _____ **b.** An overall reduction in body temperature, affecting the entire body

   _____ **c.** Transfer of body heat through direct physical contact with nearby objects

   _____ **d.** Low body temperature

   _____ **e.** Helping the body to rewarm itself by simply placing the patient in a warm environment and covering him with blankets

   _____ **f.** Conversion of a liquid or solid into a gas

   _____ **g.** The increase in rate of cooling in the presence of water or wet clothing

   _____ **h.** Loss of body heat to the atmosphere when air passes over the body

   _____ **i.** Transfer of heat from the surface of one object to the surface of another without physical contact between the objects

   _____ **j.** The combined effect of wind speed and environmental temperature

   _____ **k.** High body temperature

   _____ **l.** Damage to body tissues in a specific part of the body resulting from exposure to cold

CONTENT REVIEW

▼

1. Which of the following is NOT one of the mechanisms by which the body loses heat?
   a. Respiration
   b. Conduction
   c. Consolidation
   d. Evaporation

2. Exposure to cold can cause two kinds of emergencies:
   a. Generalized cold emergency and generalized hypothermia
   b. Generalized hypothermia and local cold injury
   c. Generalized hypovolemia and local cold injury
   d. Generalized hypovolemia and generalized hypothermia

3. Which of the following is NOT a factor that puts a patient at risk for generalized hypothermia?
   a. Medical conditions
   b. A cold environment
   c. Drugs and poisons
   d. Middle age

4. There are five stages of hypothermia. Which stage is missing from the following list?

   shivering

   decreased level of responsiveness

   decreased vital signs

   death

   a. Flushed skin
   b. High blood pressure
   c. Apathy and decreased muscle function
   d. Nausea, vomiting, and diarrhea

5. Emergency medical care for generalized hypothermia should include all of the following EXCEPT
   a. Removing the patient from the cold environment
   b. Rewarming the patient as quickly and safely as possible
   c. Having the patient walk briskly to raise body temperature
   d. Administering oxygen at 15 lpm by nonrebreather mask

6. Which of the following is true regarding the technique of active rewarming?
   a. The patient who is unresponsive or not responding appropriately is the patient who requires active rewarming.
   b. The body temperature should be increased no more than 1°F per hour.
   c. The patient should be immersed in a tub of hot water.
   d. Heat should be applied to the extremities first, then the torso.

7. Immersion hypothermia should be considered in all cases of accidental immersion. Body temperature drops to the water temperature within _____.
   a. 10 minutes
   b. 20 minutes
   c. 30 minutes
   d. 60 minutes

8. Guidelines for the emergency medical care of the patient with immersion hypothermia include all of the following EXCEPT
   a. Lift the patient from the water in a vertical position to prevent vascular collapse.
   b. Tell the patient to make as little effort as possible to stay afloat until you reach him.
   c. Remove the patient's wet clothing carefully and gently.
   d. Treatment for the patient is similar to the treatment for generalized hypothermia.

9. The stages of local cold injury are
   a. Frostbite and hypothermia
   b. Early (superficial) and late (deep)
   c. Frostnip and frostbite
   d. Generalized and local

10. All of the following are guidelines for the care of local cold injuries EXCEPT
    a. Do not rub or massage the affected skin.
    b. Quickly remove clothing that is frozen to the skin.
    c. Never initiate thawing procedures if there is a danger of refreezing.
    d. Carefully remove any jewelry or restrictive clothing.

11. Guidelines for the rapid rewarming of local cold injuries include all of the following statements EXCEPT
    a. The water temperature should be just above body temperature, or 100 to 110°F.
    b. Keep the tissue in warm water until it is soft and color and sensation return to it.
    c. Dress the area with a dry sterile dressing.
    d. Rapid rewarming is the preferred treatment for all local cold injuries.

12. Heat-related emergencies are grouped under the name
    a. Hypothermia
    b. Hyperthermia
    c. Hyperpyrexia
    d. Hypoperfusion

13. Which of the following is NOT a predisposing factor for an individual to develop a heat related emergency?
    a. Climate
    b. Inactive lifestyle
    c. Extremes of age
    d. Pre-existing illnesses

14. A patient represents a dire medical emergency if he has been exposed to heat and has which of the following signs or symptoms?
    a. Cool, pale, moist skin
    b. Dizziness
    c. Muscle cramps
    d. Hot skin, either moist or dry

15. When cooling a heat emergency patient, cooling should be slowed if
    a. The patient becomes unresponsive
    b. The skin is cool to the touch
    c. Shivering begins to occur
    d. The patient develops muscle cramps

16. A heat emergency patient with moist, pale, normal-to-cool skin who is responsive and vomiting should
    a. Be given cool water to drink
    b. Be given nothing by mouth
    c. Be given a half glass of water every 15 minutes
    d. Be given warm water to drink

17. A heat emergency patient with moist, pale, normal-to-cool skin needs transport if
    a. The patient is sweating
    b. The patient has a temperature of 99°F
    c. The patient has a headache
    d. The patient is unresponsive

18. The first step in the emergency medical care of any patient with a heat emergency is to
   a. Administer oxygen at 15 lpm via a nonrebreather mask
   b. Place the patient supine and elevate the feet
   c. Move the patient to a cool place
   d. Remove as much clothing as possible

19. Grave indications that the heat emergency patient is deteriorating are
   a. The blood pressure falls and the patient feels exhausted
   b. The capillary refill time decreases and respirations are labored
   c. The pulse rate changes rapidly and the mental status declines
   d. The patient begins to shiver and the skin becomes pale

20. Which statement is FALSE regarding bites and stings?
   a. Snakebites are relatively common and the number of people who die from snakebites each year is significant.
   b. Most insect bites are considered minor and only cause problems when the patient has an allergic reaction.
   c. Exercise caution during the scene size-up to protect you or your partner from being bitten or stung.
   d. Be especially alert when assessing the airway and breathing.

CASE STUDY 1

You are standing by to provide medical coverage during a 10-kilometer running event on a hot summer day. You have responded to a call for a runner who is disoriented. The scene appears safe as you arrive at the finish line. As an event official leads you to the patient, you ask, "Why did you call the ambulance?" He replies, "This guy just finished the race and he isn't acting right!"

As you approach the patient, you note that he looks to be about 25 years of age. He is lying next to the finish line in full sunshine. He is wearing a polyester running suit. He is lying on his back, talking incoherently. He doesn't notice you as you kneel down beside him. Your general impression is that he looks ill. His skin color is red. He responds to your questions with inappropriate statements. His respirations are rapid and shallow, his radial pulse is weak and rapid, and his skin is hot to the touch and moist. There is no sign of trauma and no bleeding is observed. You rapidly move the patient to the back of the ambulance where the air-conditioner is already turned on.

1. The next BEST action to take for this patient is to
   a. Contact medical direction for treatment options
   b. Remove as much clothing as possible
   c. Fan the patient aggressively
   d. Give the patient cool water to drink

You have removed the patient from the hot environment, performed the action in item one, and begun to administer oxygen at 15 lpm by nonrebreather mask.

2. The next BEST action to take for this patient is to
   a. Radio a report on the patient's condition to the receiving facility
   b. Place the patient in a position of comfort
   c. Pour cool water over the patient's body
   d. Obtain a SAMPLE history

You have begun rapid transport to the hospital.

3. For this patient, you should be alert and prepared to perform which of the following interventions?
   a. Establish an airway.
   b. Provide positive pressure ventilation.
   c. Manage seizures.
   d. Any of these may become necessary for a patient with severe hyperthermia.

CASE STUDY 2

You are dispatched to the scene of a possible snake bite. The scene appears safe as you arrive at a hunting lodge in the woods. A man dressed in hunting clothing meets you at the gate and escorts you to the patient. As you follow him, you ask the hunter, "Why did you call the ambulance?" He replies, "Tony just finished for the day and was walking back to the lodge. He was walking across Crooked Creek and a cotton mouth got him! I blasted it and brought it and Tony back to the lodge. Then I called you."

As you approach the patient, you note that he looks to be about 35 years of age. He is sitting in a chair holding his leg. He looks at you as you enter the room. Your general impression is that he looks well, although he appears to be in pain. His skin color is normal. He responds to your questions appropriately. His respirations are normal. His radial pulse is strong and regular. His skin is warm and dry. You examine the bite and observe two distinct puncture wounds on the lower leg. The wound is red and moderately swollen. There are no other signs of trauma and no bleeding is observed. The snake (which is obviously dead) is lying next to the patient. Tony's friend puts it into a box so you can take it along to the hospital. You are extremely careful in handling the box, even though you are sure the snake is dead.

1. Which item is an INCORRECT treatment for this patient?
   a. Wash the area around the bite with a mild agent or strong soap solution.
   b. Remove any constricting objects as soon as possible.
   c. Apply a commercial cold pack to the bite.
   d. Keep the patient calm and limit his physical activity.

2. What additional treatments should be provided for this patient?
   a. Lower the injection site slightly below the level of the heart and watch for signs of anaphylaxis.
   b. Cut and then suction the venom from the bite site.
   c. Administer epinephrine and then cut and suction the bite.
   d. Elevate the site slightly above the level of the heart and watch for signs of anaphylaxis.

CASE STUDY 3

You are dispatched to a call for a woman down. It's the middle of winter and the temperature is in the mid 20s. The scene appears safe as you arrive at a single-story residence. A well-dressed man who introduces himself as a neighbor meets you at the ambulance and escorts you to the patient. As you follow him you ask, "Why did you call the ambulance?" He replies, "Mary is in her 80s and lives by herself. I stop by to check on her when I can. I found her on the floor of her garage, and I can't wake her up!"

As you enter the garage, you note that it is quite cold inside. The patient is lying on her side next to her car. She is dressed in a nightgown and a light bathrobe and slippers. She doesn't respond as you kneel down next to her. You apply a painful stimulus and she does not respond. Your general impression is that she looks ill. Her skin color is gray. Her respirations are slow and shallow. Her radial pulse is slow and barely palpable. There is no sign of trauma and no bleeding is observed. You move the patient to the back of the ambulance where the heater is already on.

1. Assess the pulse in this patient for
   a. 10 to 20 seconds
   b. 20 to 30 seconds
   c. 30 to 45 seconds
   d. 1 to 2 minutes

2. This patient requires
   a. Active rewarming
   b. Passive rewarming
   c. Immersion in a tub of hot water or hot shower
   d. Active rewarming if more than 30 minutes from the hospital

3. When moving this patient to the ambulance, you should
   a. Move her as quickly as you can, using any possible method
   b. Try to keep her head elevated during movement if possible
   c. Hyperventilate her during movement
   d. Handle her extremely gently

CASE STUDY 4

▼

You are dispatched to a call for a child with a local cold injury. It's mid December and quite cold out. The scene appears safe as you arrive at a small convenience store. Several kids are standing next to the door as you arrive. You step out and ask, "Why did you call the ambulance?" One of the kids replies, "I think my toes are frostbit! I called my mom and she's going to meet us here." The boy is about 12 or 13 years old. He is dressed in a heavy coat and boots that look wet. He is alert and oriented to your questions. Your general impression is that he looks well. His skin color is normal. His respirations are normal. His radial pulse is strong and regular. There is no sign of trauma and no bleeding is observed. You move the patient to the back of the ambulance where the heater is already on. You remove his shoes and socks. He tells you his right great toe is numb. You examine his toe and it looks somewhat white.

1. You would expect which sign or symptom to be present if the patient has suffered an early, or superficial, local cold injury?
   a. Good feeling and sensation in the toe
   b. Firm-to-frozen feeling when the skin is palpated
   c. When you palpate the skin, the normal color does not return
   d. Swelling and blisters

2. Which item is an INCORRECT treatment method for this patient?
   a. Administer oxygen at 15 lpm.
   b. Remove any wet or restrictive clothing to prevent further injury.
   c. Splint the extremity to prevent movement.
   d. Massage the affected area.

   The toe has thawed in the warm ambulance. The tissue is soft. The color and sensation have returned to the toe.

3. It is now MOST important to
   a. Elevate the affected extremity
   b. Prevent the possibility of refreezing
   c. Dress the area with a dry sterile dressing
   d. Dress the area with a moist sterile dressing

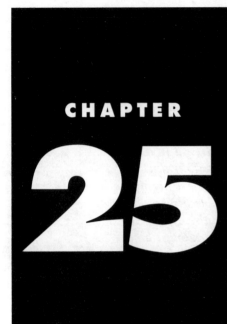

CHAPTER

25

DROWNING, NEAR-DROWNING, AND DIVING EMERGENCIES

Numbered objectives are from the United States Department of Transportation 1994 EMT-Basic National Standard Curriculum. Asterisked objectives, if any, pertain to material that is supplemental to the DOT curriculum.

4-7.6   Recognize the signs and symptoms of water-related emergencies.

4-7.7   Describe the complications of near-drowning.

KEY IDEAS

Drowning is often assumed to be the major cause of death from water-related emergencies. Drowning actually accounts for only one in twenty water-related deaths. Near-drowning, drowning, and diving emergency statistics, signs, symptoms, and management are reviewed in this chapter.

▶ Many water-related deaths could be prevented if personal flotation devices (PFDs) were utilized in and around water, adult supervision were provided around swimming pools, and pools were fenced and locked.

▶ Always suspect a spinal injury in any swimmer who is found unresponsive in or out of the water.

▶ Never enter the water to rescue a patient unless you meet all of the following criteria: You are a good swimmer, you are specially trained in water rescue techniques, you are wearing a personal flotation device, and you are accompanied by other rescuers.

▶ Use the reach, throw, row, and go strategy to reach a responsive swimmer who requires rescue.

▶ All near-drowning patients require transport even if you think they are stable.

▶ Attempt resuscitation on any pulseless, nonbreathing patient who has been submerged in cold water (68°F) for an extended time period.

▶ For the water-related-emergency patient, look for signs and symptoms of any of the following: airway obstruction, absent or inadequate breathing, pulselessness, spinal or head injury, soft tissue injuries, musculoskeletal injuries, external or internal bleeding, shock, hypothermia, or alcohol or drug abuse.

▶ The emergency care for near-drowning patients includes: If spinal injury is suspected immobilize the patient, if no spinal injury is suspected position the patient on his left side, suction as needed, rapidly establish an airway, begin positive pressure ventilation with supplemental oxygen, watch for gastric distention, and transport quickly.

TERMS AND CONCEPTS

1. **Write the number of the correct term next to each definition.**

   1. drowning
   2. gastric distention
   3. mammalian diving reflex
   4. near-drowning

   _____ a. Survival for at least 24 hours from near suffocation due to submersion
   _____ b. The body's natural response to submersion in cold water in which breathing is inhibited, the heart rate decreases, and blood vessels constrict in order to maintain cerebral and cardiac blood flow
   _____ c. Death from suffocation due to submersion
   _____ d. The filling of the stomach with water and/or air, causing an enlarged abdomen which makes ventilation difficult

CONTENT REVIEW

1. Which is NOT a true statement regarding water-related statistics?
   a. Drowning and near-drowning occur only in deep water.
   b. Drowning is responsible for one in twenty water-related deaths.
   c. Many deaths could be prevented with the wearing of personal flotation devices (PFDs).
   d. Proper adult supervision of swimming pools could reduce the number of deaths.

2. Which is NOT a major cause of drowning?
   a. Getting exhausted in the water
   b. Getting trapped or entangled while in the water
   c. Wearing a personal flotation device while in the water
   d. Using poor judgment in the water

3. You should always assume that a patient who sustained an injury when diving into a pool has
   a. Swallowed water
   b. Sustained a pelvic fracture
   c. Sustained head, neck, or spine injuries
   d. Sustained internal injuries

4. Which is NOT a true statement related to drowning or near-drowning?
   a. Near-drowning is defined as survival for at least 12 hours from near-suffocation due to submersion.
   b. Poor prognoses for near-drowning include those who struggle in the water and submersion for a long time.
   c. Poor prognoses for near-drowning include older people and people in warm, dirty, or brackish water.
   d. Panic on the part of a swimmer may contribute to a drowning death.

5. You should never go out into the water to attempt a rescue unless you meet certain criteria. Which is NOT one of these criteria?
   a. You are a good swimmer.
   b. You are trained as an EMT-Basic.
   c. You are wearing a personal flotation device.
   d. You are accompanied by other rescuers.

6. If the drowning patient is close to shore, the strategy you should use is
   a. Reach, go, row, and tow
   b. Call, throw, tow, and go
   c. Reach, throw, row, and go
   d. Go, throw, reach, and row

7. A patient is found unresponsive, floating in shallow water. Your PRIMARY suspicion should be that
   a. The patient has a spinal injury
   b. The patient is a poor swimmer
   c. The patient has been struck by a boat
   d. The patient had a seizure

8. You are evaluating a patient who, you learn, has been submerged in cold water for 30 minutes. You should
   a. Not attempt resuscitation on this patient
   b. Not attempt resuscitation until ALS arrives on scene
   c. Attempt resuscitation of the patient with full efforts
   d. Provide a brief resuscitative effort for the benefit of the family

9. Which statement is NOT true in relation to near-drowning patients?
   a. You should always transport the patient.
   b. Complications can develop up to 72 hours after the near-drowning incident.
   c. A detailed physical exam is not appropriate in near-drowning cases.
   d. You should keep the patient warm and provide high-flow oxygen.

10. When a person dives into cold water (below 68°F), this reflex can prevent death even after prolonged submersion.
    a. Human diving reflex
    b. Beck's diving reflex
    c. Mammalian diving reflex
    d. Momentary submersion reflex

CASE STUDY 1

▼

You are dispatched to a call for a possible drowning. You arrive at a small home located just outside of town. The scene appears safe as you arrive. A woman is frantically motioning to you. She screams at you as you exit the ambulance, "Please! Please! Hurry! My daughter! I just found her floating in the pool!" You follow the distraught mother to a backyard pool. As you approach the patient you note that she looks to be about 4 years of age. She is lying supine on the pool deck. CPR is being performed by a neighbor. The patient is located next to the shallow end of the pool. Your general impression is that she looks ill. Her skin color is cyanotic. She is unresponsive to pain. She has no respirations and no palpable carotid pulse. There is a small laceration on the front of her forehead with minor bleeding.

1. What is the appropriate INITIAL treatment for this patient?
   a. Determine the "down time" before beginning resuscitation
   b. Determine the "down time" and the temperature of the water before beginning resuscitation.
   c. If the "down time" is longer than 15 minutes do not begin resuscitation
   d. Begin resuscitation efforts immediately.

2. IMMEDIATE treatment for this patient should include
   a. Checking for gastric distention
   b. Treating the patient for a possible spinal injury
   c. Controlling the bleeding from the laceration
   d. Administering oxygen by nonrebreather mask

3. You have been providing positive pressure ventilation to the patient for a few minutes. You notice that the patient's abdomen is distended, and you cannot effectively ventilate the patient. You should
   a. Reduce the volume and pressure delivered during your ventilations
   b. Continue with the ventilations and advise the ALS crew of the condition when they arrive
   c. Increase the volume and pressure delivered during your ventilations
   d. Turn the patient on her left side and apply pressure over the epigastric region. Have suction available.

CASE STUDY 2

You are dispatched to the city pool for a possible drowning. On arrival, you observe a small crowd of people standing around a young boy who is sitting up in a chair. The scene appears safe as you walk to the patient. A lifeguard approaches and tells you, "I found this kid on the bottom of the pool. He couldn't have been under very long. I pulled him out and gave him one breath. He coughed and then he woke up. I called his mom to come and get him. She should be here in a few minutes." As you approach the patient, you note that he looks to be about 11 years of age. He is sitting in a chair and looks up at you as you approach. He is coughing occasionally. Your general impression is that he looks well. His skin color is normal. He answers your questions appropriately. His respirations are normal. His radial pulse is strong and regular. There is no sign of trauma, and no bleeding is observed. No other findings are made during the focused history and physical exam.

1. Should this patient be allowed to return home with his mother?
   a. Yes. The patient is stable. Allow him to return home.
   b. Yes, but only after you have described to his mother potential complications that can occur and what to watch for.
   c. No. Observe the patient at the scene for at least 30 minutes before making a decision.
   d. No. Fatal complications from a near-drowning can occur as long as 72 hours after the incident. He must be transported for evaluation by a physician.

2. Your care and treatment for this patient should include which of the following?
   a. No care is required. The patient will be allowed to return home.
   b. Administer oxygen, monitor carefully, and transport on his left side.
   c. Monitor carefully and transport sitting up.
   d. Administer oxygen, reevaluate his condition, and reach a decision following further observation.

COGNITIVE OBJECTIVES

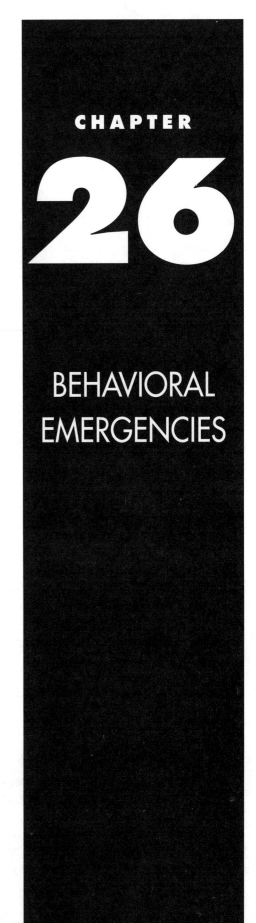

Numbered objectives are from the United States Department of Transportation 1994 EMT-Basic National Standard Curriculum. Asterisked objectives, if any, pertain to material that is supplemental to the DOT curriculum.

4-8.1 Define the term "behavioral emergency."

4-8.2 Discuss the general factors that may cause an alteration in a patient's behavior.

4-8.3 State the various reasons for psychological crises.

4-8.4 Discuss the characteristics of an individual's behavior which suggest that the patient is at risk for suicide.

4-8.5 Discuss the special medical/legal considerations for managing behavioral emergencies.

4-8.6 Discuss the special considerations for assessing a patient with behavioral emergencies.

4-8.7 Discuss the general principles of an individual's behavior which suggest he is at risk for violence.

4-8.8 Discuss methods to calm behavioral emergency patients.

KEY IDEAS

This chapter focuses on the assessment and management of behavioral emergencies. Behavioral emergencies may be manifested in a variety of ways and require special considerations from the EMT-Basic. Key concepts include:

▶ A behavioral emergency is one in which the patient exhibits behavior that may pose a danger to the patient or others and is intolerable to the patient, the family, or the community.

▶ The precipitating factor in a behavioral emergency may be extremes of emotion, a physical condition, or a psychological condition.

▶ The priority of the EMT-Basic at the scene of a behavioral emergency is to manage the patient's injuries or illness.

▶ Acts of violence, against oneself or others, are often associated with behavioral emergencies.

CHAPTER
26

BEHAVIORAL EMERGENCIES

► Every suicidal act or gesture should be taken seriously and the patient should be transported for evaluation by a physician.

► When managing behavioral emergencies, the EMT-Basic should remember that interpersonal communications may have more impact on the outcome of the situation than emergency medical skills.

► Behavioral emergencies require special assessment and medical legal considerations on the part of the EMT-Basic.

TERMS AND CONCEPTS

1. **Write the number of the correct term next to each definition.**

    1. behavior
    2. behavioral emergency
    3. humane restraints
    4. reasonable force
    5. suicide

    _____ **a.** The minimum amount of force required to prevent the patient from harming himself or others
    _____ **b.** The way a person acts or performs
    _____ **c.** A willful act designed to end one's own life
    _____ **d.** Padded leather or cloth straps used to tie a patient down to keep him from hurting himself or others
    _____ **e.** A situation in which a person exhibits "abnormal" behavior

CONTENT REVIEW

1. List three clues that a behavioral emergency may be due to a physical cause.

2. _____ often presents as an overwhelming fear that is accompanied by rapid breathing, palpitations, and dizziness.

3. Deep feelings of sadness and worthlessness accompanied by fatigue, loss of appetite, and a sense of hopelessness may be due to a common psychiatric disorder known as _____

4. _____ is a group of psychiatric disorders characterized by distortions of thought or speech, bizarre delusions, and inappropriate emotional responses.

5. All of the following patients exhibit characteristics that indicate a high suicide risk EXCEPT
   a. 50-year-old married female with a history of previous suicidal attempts
   b. 60-year-old widowed male recently diagnosed with terminal cancer
   c. 45-year-old single female with a history of chronic depression
   d. 35-year-old married male who recently had gall bladder surgery

6. You respond to a call at a movie theater. Your patient is pacing back and forth in the lobby, shouting loudly, and threatening harm to anyone who comes near him. You recognize that this behavior may be
   a. A sign that this person may become violent
   b. Due to a psychiatric disorder
   c. A result of physical trauma or illness
   d. Any of these

7. _____ is your best protection against legal problems or false accusations when dealing with emotionally disturbed patients.

8. Which of the following best describes the guidelines that apply when restraining a combative patient?
   a. Use as much force as possible.
   b. Never attempt restraint until you have sufficient help and an appropriate plan.
   c. Once you have determined that restraint is necessary, move slowly to avoid agitating the patient.
   d. Police-style metal handcuffs are a good way to restrain a combative patient to the stretcher.

9. The first priority in dealing with a behavioral emergency is to
   a. Determine if the behavior is caused by a medical condition
   b. Establish and maintain an airway and oxygenation
   c. Protect yourself and others at the scene from harm
   d. Restrain the patient to protect him from harming himself

10. All of the following are appropriate methods to use to calm behavioral emergency patients EXCEPT
    a. Maintain good eye contact with the patient.
    b. "Play along" with the patient's auditory and visual hallucinations.
    c. Avoid unnecessary or uninvited physical contact.
    d. Respond honestly to questions but don't foster false expectations.

CASE STUDY

You have been called to a dormitory at the local college. Your patient is a 20-year-old male who is cowering in the corner of the lobby. Bystanders report that his name is Jim, and that just before your arrival he was shouting "Go away, leave me alone," and gesturing at someone or something that isn't there.

1. What should you do first?

Jim allows you to come within 3 feet of his location. You notice that he seems frightened. His hands are trembling slightly, and his breathing is rapid. You note that his skin is pink and dry, and you observe no obvious injuries. He tells you that he's hearing voices who are telling him to do "bad things."

2. What should you do now?

3. What should your partner be doing?

After 15 minutes of quiet conversation, you find that Jim has no past medical history but has had trouble concentrating and sleeping over the past several weeks. He denies that he has been injured recently. You ask Jim if he'll let you take him to the hospital to see the doctor. Jim agrees to accompany you. You help Jim to his feet and lead him out of the lobby and to your ambulance.

4. What should you do while en route to the hospital?

COGNITIVE OBJECTIVES

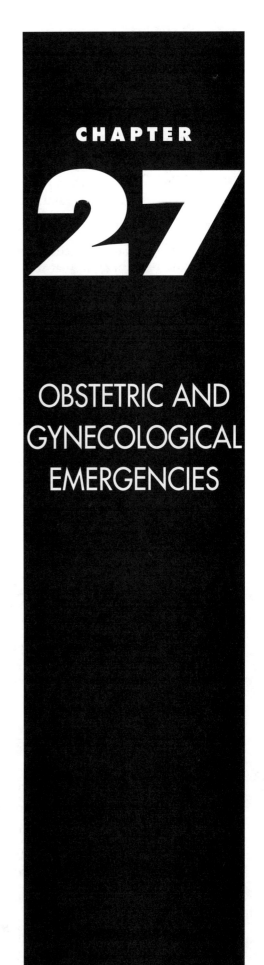

4-9.1 Identify the following structures: uterus, vagina, fetus, placenta, umbilical cord, amniotic sac, perineum.

4-9.2 Identify and explain the use of the contents of an obstetrics kit.

4-9.3 Identify predelivery emergencies.

4-9.4 State indications of an imminent delivery.

4-9.5 Differentiate the emergency medical care provided to a patient with predelivery emergencies from a normal delivery.

4-9.6 State the steps in the predelivery preparation of the mother.

4-9.7 Establish the relationship between body substance isolation and childbirth.

4-9.8 State the steps to assist in the delivery.

4-9.9 Describe care of the infant as the head appears.

4-9.10 Describe how and when to cut the umbilical cord.

4-9.11 Discuss the steps in the delivery of the placenta.

4-9.12 List the steps in the emergency medical care of the mother post-delivery.

4-9.13 Summarize neonatal resuscitation procedures.

4-9.14 Describe the procedures for the following abnormal deliveries: breech birth, prolapsed cord, limb presentation.

4-9.15 Differentiate the special considerations for multiple births.

4-9.16 Describe special considerations of meconium.

4-9.17 Describe special considerations of a premature baby.

4-9.18 Discuss the emergency medical care of a patient with a gynecological emergency.

CHAPTER 27

OBSTETRIC AND GYNECOLOGICAL EMERGENCIES

KEY IDEAS

This chapter focuses on the assessment and management of obstetric and gynecologic emergencies. The EMT-Basic does not frequently encounter emergencies related to the reproductive organs, so these are often stressful calls. In this chapter you will learn how to recognize and provide emergency care for obstetric and gynecologic emergencies. Key concepts include:

▶ The anatomic structures associated with pregnancy include the uterus, placenta, amniotic sac, umbilical cord, cervix, and vagina.

▶ The three stages of labor are dilation, expulsion, and placental.

▶ Recognition of a predelivery emergency is based on information obtained from the focused history and physical exam that relates to the reported abnormality, such as pain, discomfort, or bleeding.

▶ The priorities for care do not change at the scene of an obstetric or gynecologic emergency. Use the same assessment and treatment techniques as you would use on any patient who is not pregnant.

▶ Imminent delivery is recognized by crowning, the frequency and duration of contractions, and the sensation of bowel movement (urge to push).

▶ The role of the EMT-Basic during childbirth is to assist in the delivery and to recognize and treat life-threatening problems for the mother or baby.

▶ Delivery emergencies include: abnormal presentation, prematurity, meconium staining, and multiple births.

▶ The essential emergency care of the newborn includes the establishment and maintenance of an adequate airway and breathing status and the prevention of heat loss.

▶ The goals for the emergency management of gynecologic emergencies are to ensure an adequate airway, breathing, and circulation; to control vaginal bleeding; and treat for shock (hypoperfusion).

TERMS AND CONCEPTS

1. Write the number of the correct term next to each definition.

   1. amniotic sac
   2. embryo
   3. fetus
   4. placenta
   5. umbilical cord

   _____ a. Unborn infant from the third month of pregnancy to birth
   _____ b. Placental extension that supplies nourishment to the fetus
   _____ c. Organ of pregnancy for the exchange of oxygen and waste products
   _____ d. Transparent membrane forming the sac which holds fluid and the fetus
   _____ e. Unborn infant from conception to the third month of pregnancy

CONTENT REVIEW

1. The _____ is the lowest portion of the birth canal.
   a. Cervix
   b. Uterus
   c. Vagina
   d. Perineum

2. _____ consists of uterine contractions that expel the fetus and placenta.

3. Define the three stages of labor.

4. When performing a focused history on a 24-year-old female patient who is pregnant, which of the following questions would be appropriate?
   a. Are you experiencing any pain or discomfort?
   b. Have you had any vaginal discharge or bleeding?
   c. When is your due date?
   d. All of these

5. All of the following may be signs or symptoms of a predelivery emergency EXCEPT
   a. Abdominal pain or trauma
   b. Vaginal bleeding or discharge
   c. Headache with numbness in arms
   d. Altered mental status or seizures

6. Your supine pregnant patient is noted to have a low blood pressure. You suspect that this may be due to _____.

7. Management specific to the situation noted above (item 6) should include
   a. Inserting a nasopharyngeal airway
   b. Beginning chest compressions
   c. Positioning the patient on her left side
   d. Applying the AED

8. Your 30-year-old female patient is four months pregnant. She complains of cramping abdominal pain and bright red vaginal bleeding. Your treatment of this patient should include all of the following EXCEPT
   a. Pack the vagina to control bleeding.
   b. Place a sanitary pad over the vaginal opening.
   c. Elevate the lower extremities 8 inches.
   d. Administer oxygen at 15 lpm by nonrebrether mask.

9. Your 20-year-old patient is eight months pregnant. Prior to your arrival she had a seizure, which lasted 2 minutes. You find her to have an altered mental status, with a patent airway and adequate respirations and perfusion. Care of this patient should include all of the following EXCEPT
   a. Administer high-flow oxygen via a nonrebreather mask.
   b. Be prepared to administer positive pressure ventilation.
   c. Transport on the left side.
   d. Minimize noise, light, and movement to help prevent seizures.

10. All of the following are signs and symptoms of an imminent delivery EXCEPT
    a. The presence of crowning
    b. Contractions occurring every 2 minutes which last 30 to 90 seconds
    c. Passage of a slight amount of blood and mucus
    d. Sensation of an urge to have a bowel movement

11. After taking appropriate BSI precautions and positioning the patient, arrange in the proper sequence (1–5), the emergency care of a patient during active labor for a normal delivery.

    _____ Suction the infant's mouth and nose. Support the body as it delivers, then again suction the mouth and nose. Dry and wrap the infant.

    _____ Observe for the delivery of the placenta. As it delivers, grasp it gently and rotate. Place in a towel and bag it for transport to the hospital.

    _____ Support the bony part of the infant's skull and exert gentle pressure against the perineum as the head delivers. Determine the position of the umbilical cord.

    _____ Keep the infant level with the vagina. Have your partner assume care of the infant. When the pulsations cease, clamp, tie, and cut the umbilical cord.

    _____ Place a sanitary napkin at the vaginal opening. Record the time of delivery and transport. Keep mother and infant warm en route.

12. Your patient has just delivered a healthy baby boy. Following the delivery of the placenta, her vaginal bleeding seems to increase. Which of the following best describes what you should do to provide emergency care for this patient?
    a. Massage the uterus and position your patient on her left side.
    b. Administer oxygen and firmly massage the uterus.
    c. Massage the uterus and pack the vagina to control bleeding.
    d. Administer oxygen and pack the vagina with sanitary napkins.

13. Which of the following is NOT a sign or symptom of an abnormal delivery emergency?
    a. Presentation of any part of the fetus other than its head
    b. Cessation of contractions after delivery of the infant
    c. Green color of the amniotic fluid
    d. Labor that occurs before the 38th week of pregnancy

14. Management of a breech or limb presentation should include
    a. Administer high-flow oxygen to the mother
    b. Immediate transport to the hospital
    c. Position mother with her head down and pelvis elevated
    d. All of these

15. _____ is an abnormal delivery situation where there may be compression of the cord against the vaginal walls by the pressure of the infant's head.

16. How should you manage the situation above (item 15)?
    a. Immediately push the cord back into the vagina.
    b. Insert a gloved hand into the vagina to relieve pressure on the cord.
    c. Cover the cord with a dry sterile towel to prevent infection.
    d. Push on the mother's abdomen to expedite delivery.

17. Meconium staining of the amniotic fluid should be managed by
    a. Immediate transport to the hospital for evaluation by a physician
    b. Administration of oxygen to the mother to resolve fetal distress
    c. Suctioning mouth and nose before the infant takes his first breath
    d. Stimulating the infant to cough to clear meconium from airway

18. In addition to the usual care for a newborn, care of the premature infant requires
    a. Vigorous suctioning to maintain airway
    b. Direct administration of supplemental oxygen by a face mask
    c. Immediate transport for resuscitation
    d. Vigilant attention to prevent heat loss or contamination

19. Briefly explain the purpose of the Apgar scoring assessment of the newborn and list the components of Apgar scoring.

20. Which of the following is NOT a sign of a severely depressed newborn?
    a. Shallow, gasping respirations
    b. Cyanotic extremities
    c. Weak, irregular pulses
    d. Poor muscle tone

21. You have just assisted with the delivery of a baby girl. She has shallow, gasping respirations and a heart rate that is less than 90 beats per minute. Which of the following best describes your emergency care for this patient?
    a. Administer "blow by" oxygen and monitor pulse for 60 seconds.
    b. Assist ventilations with a bag-valve mask and reassess in 30 seconds.
    c. Administer high-flow oxygen with a nonrebreather mask.
    d. Assist ventilations with a bag-valve mask and begin chest compressions.

22. You have responded to the scene of a sexual assault. After taking appropriate BSI precautions and completing the initial assessment, your focused history and physical exam should include
    a. Direct examination of the genitalia to verify injury
    b. Cleaning and dressing the patient's wounds
    c. Questioning the patient about other potential injuries
    d. Placing any clothing that is removed in one bag to preserve evidence

23. The victim of a sexual assault has a need for emergency medical care and

_____.

24. Emergency management of the situation above (items 22 and 23) should include
   a. Ensuring maintenance of airway, breathing, and circulation
   b. Controlling bleeding from the vagina with a sanitary napkin
   c. Treating any other signs and symptoms as you would any other patient
   d. All of these

CASE STUDY
▼

You have been dispatched to the scene of a single vehicle accidentally driven into the river. A jogger and another bystander dove into the river and were able to rescue the driver. Your patient is a woman in her 30s who is obviously pregnant. By the size of her abdomen, you suspect that she is near term. Your initial assessment reveals an unresponsive female with rapid, shallow respirations. Her pulse is slow and irregular. Her skin is cool and dry. There are no obvious signs of injury.

1. What should you do?

You have moved the patient to the ambulance. Without assistance her baseline vital signs are BP 90/76; pulse 52 and irregular, respirations 28, shallow and gasping.

2. How can you position your patient to minimize supine hypotensive syndrome?

3. What care should your patient receive en route?

Two blocks from the hospital your patient stops breathing and becomes pulseless.

4. What should you do now?

Your patient is resuscitated at the hospital and undergoes surgical delivery of a baby girl.

MODULE 4 REVIEW
MEDICAL, BEHAVIORAL, AND OBSTETRICS/GYNECOLOGY: CHAPTERS 13-27

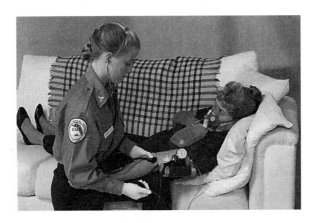

Medical emergencies are usually the result of something that goes wrong inside the body — as opposed to traumatic injuries, which are usually the result of some outside force.

Q **Why is it important to look for a mechanism of injury at the scene of a medical call?**

A It is important to rule out trauma. Sometimes the only clue that the patient's signs and symptoms are due to a medical cause is the absence of a mechanism of injury. It is also possible that a patient with a medical condition may also be suffering from trauma. For example, the patient may have become dizzy because of a breathing problem, then fallen and sustained an injury. (Conversely, a patient who has sustained an injury may also be suffering from a medical condition — for example, a heart attack brought on by the trauma.) Never assume that this is "only" a medical call until you have ruled out any mechanism of injury or sign of trauma.

Q **Why is there so much emphasis on altered mental status for a wide variety of medical conditions?**

A Partly because an altered mental status — which may range from confusion to complete unresponsiveness — may be a sign of a serious condition. Mostly, however, it is emphasized because a patient with an altered mental status may lose the ability to protect his own airway, and — as you learned in the Airway module — without a patent airway, all other assessments and treatments are worthless. So mental status and airway must be monitored on every medical call.

Q **Why does the emergency care for almost any medical condition include providing oxygen?**

A The body requires oxygen to function. In many conditions, something is preventing enough oxygen from entering the body or the bloodstream or is preventing it from being carried adequately to all the body's cells, and especially to the brain. Even if the body is receiving its normal supply of oxygen, extra oxygen can help to support the functions of body and brain and will help to prevent many conditions from getting worse. In other words, oxygen is a medication that is almost always good for any medical condition and will almost never be harmful if given to the patient.

(Module 4 Review continued)

Q What other medications, besides oxygen, are EMT-Bs allowed to administer to patients?

A Oral glucose (used in certain diabetic emergencies) and activated charcoal (administered in some ingested poisonings) are carried on the ambulance and may be administered by the EMT-B under certain circumstances with on-line or off-line approval from medical direction. Three medications that may have been prescribed to the patient and may be found in his possession may also be administered by the EMT-B under certain circumstances with on-line or off-line approval of medical direction. These are the metered-dose inhaler (for certain respiratory emergencies), nitroglycerin (for chest pain), and epinephrine (administered by auto-injector for severe allergic reactions). *Detailed information on these medications is found on the Medication Cards at the back of this book.*

Q What are the chief functions of the EMT-B at the scene of a medical emergency?

A Chief functions are to assess the patient, gathering as much information as possible from the environment and the SAMPLE history, to monitor the patient's mental status and protect the airway, to administer oxygen or positive pressure ventilation as appropriate, to administer medications as appropriate and permitted by medical direction, to position the patient (often in a position of comfort), and to transport.

Q What are the key functions of the EMT-B in a behavioral emergency?

A Key functions are to protect your safety and that of your partner, to treat the patient's medical condition or injuries, to calm and reassure the patient to the degree possible, and to transport the patient, with humane restraints if necessary.

Q What are the key functions of the EMT-B at the scene of an obstetrical or gynecological emergency?

A Key functions are to treat the medical condition or injuries of the patient as for any patient, to transport a pregnant patient if delivery is not imminent, to assist the mother in delivering the baby if transport cannot be accomplished before delivery, and to care for both the mother and the newborn (or newborns!).

Numbered objectives are from the United States Department of Transportation 1994 EMT-Basic National Standard Curriculum. Asterisked objectives, if any, pertain to material that is supplemental to the DOT curriculum.

3-1.4   Discuss common mechanisms of injury/nature of illness.

*   Explain how the following affect the force of impact: mass and velocity, acceleration and deceleration, energy changing form and direction.

*   Describe the three main impacts that occur in a vehicle collision.

*   Discuss the following mechanisms of injury and their effects on the human body: motor vehicle collisions, vehicle pedestrian collisions, motorcycle collisions, falls, penetrating injuries, and blast injuries.

*   Discuss the steps of patient assessment, including the priority decision, as they relate to and are guided by the mechanism of injury.

KEY IDEAS

Maintaining a high index of suspicion for hidden injuries in the trauma patient is just as important as identifying obvious injuries. An understanding of the mechanism of injury (how the patient was injured) is the chief component of this crucial assessment skill.

▶ The amount of kinetic energy contained in a moving body depends on the body's mass (weight) and velocity (speed). Velocity is the more significant factor when evaluating the mechanism of injury.

▶ Motor vehicle collisions can be classified as frontal, rear-end, lateral, or rotational. Each type involves characteristic injuries.

▶ In a vehicle-pedestrian collision, the extent of injury depends on the speed of the vehicle, what part of the pedestrian's body was struck, how far he was thrown, the surface he lands on, and the body part that first impacts the ground.

▶ Motorcycle collisions are classified as head-on impact, angular impact, or ejection. Incidence of injury and death is greatly increased when the rider does not wear a helmet.

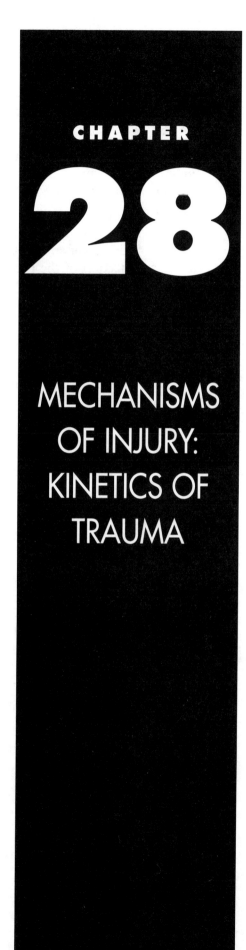

CHAPTER

28

MECHANISMS OF INJURY: KINETICS OF TRAUMA

► Falls are the most common mechanism of injury. The severity of injury depends on the falling distance, landing surface, and the body part that impacts first. A fall of 15 feet or more onto an unyielding surface is considered severe for an adult. A fall greater than 10 feet is considered severe for a child.

► Penetrating injuries are classified as low-velocity (knives), medium-velocity (shotgun and handgun pellets or bullets), or high-velocity (high-speed rifles). Assess the patient for both entrance and exit wounds.

► Blast injuries are classified as primary-phase (injuries due to the pressure wave), secondary-phase (injuries due to flying debris), and tertiary-phase injuries (patient is thrown from source of blast). Keep a high index of suspicion for all three types of injuries when a patient has been involved in a blast.

► Start to evaluate the mechanism of injury during your scene size-up. Rely on it when making decisions regarding patient priorities; determine what injuries are possible, even when they are not apparent. During patient assessment, the mechanism of injury will help you determine if manual in-line stabilization of the patient's head and neck is necessary, how to proceed with the focused history and physical exam, and what problems may arise during transport. Be sure to give the hospital staff all relevant information about the patient's mechanism of injury.

TERMS AND CONCEPTS

1. **Write the number of each term next to its definition.**

    1. cavitation
    2. dissipation of energy
    3. drag
    4. kinetic energy
    5. kinetics of trauma
    6. mechanism of injury
    7. profile
    8. trajectory

    _____ **a.** A cavity formed by a pressure wave resulting from the kinetic energy of a bullet traveling through body tissue; also called pathway expansion

    _____ **b.** Refers to the size and shape of a bullet's point of impact; the greater the point of impact the greater the injury

    _____ **c.** The energy contained by an object in motion

    _____ **d.** The factors and forces that cause traumatic injury

    _____ **e.** The factors that slow a projectiles

    _____ **f.** The path of a projectile during its travel; it may be flat or curved

    _____ **g.** The science of analyzing mechanisms of injury

    _____ **h.** The way energy is transferred to the human body by the forces acting upon it

CONTENT REVIEW

1. The amount of kinetic energy a moving body contains depends on what two factors?
   a. Mass and weight
   b. Rate of acceleration and mass
   c. Rate of acceleration and velocity
   d. Mass and velocity

2. Identify the factor that is MOST significant when evaluating the mechanism of injury.
   a. Mass
   b. Rate of acceleration
   c. Velocity
   d. Rate of deceleration

3. The rate at which a body in motion INCREASES its speed is known as
   a. Mass
   b. Deceleration
   c. Velocity
   d. Acceleration

4. The typical vehicular collision involves
   a. One impact (vehicle)
   b. Two impacts (vehicle and body)
   c. Three impacts (vehicle, body, and organs)
   d. Two or more impacts (two or more vehicles)

5. What is the most COMMON mechanism of injury?
   a. Vehicular collisions
   b. Falls
   c. Penetrating gunshots
   d. Explosions

6. What is the most LETHAL mechanism of injury?
   a. Vehicular collisions
   b. Falls
   c. Penetrating gunshots
   d. Explosions

7. List three situations or findings at the scene of a motor vehicle collision that would cause you to have a high index of suspicion of serious injury.

8. In a motor vehicle collision, the "up and over" and "down and under" pathways are examples of injury patterns associated with _____ impact.

9. When a passenger's head strikes the car windshield, the glass may crack in a typical _____ pattern.

10. The automobile driver's neck whips back, and the body is propelled forward even while the head seems to remain at rest. This BEST describes
   a. A rotational impact
   b. A rear-end impact
   c. A lateral impact
   d. A frontal impact

11. In this type of motor vehicle collision, the body is struck from the side. This BEST describes
   a. A rotational impact
   b. A rear-end impact
   c. A lateral impact
   d. A frontal impact

12. Injuries due to rotational or rollover impact are difficult to predict, but typically affect multiple systems.
   a. True
   b. False

13. A child who is about to be struck by an auto generally
   a. Turns away from the oncoming auto
   b. Turns to the side of the oncoming auto
   c. Turns to face the oncoming auto
   d. Does not turn at all

14. A common pattern of injuries to a child struck by an auto is injuries to the
   a. Upper and lower extremities
   b. Femur, chest, abdomen, and head
   c. Phalanges, radius, and ulna
   d. Pelvis, chest, skull, and face

15. Which of the following is NOT a true statement about motor vehicle restraints?
   a. In a collision, a seat belt worn too low can dislocate the hips.
   b. Properly applied lap belts and shoulder straps do not protect the head and neck.
   c. Air bags don't work well in multiple collision events.
   d. A deployed airbag should not be lifted from the steering wheel.

16. "Laying the bike down" is an evasive action meant to prevent ejection or separation of a motorcycle rider from his bike.
   a. True
   b. False

17. A fall of _____ feet onto an unyielding surface is considered severe for an adult. A fall of more than _____ feet can cause severe injuries in a child.
   a. 5, 10
   b. 10, 5
   c. 15, 10
   d. 10, 15

18. Experts say that a patient in a feet-first fall who falls _____ or more probably will have a spinal injury.
   a. Two times his height
   b. Three times his height
   c. Four times his height
   d. Five times his height

19. In a gunshot incident, the EMT-B should suspect both thoracic and abdominal injury if the entrance wound is
   a. Between the nipple line and the waist
   b. Between the navel and the waist
   c. Between the trachea and the clavicle
   d. Between the nipple line and the sternum

20. Primary-phase, secondary-phase, and tertiary-phase injuries are related to
   a. Motor vehicle collisions
   b. Blasts and explosions
   c. Low- and medium-velocity weapons
   d. Head-first falls

CASE STUDY 1

You are at the scene of a one-car, high-speed motor vehicle collision. The driver is dead, ejected from the vehicle sometime during several rollovers. A woman about 20 years of age approaches you and identifies herself as a passenger in the vehicle. She tells you she walked to a gas station to call for help, then returned. Your general impression is that she looks well, although she has a small laceration over her left eye. She is holding her left upper abdominal and chest region. Her skin color appears to be normal. She responds to your questions appropriately although somewhat slowly.

1. Which statement BEST describes the appropriate treatment for the female patient?
   a. The patient should be assessed for any injuries.
   b. The patient should be advised of potential serious signs and symptoms to watch for and released.
   c. The patient should be assessed, immobilized, monitored carefully, and transported.
   d. The patient should be transported by a family member for evaluation at a local hospital.

2. In your opinion, the patient's mental status
   a. Should concern you, but only if her mental status deteriorates further
   b. Should concern you, since an altered mental status is one of the earliest signs of brain injury
   c. Should not concern you since it appears to be normal or only slightly altered
   d. Should not concern you, since the mechanism of injury has been identified

CASE STUDY 2

You have been dispatched to a residential area to assist a worker who fell from a tree. The 35-year-old patient is lying on his right side in a soft grassy area. His eyes are open. You ask him, "What happened?" He tells you that he was trimming the tree when the branch he was standing on gave way.

1. Which of the following questions will BEST help you determine the patient's condition?
   a. How long have you been lying here?
   b. Where do you hurt the most?
   c. What is your doctor's name?
   d. How did you land?

2. The patient tells you that he landed feet first with his knees locked and then broke his forward fall with his hands. What potential injuries should you suspect?
   a. Spine injury in the lumbar, midthoracic, and cervical regions; and head trauma
   b. Injuries to the femur, hips, pelvis, spine, midthoracic and cervical regions, and wrists
   c. Spinal injury in the cervical and lumbar region, plus chest and shoulder injury
   d. Injuries to the hands and knees

CASE STUDY 3

A teenage gunshot victim is lying on her back next to the front door of her house. Her eyes are open. You ask, "What happened?" She replies, "I was just standing here and these guys drive by and shoot me." There is noticeable bleeding to her left chest, and she is holding the area with her right hand. Her skin is pale, cool, and moist. Respirations are normal, and radial pulse is weak, rapid, and regular.

1. Which of the following questions, if it can be answered, will provide important information about the mechanism of injury?
   a. What kind of gun was used (e.g., shotgun, handgun, high-speed rifle?)
   b. Was the patient shot from a distance or at close range?
   c. How many shots were fired? (Does the patient have multiple wounds?)
   d. All of these will provide important information about the mechanism of injury.

2. You determine that only one shot was fired. You dress the wound to the patient's chest. What have you forgotten to do?
   a. Look for and treat any additional (entrance or exit) wounds.
   b. Probe the wound to see if the bullet has lodged in the body.
   c. Pour an antiseptic solution into the wound.
   d. Support the patient's breathing with positive pressure ventilation.

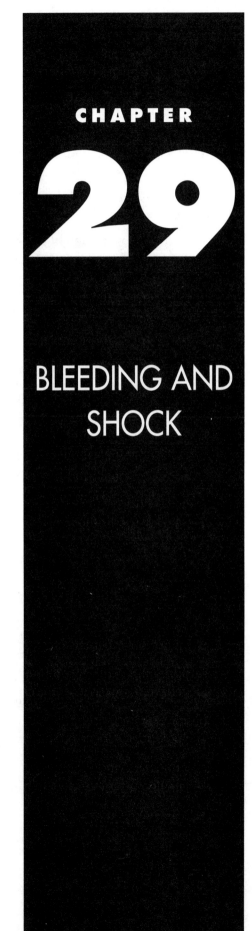

CHAPTER 29

BLEEDING AND SHOCK

COGNITIVE OBJECTIVES

Numbered objectives are from the United States Department of Transportation 1994 EMT-Basic National Standard Curriculum. Asterisked objectives, if any, pertain to material that is supplemental to the DOT curriculum.

5-1.1   List the structure and function of the circulatory system.

5-1.2   Differentiate between arterial, venous, and capillary bleeding.

5-1.3   State methods of emergency medical care of external bleeding.

5-1.4   Establish the relationship between body substance isolation and bleeding.

5-1.5   Establish the relationship between airway management and the trauma patient.

5-1.6   Establish the relationship between mechanism of injury and internal bleeding.

5-1.7   List the signs of internal bleeding.

5-1.8   List the steps in emergency medical care of the patient with signs and symptoms of internal bleeding.

5-1.9   List signs and symptoms of shock (hypoperfusion).

5-1.10 State the steps in the emergency medical care of the patient with signs and symptoms of shock (hypoperfusion).

KEY IDEAS

This chapter focuses on the emergency management of bleeding and shock (hypoperfusion). As an EMT-Basic you must be able to recognize the signs and symptoms of internal and external bleeding. Failure to treat bleeding of either type has the potential to lead to rapid patient deterioration, shock, and death.

▶ It is imperative that the EMT-Basic always take all appropriate BSI precautions and practice good hand washing when caring for any patient.

▶ Differentiation of the type of bleeding (arterial, venous, or capillary) is based on the color of the blood and the nature of blood flow. Each type can be life-threatening.

► Only airway and breathing have a higher priority than the control of severe bleeding.

► Control of severe external bleeding is performed during the initial assessment, while the treatment of internal bleeding and shock is accomplished immediately following the initial assessment.

► External bleeding may be controlled by a variety of methods including direct pressure and elevation, pressure points, splints, pressure splints, and tourniquets.

► Always suspect internal bleeding in cases of unexplained shock.

► The goal of emergency medical care for internal bleeding is to recognize its presence quickly, maintain the body's perfusion, and provide rapid transport to an appropriate medical facility.

► Shock is the direct result of inadequate perfusion. If allowed to persist, cell failure, organ failure, and death will follow.

► No matter what kind of bleeding has caused shock, rapid transport to a medical facility is an important element of the emergency medical care.

TERMS AND CONCEPTS

1. _____ is the insufficient supply of oxygen and other nutrients to the body's cells, which results from inadequate circulation of blood.

2. The medical term for a nosebleed is _____.

3. By compressing an artery at a _____ _____, arterial blood flow can be reduced in an extremity.

CONTENT REVIEW

1. Define the role of the circulatory system in the human body.

2. The three main components of the circulatory system are:

3. _____ and _____ are two measures of heart and circulatory system function.
    a. Respiratory rate/quality
    b. Pupil size/reactivity
    c. Pulse/blood pressure
    d. Blood color/flow

4. Write the number of the correct term beside its description.

　　1. arterial bleeding
　　2. venous bleeding
　　3. capillary bleeding

　____ a. Dark red blood that flows steadily from a wound
　____ b. Dark red blood that slowly oozes from a wound
　____ c. Bright red blood that spurts from a wound

5. Life-threatening bleeding takes precedence over all other emergency medical care INCLUDING that for airway or breathing.
　　a. True
　　b. False

6. Your patient has a large wound to his right lower leg which is bleeding profusely. There is no deformity of the extremity. After taking appropriate BSI precautions, which of the following best describes the FIRST steps in emergency management of this injury?
　　a. Use a tourniquet and elevation.
　　b. Use a sling, swathe, and elevation.
　　c. Use direct pressure and elevation.
　　d. Use the femoral pressure point and elevation.

7. Label each photograph with the name of the major pressure point that is illustrated.

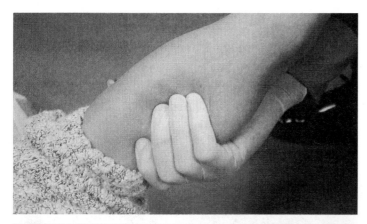

a. _____

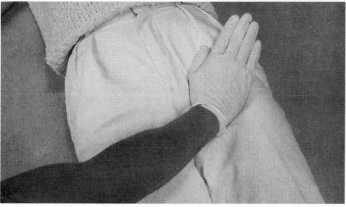

b. _____

8. The only circumstance in which a tourniquet should be CONSIDERED as a way to control bleeding is
   a. When there is spurting arterial bleeding
   b. When there is an amputated extremity
   c. When nerves, muscles, and blood vessels are damaged
   d. When pressure is also needed to stabilize bones

9. List at least three mechanisms of injury that can cause internal bleeding.

10. Describe the emergency medical care of internal bleeding.

11. Shock (hypoperfusion) should be suspected in patients who have suffered which of the following injuries?
    1. Penetrating injury
    2. Burns
    3. Organ rupture or laceration
    4. Crush injury
    5. Blunt trauma

    a. 2, 3
    b. 1, 3, 4
    c. 1, 2, 4, 5
    d. 1, 2, 3, 4, 5

12. _____ and _____ and other signs of altered mental status are early signs of shock.

13. The following items reflect the progressive nature of shock (hypoperfusion). Write the numbers 1 to 5 to rank them in the general order in which they occur.

    _____ Leaking capillaries cause loss of vital blood plasma; unresponsiveness and death may result.

    _____ Blood vessels constrict in extremities to conserve blood causing cold, clammy skin.

    _____ Low oxygen levels to breathing control centers of the brain make respirations rapid and shallow; nervous system reaction results in profuse sweating.

    _____ Vasoconstriction fails, and blood pressure drops.

    _____ Blood loss causes rapid heart rate and weak pulse.

14. Describe the emergency medical care of shock.

CASE STUDY

▼

You are on scene with a 28-year-old male who put his hands through a window while attempting to open it. Your initial assessment reveals that he is responsive and alert with a patent airway and adequate respirations. He has numerous lacerations on both hands and forearms, which are bleeding steadily, as well as a very large wound on the inside of his right wrist, which is spurting bright red blood. His skin is pale, cool, and clammy.

1. What should you do?

After taking the steps you have just described, you note that the patient seems more anxious and restless than when you arrived several minutes ago. He continues to talk coherently and answers your questions.

2. What is the significance of his increasing agitation? What should you do?

You move him to your ambulance and prepare to begin transport. You have learned that he has no allergies and he takes AZT because he is HIV positive. He says that he's been feeling fine and has no other medical problems. He ate a sandwich and had a soda for lunch about an hour ago. He says that the window was stuck and he was trying to pull it open when he lost his balance, put his hands up to catch himself, and shattered the window.

3. Given his health history, what other precautions should you take?

4. What care should your patient receive en route to the hospital?

COGNITIVE OBJECTIVES

Numbered objectives are from the United States Department of Transportation 1994 EMT-Basic National Standard Curriculum. Asterisked objectives, if any, pertain to material that is supplemental to the DOT curriculum.

5-2.1   State the major functions of the skin.

5-2.2   List the layers of the skin.

5-2.3   Establish the relationship between body substance isolation (BSI) and soft tissue injuries.

5-2.4   List the types of closed soft tissue injuries.

5-2.5   Describe the emergency medical care of the patient with a closed soft tissue injury.

5-2.6   State the types of open soft tissue injuries.

5-2.7   Describe the emergency medical care of the patient with an open soft tissue injury.

5-2.8   Discuss the emergency medical care considerations for a patient with a penetrating chest injury.

5-2.9   State the emergency medical care considerations for a patient with an open wound to the abdomen.

5-2.10 Differentiate the care of an open wound to the chest from an open wound to the abdomen.

5-2.21 List the functions of dressing and bandaging.

5-2.22 Describe the purpose of a bandage.

5-2.23 Describe the steps in applying a pressure dressing.

5-2.24 Establish the relationship between airway management and the patient with chest injury, burns, blunt, and penetrating injuries.

5-2.25 Describe the effects of improperly applied dressings, splints, and tourniquets.

5-2.26 Describe the emergency medical care of a patient with an impaled object.

5-2.27 Describe the emergency medical care of a patient with an amputation.

KEY IDEAS

A soft tissue injury is an injury to skin, muscles, nerves, blood vessels, or organs. The general goals of the emergency medical care of such injuries are to control bleeding, to prevent further injury, and to reduce the risk of infection.

▶ Soft tissue injuries are categorized as closed, open, single, or multiple.

▶ In general, emergency care of closed injuries includes taking BSI precautions; ensuring an open airway and adequate breathing; treating for shock; and splinting painful, swollen, or deformed extremities.

▶ In general, emergency care of open injuries includes taking BSI precautions; ensuring an open airway and adequate breathing; exposing the wound; controlling bleeding; preventing further contamination; and treating for shock.

▶ Special considerations for the emergency care of soft tissue injuries include using occlusive dressings on open chest wounds, abdominal eviscerations, and large open neck injuries; securing objects impaled in the body (except the cheek); and caring for amputated parts.

▶ Dressings cover open wounds, and bandages hold dressings in place. A pressure (or bulky) dressing can be used to control bleeding. General principles of dressing and bandaging include: using materials that are sterile or at least clean; bandaging only when bleeding has stopped; adequately covering the entire wound with a dressing and the entire dressing with a bandage; applying a bandage from distal to proximal; removing all jewelry from injured parts; bandaging not too loosely or tightly (checking distal pulses, motor, and sensory function before and after bandage application); on an extremity, bandaging a larger area than the wound to avoid creating a pressure point; and applying a tourniquet only as a last resort.

TERMS AND CONCEPTS

1. **Write the number of the correct term next to each definition.**

1. abrasion	6. evisceration
2. air embolism	7. hematoma
3. avulsion	8. laceration
4. contusion	9. occlusive dressing
5. crush injury	10. penetration/puncture

_____ **a.** An open injury usually caused by forceful impact with a sharp object and characterized by a wound whose edges may be linear or stellate in appearance

_____ **b.** A protrusion of organs from a wound

_____ **c.** A closed or open injury to soft tissues and underlying organs that is the result of a crushing force applied to the body

_____ **d.** An open injury to the outermost layer of the skin caused by a scraping, rubbing, or shearing away of the tissue

_____ **e.** An open injury caused by a sharp, pointed, object being forced into the soft tissues

_____ **f.** An air bubble that obstructs a blood vessel

_____ g. A closed injury to the cells and blood vessels contained within the dermis that is characterized by discoloration, swelling, and pain; a bruise

_____ h. A closed injury to the soft tissues characterized by swelling and discoloration caused by a mass of blood beneath the epidermis

_____ i. A dressing that can form an airtight seal over a wound

_____ j. An open injury characterized by a loose flap of skin and soft tissue that has been torn loose or pulled completely off

CONTENT REVIEW

1. The layers of the skin from the outside in are
   a. Dermis, epidermis, and subcutaneous layer
   b. Subcutaneous, epidermis, and dermis layer
   c. Subcutaneous, dermis, and epidermis layer
   d. Epidermis, dermis, and subcutaneous layer

2. Identify the description that is NOT a function of the skin.
   a. Aids in the elimination of water and various salts
   b. Serves as a receptor organ
   c. Produces white blood cells
   d. Protects the body from the environment

3. Which of the following is NOT a closed injury?
   a. Contusion
   b. Amputation
   c. Hematoma
   d. Crush injury

4. Body substance isolation (BSI) precautions are almost never required with closed injuries.
   a. True
   b. False

5. Select the correct order for treatment of closed soft tissue injuries.
   a. Airway and breathing, BSI precautions, shock, injured extremities
   b. BSI precautions, shock, airway and breathing, injured extremities
   c. BSI precautions, airway and breathing, shock, injured extremities
   d. Injured extremities, BSI precautions, airway and breathing, shock

6. What type of dressing is used on a chest wound to prevent air from entering the chest cavity?
   a. Nonelastic, self-adhering
   b. Multi-trauma
   c. Universal
   d. Occlusive

7. How should you tape the dressing for an open chest wound?
   a. On the top and bottom only
   b. On three sides only
   c. On all four sides
   d. Down the middle only

8. List the steps of emergency medical care for open injuries.

9. Identify the correct order of steps for emergency care of a patient with an impaled object.

   1. Use a bulky dressing to help stabilize the object.

   2. Manually secure the object.

   3. Control bleeding.

   4. Expose the wound area.

   a. 2, 4, 3, 1

   b. 4, 3, 2, 1

   c. 3, 1, 2, 4

   d. 4, 2, 3, 1

10. Which item is NOT an appropriate treatment for an amputated part?
    a. Immerse it in cool sterile water.
    b. Wrap the part in dry sterile dressing.
    c. Wrap or bag the part in plastic.
    d. Keep the amputated part cool.

11. Bleeding control and prevention of an air embolism are the major goals of emergency care
    of a large open neck wound.
    a. True
    b. False

12. Write the steps for applying a pressure dressing.

13. When applying a bandage, proceed from
    a. Medial to lateral
    b. Superior to inferior
    c. Distal to proximal
    d. Proximal to distal

14. For circumferential bandages, check _____ before and after bandaging.
    a. Distal pulses, skin color, and temperature
    b. Capillary refill, skin color, and temperature
    c. Distal pulses, motor function, and sensory function
    d. ABCs, motor function, and sensory function

15. Identify the proper dressings for an abdominal evisceration.
    a. Sterile moist gauze, then an occlusive dressing
    b. Self-adhering roller bandage, then an occlusive dressing
    c. Any sterile absorbent material, then an occlusive dressing
    d. Bulky dressing, then an occlusive dressing

16. You have ruled out potential spinal injury in a patient with abdominal evisceration. Your partner asks you to flex the patient's hips and knees during transport. Why?
    a. It helps stabilize the abdominal organs.
    b. It will prevent the development of an embolism.
    c. It reduces the tension on the abdominal muscles.
    d. It helps to increase oxygen to the vital organs.

CASE STUDY 1

You are dispatched to a local bar for a stabbing. The patient is a female, about 25 years of age. She is sitting at a table, her hand to her neck, with dark red blood flowing steadily through her fingers. Your general impression of her is good; however, her skin is pale, warm, and slightly moist. As your partner begins to control the bleeding, you find that respirations are full and regular and radial pulse is strong and regular. There are no other obvious signs of trauma or bleeding present.

1. The bleeding from the patient's neck wound probably is
    a. Capillary bleeding
    b. Arterial bleeding
    c. Venous bleeding
    d. Combination of arterial/capillary bleeding

2. Emergency care for this wound is described in the following items. Which lists the correct procedures in the correct order?
    a. Gloved hand over the wound, then an occlusive dressing, and finally a pressure dressing
    b. Occlusive dressing over the wound, then a pressure dressing, and finally your gloved hand
    c. Pressure dressing over the wound, then an occlusive dressing, and finally your gloved hand
    d. Gloved hand over the wound, then a pressure dressing, and finally an occlusive dressing

CASE STUDY 2

▼

You are at the scene of a shooting. The 20-year-old patient is supine and responsive. A law enforcement officer has told you that three shots were fired, the weapon was a .357 caliber handgun, and the patient was shot from about 30 to 40 yards. There is obvious bleeding coming from the patient's right upper chest region and a sucking sound is heard with each breath. As your partner proceeds to control bleeding, you find that the patient is cyanotic, respirations are shallow and rapid, radial pulse is weak and regular, and skin is cool and slightly moist.

1. In addition to this patient's obvious injury, you should suspect
    a. Ring avulsion
    b. Spinal injury
    c. Lower airway obstruction
    d. Cardiac tamponade

2. In addition to treatment for this patient's obvious injury, treatment also includes
    a. Splinting of upper extremities
    b. Care of large open neck injuries
    c. Methodically assessing for closed wounds
    d. Assessing for other entry and exit wounds

CHAPTER

31

BURN EMERGENCIES

Numbered objectives are from the United States Department of Transportation 1994 EMT-Basic National Standard Curriculum. Asterisked objectives, if any, pertain to material that is supplemental to the DOT curriculum.

5-2.1 State the major functions of the skin.

5-2.2 List the layers of the skin.

5-2.11 List the classifications of burns.

5-2.12 Define superficial burns.

5-2.13 List the characteristics of a superficial burn.

5-2.14 Define partial thickness burn.

5-2.15 List the characteristics of a partial thickness burn.

5-2.16 Define full thickness burn.

5-2.17 List the characteristics of a full thickness burn.

5-2.18 Describe the emergency medical care of a patient with a superficial burn.

5-2.19 Describe the emergency medical care of a patient with a partial thickness burn.

5-2.20 Describe the emergency medical care of a patient with a full thickness burn.

5-2.24 Establish the relationship between airway management and the patient with chest injury, burns, blunt and penetrating injuries.

5-2.28 Describe the emergency care for a chemical burn.

5-2.29 Describe the emergency care for an electrical burn.

KEY IDEAS

▼

Burn injuries can do more than burn the skin. They can impair the body's fluid and chemical balance, its temperature regulation, and its musculoskeletal, circulatory, and respiratory functions. In order to care for burns properly, you need to have a basic understanding of the kinds of burns; how burn injuries are classified; and how they affect adult, child, and infant patients.

► Burns are classified according to the depth of the injury. A superficial burn affects the epidermis. A partial thickness burn affects the epidermis and portions of the dermis. A full thickness burn involves all layers of the skin and can extend into the muscle, bone, or organs below.

► Burns are also classified by severity of injury – critical, moderate, or minor. The most important factors in determining burn severity are percentage and location of body surface area involved, the patient's age, and preexisting medical conditions.

► Assessment and emergency care of burn patients includes removing the patient from the source of the burn and stopping the burning process, being especially alert for compromise of the airway, estimating severity of the burns, and determining whether or not the patient is a priority for transport.

► When called to care for chemical burns, be prepared to protect yourself from exposure to hazardous materials. Remember to flush chemicals from the patient, when appropriate, for at least 20 minutes. Brush off dry chemicals before flushing.

► Special considerations for care of electrical burns include making sure power sources have been shut down before rescue and emergency care, monitoring the patient for respiratory and cardiac arrest, and assessing for both entrance and exit wounds.

TERMS AND CONCEPTS

▼

1. **Write the number of each term next to its definition.**

    1. circumferential burn
    2. eschar
    3. full thickness burn
    4. partial thickness burn
    5. rule of nines
    6. superficial burn

_____ **a.** Standardized format used to quickly identify the amount or percentage of skin or body surface area that has been burned

_____ **b.** Burn that involves all of the layers of the skin and can extend beyond the subcutaneous layer into the muscle, bone, or organs below

_____ **c.** The hard, tough, leathery, dead soft tissue formed as a result of a full thickness burn

_____ **d.** A burn that encircles a body area

_____ **e.** A burn that involves only the epidermis

_____ **f.** A burn that involves the epidermis and portions of the dermis

CONTENT REVIEW

1. List six functions of the skin.

2. In discussing burn assessment, the letters "BSA" stand for
   a. Body surface area
   b. Burn severity assessment
   c. Blistered surface area
   d. Burn surface analysis

3. Which classification of burn is usually caused by a flash flame or hot liquid?
   a. Superficial burn
   b. Partial thickness burn
   c. Full thickness burn
   d. Circumferential burn

4. What kind of burn damages the blood vessels, causing plasma and tissue fluid to collect between layers of the skin?
   a. Superficial burn
   b. Partial thickness burn
   c. Eschar
   d. Circumferential burn

5. Burns to the face are considered
   a. Minor
   b. Moderate
   c. Critical
   d. Fatal

6. In a child, partial thickness burns of 10% to 20% BSA are considered
   a. Minor
   b. Moderate
   c. Critical
   d. Fatal

7. Which age groups are less tolerant of burn injuries?
   a. Children under 3 and adults over 33
   b. Children under 4 and adults over 44
   c. Children under 5 and adults over 55
   d. Children under 6 and adults over 66

8. Briefly list the steps of emergency medical care of burn injuries.

9. Separate burned fingers or toes with dry sterile dressings to prevent
   a. Scarring of burned areas
   b. Adherence of burned areas
   c. Further contamination of burned areas
   d. Potential blistering of burned areas

10. The patient should be allowed to use the unburned eye once the burned eye is covered by a dressing and a bandage.
   a. True
   b. False

11. Which of the following is NOT true about the care of patients with chemical burns?
   a. Chemical burns may involve hazardous materials, so protect yourself first.
   b. Dry chemicals should be immediately flushed off the patient.
   c. Some chemicals may produce combustion when in contact with water.
   d. Chemical burns require immediate care.

12. Which of the following is true about the assessment and care of an electrical burn patient?
   a. Always assume that the power source has been shut down.
   b. Rescue all victims in contact with an electrical source.
   c. All tissues between the entrance and exit wounds may be injured.
   d. Injuries caused by an electrical burn always have a rapid onset.

CASE STUDY

You are called to the scene of a burned child. You note that the patient's pajamas are still smoldering. The patient is crying loudly.

1. After soaking the pajamas with water, you try to remove them. However, the plastic booties have adhered to the patient's feet. You should
   a. Gently try to remove the plastic from the skin
   b. Gently cut around the area with bandage scissors
   c. Transport to the hospital with the clothes left on
   d. Call medical direction for help with this situation

2. Your partner notices singed nasal hairs in the patient. You should provide
   a. Oxygen via nasal cannula at 6 lpm
   b. Oxygen via simple mask at 8 lpm
   c. Oxygen via nonrebreather mask at 15 lpm
   d. Positive pressure ventilations with oxygen

The mother tells you that she heard the 4-year-old child's screams and found him in the garage on fire. She suspects that lighter fluid may have been involved. You determine that the burns are all partial thickness burns that cover the entire right leg and foot. You begin to transport to the hospital, which is also a burn center.

3. What is the estimated body surface area affected by the burn, and what is the severity classification?
   a. 1% and moderate
   b. 9% and critical
   c. 14% and critical
   d. 18% and moderate

4. You continue the emergency care en route to the hospital. Which of the following is most appropriate?
   a. Cover the burned area with a sterile dry dressing, and keep the patient cool.
   b. Cover the burned area with a sterile dry dressing, and keep the patient warm.
   c. Cover the burned area with a sterile moist dressing, and keep the patient cool.
   d. Cover the burned area with a sterile moist dressing, and keep the patient warm.

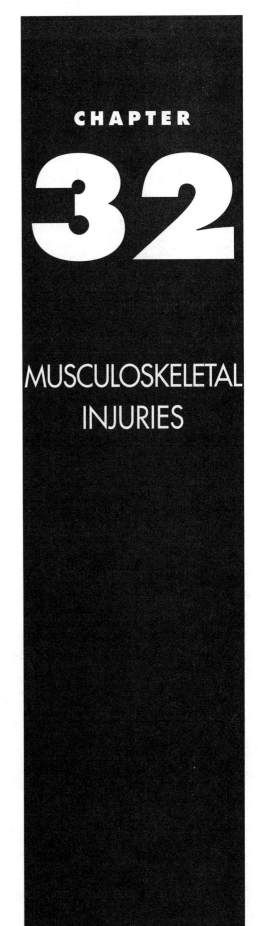

COGNITIVE OBJECTIVES

CHAPTER 32

MUSCULOSKELETAL INJURIES

Numbered objectives are from the United States Department of Transportation 1994 EMT-Basic National Standard Curriculum. Asterisked objectives, if any, pertain to material that is supplemental to the DOT curriculum.

5-3.1 Describe the function of the muscular system.

5-3.2 Describe the function of the skeletal system.

5-3.3 List the major bones or bone groupings of the spinal column, the thorax, the upper extremities, and the lower extremities.

5-3.4 Differentiate between an open and a closed painful, swollen, and deformed extremity.

5-3.5 State the reasons for splinting.

5-3.6 List the general rules of splinting.

5-3.7 List the complications of splinting.

5-3.8 List the emergency medical care for a patient with a painful, swollen, and deformed extremity.

KEY IDEAS

Musculoskeletal injuries are frequently encountered in the field. Most of these injuries are simple and not life threatening. Appropriate management can prevent further painful injury and even prevent permanent disability or death. This chapter provides a review of the musculoskeletal system and discusses musculoskeletal injuries and their appropriate management.

▶ The functions of the musculoskeletal system are to give the body shape, to protect the internal organs, and to provide for movement.

▶ The six basic components of the skeletal system are the skull, spinal column, thorax, pelvis, lower extremities, and upper extremities.

▶ The forces that may cause bone and joint injuries are direct, indirect, and twisting forces.

▶ Bone and joint injuries can be either open or closed.

▶ Any painful, swollen, or deformed extremity should be immobilized.

▶ Splinting prevents movement of bone fragments, bone ends, or dislocated joints, thereby reducing the chance for further injury; and it reduces pain and minimizes complications.

▶ The general rules of splinting include: Check pulse, motor function, and sensation (PMS) before and after splinting; immobilize the joints above and below a long-bone injury site, or immobilize the bones above and below a joint injury; remove clothing and jewelry; cover all wounds before splinting; never replace bone ends; splint before moving the patient; when in doubt, splint the injury; and pad splints.

▶ If there is severe deformity or the distal extremity is cyanotic or pulseless, then make one attempt to realign the limb. If pain, resistance, or crepitus increase, stop and transport immediately.

▶ If a patient shows signs of shock, care for shock and transport without taking time to splint.

▶ The general types of splints are rigid, traction, pressure, improvised, and sling and swathe.

TERMS AND CONCEPTS

1. Write the number of each term next to its definition.

   1. crepitus
   2. direct force
   3. indirect force
   4. paresthesia
   5. splint
   6. twisting force

   _____ **a.** A force that rotates a bone while one end is held stationary

   _____ **b.** The sound or feel of broken fragments of bone grinding against each other

   _____ **c.** A force that causes injury some distance away from the point of impact

   _____ **d.** A force that causes injury at the point of impact

   _____ **e.** Any device used to immobilize a body part

   _____ **f.** A prickling or tingling feeling that indicates some loss of sensation

CONTENT REVIEW

1. Which of the following is NOT a function of the musculoskeletal system?
   a. Gives the body shape
   b. Produces platelets
   c. Protects the internal organs
   d. Provides for movement

2. List the six basic components of the skeletal system.
   a.
   b.
   c.
   d.
   e.
   f.

3. The forces that cause bone and joint injury are
   a. Direct, partial, and indeterminate
   b. Direct, indirect, and frontal
   c. Direct, indirect, and twisting
   d. Direct, primary, and secondary

4. _____ and ____ distal to an injured extremity is considered to be a serious condition.
   a. Swelling, tenderness
   b. Coolness, paleness
   c. Pain, flushing
   d. Pulselessness, cyanosis

5. A patient has an injured extremity. This patient is unresponsive and has a suspected spinal injury and other life-threatening injuries unrelated to the extremity injury. You and your partner have established manual in-line stabilization of the head and spine, assured an open airway and adequate breathing, controlled major bleeding, and completed a rapid trauma assessment. There is no one at the scene who can provide a history, and you will assess vital signs en route. In addition, you perform the steps listed below. Number the steps 1 to 4 to indicate the order of priority for performing these steps.

   _____   Splint the injured extremity.
   _____   Perform further management of the life-threatening injuries and ongoing assessments every 5 minutes.
   _____   Immobilize the patient to a spine board.
   _____   Initiate transport.

6. The skin over the fracture site has been broken. The bone may or may not protrude through the skin. This statement best describes
   a. A spiral injury
   b. An open injury
   c. A closed injury
   d. A multiple injury

7. List at least five signs and symptoms of bone or joint injury.

8. If an injured extremity is painful, swollen, and deformed
   a. Apply warm packs to the site
   b. Restrict blood flow
   c. Splint the extremity
   d. Position the extremity below the heart

9. The patient's distal pulses, sensation, and motor function should be checked
   a. Before splinting
   b. After splinting
   c. Before and after splinting
   d. Just before arrival at the hospital

10. A general rule for the immobilization of an injury to a long bone is to immobilize
    a. The joints above and below the injury site
    b. The joint above the injury site only
    c. The joint below the injury site only
    d. Only the bone, never an adjacent joint

11. If there is severe deformity in an extremity, the distal pulses are absent, or the extremity is cyanotic you should
    a. Make no attempt to align the extremity
    b. Make one attempt to align the extremity
    c. Persist until the extremity is aligned
    d. Apply the splint before attempting to align

12. Which of the following is NOT an appropriate action when splinting an injured extremity?
    a. Maintain manual traction until after the splint has been applied.
    b. Push protruding bones back into the skin.
    c. Cover all open wounds before splinting.
    d. Cut clothing away and remove jewelry from the site.

13. When forced to use an improvised splint, ensure that the splint is
    a. Heavy, but flexible and soft
    b. Short, extending just the length of the bone
    c. Narrower than the thickest part of the injured limb
    d. Well padded on the inner surface

14. Which of the following is a hazard of improper splinting?
    a. Stabilizes broken bone ends
    b. Compresses nerves, tissues, and blood vessels
    c. Reduces pain associated with the fracture
    d. Prevents a reduction in distal circulation

15. A "sling and swathe" is commonly used to provide stability to a painful and tender
    a. Leg injury
    b. Shoulder injury
    c. Cervical spine injury
    d. Pelvic injury

16. When splinting an extremity, the hand or foot must be immobilized in the position of function. The position of function for the hand can be attained by
    a. Extending the hand over the end of the splint
    b. Securing the hand to the splint in a palm-up position
    c. Bandaging the hand in a clenched-fist position
    d. Putting a roll of bandage in the patient's hand

17. Which of the following describe(s) situations in which you should NOT use a traction splint?

    1. The injury is within 1 or 2 inches of the knee

    2. The knee has been injured

    3. The thigh is painful, swollen, or deformed

    4. The hip or pelvis has been injured

    a. 3

    b. 2 and 4

    c. 2, 3, and 4

    d. 1, 2, and 4

18. Which statement BEST describes how the traction splint achieves stabilization?
    a. It applies circumferential pressure to the femur.
    b. It stabilizes the bone ends by producing negative torque.
    c. It pulls on the thigh and realigns the broken femur.
    d. It pushes the bones together and "resets" the fracture.

CASE STUDY 1

▼

You are dispatched to a high school to assist a 17-year-old soccer player who is injured. The patient is sitting on a bench on the sideline of the field, holding his left shoulder and leaning forward. You sit down next to him and ask, "What happened?" He replies, "I was moving down to score and tripped in a hole. I put my arm out to catch myself and I felt something snap in my shoulder." Your general impression is a non-critical injured patient. He responds to your questions appropriately and is alert and oriented. His respirations are normal; radial pulse is strong and regular; and skin is a good color, warm, and dry. You examine his shoulder and observe deformity over his left clavicle. The area is tender to touch and obviously swollen. He denies any other complaints or injuries.

1. What is the next BEST IMMEDIATE action to take for this patient?
    a. Immobilize the shoulder with an air splint on the entire arm.
    b. Evaluate the pulse, motor function, and sensation.
    c. Immobilize the shoulder with a sling and swathe.
    d. Immobilize the shoulder with a rigid splint on the entire arm.

2. What is the best way to evaluate this patient's sensory function?
   a. Ask if he can feel you pinch him on the back.
   b. Ask him to wiggle his fingers without looking.
   c. Ask him to tell you which finger you are touching without looking.
   d. Ask him if he can feel you jab him with a sharp object.

3. This patient's injury is most likely due to what type of force?
   a. Direct
   b. Indirect
   c. Twisting
   d. Secondary

CASE STUDY 2

You are at the scene of a motorcycle collision with a car. About 20 yards from the vehicles, a male biker is sitting holding his right leg. He looks to be about 30 years old. You ask, "What happened?" He replies, "That car stopped in front of me. I hit the rear, flew off the bike, and landed on my leg." Respirations are normal; radial pulse is strong and regular; skin is a good color, warm, and dry. You cut away his pant leg so you can evaluate his injury. The thigh region is deformed, swollen, and tender to touch. He denies any other complaints or injuries. You ask you partner to initiate manual traction to the right leg.

1. Manual traction on the patient's leg
   a. Should be continued until you arrive at the hospital
   b. Should be continued until you are ready to position the splint
   c. Should be continued until the splint is applied
   d. Should not have been requested

2. When checking the pulse distal to the injury site on this patient, use the
   a. Pedal or posterior tibial pulse
   b. Radial or brachial pulse
   c. Popliteal or femoral pulse
   d. Carotid or femoral pulse

CASE STUDY 3

▼

You are dispatched to a call for an elderly patient who is lying on the kitchen floor. She is 70 years of age and in severe pain. She tells you that when she fell she heard a "loud pop." There is bruising to the right hip region, and the patient complains of severe pain there upon palpation. She also tells you that her leg feels numb and is tingling. She denies any additional complaints or injuries. You apply a padded rigid splint that extends from below the foot to above the hip.

1. The patient's complaint of numbness and tingling in her right leg
   a. May indicate some loss of sensation
   b. May indicate an additional injury to the lower leg
   c. May require the application of a full leg air splint
   d. Is to be expected after this type of injury

2. The patient's foot should be immobilized in a position of function. Which statement best describes the position of function for the foot?
   a. Toes curled toward the sole of the foot
   b. Foot bent at a normal angle to the leg
   c. Foot pushed downward to align with the shin
   d. Foot bent upward toward the shin

3. To evaluate this patient's motor function
   a. Ask her to lift the leg and rotate it outward
   b. Ask her to rotate the leg outward and tense the foot
   c. Ask her to tighten the kneecap and move the foot up and down
   d. Ask her to tighten the buttocks and lift the leg

COGNITIVE OBJECTIVES

Numbered objectives are from the United States Department of Transportation 1994 EMT-Basic National Standard Curriculum. Asterisked objectives, if any, pertain to material that is supplemental to the DOT curriculum.

5-4.1   State the components of the nervous system.

5-4.2   List the functions of the central nervous system.

5-4.3   Define the structure of the skeletal system as it relates to the nervous system.

5-4.4   Relate mechanism of injury to potential injuries of the head and spine.

5-4.11 Establish the relationship between airway management and the patient with head and spine injuries.

KEY IDEAS

Injury to the skull, which contains the brain, can have severe consequences for the patient. Since head injuries may occur weeks before signs and symptoms appear, it is important to recognize both potential and actual injury at the scene.

▶ The brain and spinal cord make up the central nervous system, which controls the body's systems.

▶ The skull, which protects the brain, is made up of the cranial skull, the facial bones, and the basilar skull. Cerebrospinal fluid and the meninges help protect the brain inside the skull.

▶ The brain is made up of three parts: the cerebrum (conscious and sensory functions), cerebellum (muscle movement and coordination), and brain stem (most automatic and vital functions).

▶ Head injuries may involve the scalp, skull, and/or brain and are classified as open or closed. Both open and closed injuries of the head may involve extensive damage to the brain.

▶ Brain injury may be direct (from penetrating trauma), indirect (from a blow to the skull), or secondary (for example, from lack of oxygen, build-up of carbon dioxide, or a change in blood pressure).

▶ Unresponsiveness or an altered mental status, especially in trauma patients, should always suggest the possibility of head injury. Nontraumatic injury may be caused by clots or hemorrhaging and also may result in an altered mental status.

▶ Emergency medical care of head injury includes taking in-line spinal stabilization; maintaining a patent airway; administering adequate oxygenation; providing hyperventilation, if possible; monitoring airway, breathing, pulse, and mental status for deterioration; and immediate transport.

TERMS AND CONCEPTS

1. **Write the number of each term next to its definition.**

   1. Battle's sign
   2. cerebrospinal fluid
   3. concussion
   4. decerebrate posturing
   5. decorticate posturing
   6. raccoon sign

   _____ **a.** The patient extends arms and legs and sometimes arches the back, which may be a sign of serious brain injury

   _____ **b.** Discoloration of the mastoid suggesting basilar skull deformation

   _____ **c.** Discoloration of tissue around the eyes

   _____ **d.** Serous substance that protects the brain

   _____ **e.** The patient flexes arms across the chest and extends legs, which may be a sign of serious brain injury

   _____ **f.** Temporary loss of brain function

CONTENT REVIEW

1. The brain may be injured by any of the following EXCEPT
   a. Blunt force applied to the skull
   b. Penetrating trauma
   c. Elevated carbon dioxide levels
   d. Elevated oxygen levels

2. All of the following usually are observed during the scene size-up EXCEPT
   a. Unresponsiveness
   b. Pupillary changes
   c. Bleeding from the scalp
   d. Apparent mechanism of injury

3. Describe the first step in the initial assessment of the patient with a possible head injury.

4. Which technique should be used to maintain the airway of a possible head-injured patient who has a decreased level of responsiveness?
   a. Head-tilt, chin-lift maneuver
   b. Jaw-thrust maneuver
   c. Crossed-finger technique
   d. Two-rescuer ventilation

5. The mental status response that is likely to indicate the most serious head injury is
   a. Alertness
   b. Responsiveness to verbal stimulus
   c. Responsiveness to painful stimulus
   d. Unresponsiveness

6. Any patient whose mental status worsens at any stage of the assessment or treatment process needs
   a. Treatment for anaphylactic shock
   b. Palpation of the head and neck
   c. Immediate transport and monitoring
   d. SAMPLE history and rapid trauma assessment

7. List the parts of the rapid trauma assessment to which you should pay particular attention in cases of suspected head injury.

8. A patient with suspected head injury is unresponsive and has a breathing rate above the normal range. After taking BSI precautions and establishing in-line stabilization of the head and neck, explain what your next step should be.

9. Which of the following questions would be LEAST helpful in providing you with pertinent information about a possible head injury?
   a. Did the patient lose consciousness?
   b. Does the patient have any allergies?
   c. Did the patient strike his head within the past month or so?
   d. Did the patient lose consciousness, regain it, and lose it again?

10. Emergency care of a patient with a head injury should include all of the following EXCEPT
    a. Vigilant attention to maintaining an open airway
    b. Hyperventilation at 24 to 30 breaths if necessary
    c. Application of a pressure dressing to any open skull injury
    d. Anticipation of potential seizure activity

CASE STUDY

You have been called to the scene of a fall. The caller, who is the patient's nephew, says he found the 70-year-old female, Mrs. McDonnell, lying at the bottom of her basement stairs. He has not moved her. She is unresponsive with slow snoring respirations, pulse is slow and strong, skin is warm and dry. There are no obvious injuries or bleeding noted.

1.   What should you do?

You observe a large deformity at the back of Mrs. McDonnell's head, dilated and equal pupils sluggishly reactive to light, and bruising around both eyes and mastoid process. You find no blood or clear fluid in the nose or ears. She is unresponsive to all stimuli. You find no other evidence of injury. Baseline vital signs are blood pressure 178/ 72, pulse 68, and strong respirations deep and regular at 6 per minute.

2.   What is the significance of the bruising?

3.   What is the significance of the patient's vital signs?

CHAPTER

34

INJURIES TO THE SPINE

Numbered objectives are from the United States Department of Transportation 1994 EMT-Basic National Standard Curriculum. Asterisked objectives, if any, pertain to material that is supplemental to the DOT curriculum.

5-4.1   State the components of the nervous system.

5-4.2   List the functions of the central nervous system.

5-4.3   Define the structure of the skeletal system as it relates to the nervous system.

5-4.4   Relate mechanism of injury to potential injuries of the head and spine.

5-4.5   Describe the implications of not properly caring for potential spine injuries.

5-4.6   State the signs and symptoms of a potential spine injury.

5-4.7   Describe the method of determining if a responsive patient may have a spine injury.

5-4.8   Relate the airway emergency medical care techniques to the patient with a suspected spine injury.

5-4.9   Describe how to stabilize the cervical spine.

5-4.10 Discuss indications for sizing and using a cervical spine immobilization device.

5-4.11 Establish the relationship between airway management and the patient with head and spine injuries.

5-4.12 Describe a method for sizing a cervical spine immobilization device.

5-4.13 Describe how to log roll a patient with a suspected spine injury.

5-4.14 Describe how to secure a patient to a long spine board.

5-4.15 List instances when a short spine board should be used.

5-4.16 Describe how to immobilize a patient using a short spine board.

5-4.17 Describe the indications for the use of rapid extrication.

5-4.18 List steps in performing rapid extrication.

5-4.19 State the circumstances when a helmet should be left on the patient.

5-4.20 Discuss the circumstances when a helmet should be removed.

5-4.21 Identify different types of helmets.

5-4.22 Describe the unique characteristics of sports helmets.

5-4.23 Explain the preferred methods to remove a helmet.

5-4.24 Discuss alternative methods for removal of a helmet.

5-4.25 Describe how the patient's head is stabilized to remove the helmet.

5-4.26 Differentiate how the head is stabilized with a helmet compared to without a helmet.

KEY IDEAS

As an EMT-Basic you may encounter patients with potential spinal injuries in a wide variety of settings. Each encounter must be grounded in the recognition that improper movement and handling of such patients could easily lead to permanent disability or even death. This chapter focuses on the assessment and management of spinal injuries.

▶ The spinal column, which serves to protect the spinal cord, is the principal support system of the body. It is made up of 33 vertebrae, each pair of vertebrae separated by a disc.

▶ Common mechanisms of spinal injury include compression, flexion, extension, rotation, lateral bending, distraction, and penetration which may occur as a result of collisions, falls, diving accidents, and so on.

▶ Even in the absence of obvious trauma or patient complaints, when the mechanism of injury suggests possible spinal injury, every care must be taken and immediate manual in-line spinal stabilization must be established.

▶ Once established, manual stabilization must not be released until the patient is securely strapped to a backboard with head and neck immobilized.

▶ The goal of emergency management of suspected spinal cord injury is to ensure that life-threatening conditions are cared for, that the possibility of further injury is reduced through careful handling, and that the patient is properly immobilized and expeditiously transported.

▶ The tools associated with spinal immobilization include cervical spinal immobilization collars, full-body spinal immobilization devices, and short spinal immobilization devices.

TERMS AND CONCEPTS

1. **Write the number of each term next to its definition.**

    1. autonomic nervous system
    2. central nervous system
    3. peripheral nervous system
    4. voluntary nervous system

    _____   **a.** The portion of the nervous system that influences deliberate muscle movement
    _____   **b.** The structures of the nervous system located outside the brain and spinal cord
    _____   **c.** The portion of the nervous system that influences involuntary muscles and glands
    _____   **d.** The portion of the nervous system consisting of the brain and the spinal cord

2. Label the diagram with the following spinal column divisions:

cervical spine

coccyx

lumbar spine

sacral spine

thoracic spine

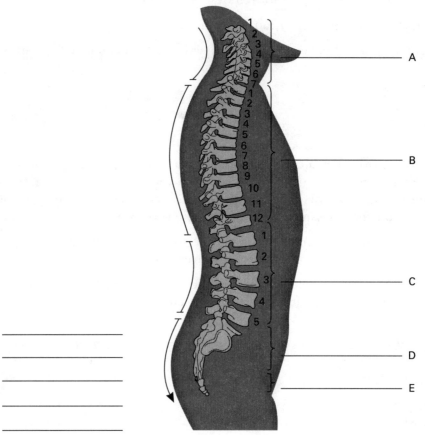

A _____

B _____

C _____

D _____

E _____

CONTENT REVIEW

1. List at least five types of emergency scenes or mechanisms of injury that warrant a high index of suspicion for spinal injury.

2. Which of the following would apply to a patient who is found lying unresponsive in an alley beside an apartment building?
   a. Assume the patient has a medical condition.
   b. Maintain a high index of suspicion for spinal injury.
   c. If the patient can move his extremities, there is no spinal injury.
   d. Place him in a lateral recumbent position.

3. All of the following would be appropriate actions for airway management of the unresponsive patient who has possible spinal injury EXCEPT
   a. Initiate and maintain manual in-line spinal stabilization.
   b. Use the jaw-thrust maneuver to open the airway.
   c. To facilitate drainage of vomitus, place the patient in a lateral recumbent position.
   d. Insert an oropharyngeal or nasopharyngeal airway.

4. List three major complications of spinal injury.

5. When would you NOT assess the pulse, motor function, and sensation in the extremities of the suspected spine-injured patient?
   a. During the initial assessment
   b. During the rapid trauma assessment
   c. During the detailed physical exam
   d. After immobilization on a long backboard

6. When positioning the patient for manual spinal stabilization, the nose should be aligned with the navel and the head should be
   a. Slightly flexed forward in a "sniffing" position
   b. Slightly extended with chin pointing up
   c. Neither flexed nor extended
   d. Both flexed and extended

7. Which statement about cervical spine immobilization collars is correct?
   a. Soft collars permit needed lateral movement.
   b. The collar provides complete immobilization of the spine.
   c. The size of the collar is important but not critical.
   d. The collar should be applied by two rescuers.

8. Which of the following immobilization devices is indicated for the non-critically injured seated patient with suspected spinal injury?
   a. Long backboard only
   c. Cervical spine immobilization collar only
   b. Short spinal immobilization device only
   d. Cervical spine immobilization collar, short spinal immobilization device, and long backboard

9. Immobilization is complete once the patient has been placed on the long backboard.
   a. True
   b. False

10. Define the term "log rolling" as it applies to spinal immobilization.

11. The items below describe the procedure for immobilizing a supine or prone patient. Identify the correct order by numbering the steps 1 to 7.

_____ Place pads in the spaces between the patient and the board.

_____ Establish and maintain in-line manual stabilization.

_____ Apply a cervical spine immobilization collar.

_____ Immobilize the patient's torso to the board with straps.

_____ Log roll the patient onto the long spine board.

_____ Secure the patient's legs to the board.

_____ Immobilize the patient's head to the board.

12. Identify the best description of immobilization of a standing patient.
    a. Walk him to the cot, and have him lie on the backboard placed there.
    b. Immobilize him from a standing position while maintaining alignment.
    c. Have him sit on the backboard, and then carefully help him lie down.
    d. Patients who are able to stand or walk do not require immobilization.

13. All of the following are points to consider when using a short spinal immobilization device EXCEPT
    a. Always use a chin strap to help maintain neutral spinal alignment.
    b. Always assess the patient's back for injury before applying the board.
    c. Never pad between the cervical collar and the board.
    d. Never allow strap buckles to be placed at midsternum.

14. List three indications for the use of rapid extrication.

15. Safe and effective rapid extrication requires
    a. Constant cervical spine stabilization
    b. Application of a short spine board or vest-type immobilization device
    c. Application of only a cervical spine immobilization collar with no manual stabilization
    d. At least one rescuer

16. List five criteria for leaving the helmet in place on the patient with potential spine injury.

17. Which of the following describes what is generally the best care for a football player with potential spinal injury?
    a. Leave the helmet and shoulder pads in place.
    b. Remove the helmet, but leave the shoulder pads in place.
    c. Leave the shoulder pads, but remove the helmet.
    d. Remove both the helmet and the shoulder pads.

18. Identify the proper sequence of steps necessary to immobilize an infant in a car seat by writing the numbers 1 to 5.

_____ Transport in the normal seated position after securing the car seat to the ambulance seat.

_____ Assess the infant to ensure there are no life-threatening injuries or other reasons for removal from the car seat.

_____ Determine if padding is required between the infant's body and the car seat.

_____ Apply manual in-line spinal stabilization.

_____ Support the head in a neutral position using towel rolls and tape.

CASE STUDY

You and your partner are at the scene, the bleachers at the sports arena of the local college. A witness reports that your patient fell while being "body-passed" and that her name is Lori. You find the patient, a young woman, nearly supine on the concrete with her neck hyperflexed so that her chin touches her chest.

1. What should you do first?

2. During the initial assessment, how will you care for the airway and breathing?

3. What should you do in order to transport the patient safely?

CHAPTER

35

EYE, FACE, AND NECK INJURIES

COGNITIVE OBJECTIVES

Numbered objectives are from the United States Department of Transportation 1994 EMT-Basic National Standard Curriculum. Asterisked objectives, if any, pertain to material that is supplemental to the DOT curriculum.

* List the major anatomical structures of the eye, face, and neck.

* Describe the relationship between eye, face, and neck injuries and the personal protection and safety of the EMT-B.

* List the overall assessment procedures for eye, face, and neck injuries.

* Describe the general assessment procedures for eye injuries, including use of the penlight.

* List the basic rules for emergency medical care for eye injuries.

* List specific common eye injuries and describe their appropriate emergency medical care.

* Describe emergency medical care for eye-injured patients wearing contact lenses.

* Describe the general assessment and care guidelines for face injuries.

* List the signs and symptoms and describe the emergency medical care for injuries to the mid-face, upper jaw, and lower jaw.

* Describe the emergency medical care for an object impaled in the cheek.

* Describe the emergency medical care for injuries to the nose and ear.

* List special signs and symptoms of injury to the neck.

* Describe the emergency medical care for injuries to the neck.

KEY IDEAS

Injuries to the eyes, face, or neck have a high probability of causing airway compromise, severe bleeding, and shock. Injuries to the face and neck also are associated with spinal injury. When the potential for these life-threatening conditions exists, establish manual stabilization of the head and neck, open the airway with the jaw-thrust maneuver, and suction as needed. Consider ALS back-up for advanced airway care, and provide oxygen.

▶ Basic rules for emergency care of eye injuries include: Consult medical direction before irrigating foreign objects from the eye and before removing contact lenses; do not remove blood or blood clots from the eye; do not apply salve or medicine; do not try to force the eyelid open unless chemicals must be flushed out; flush a chemically burned eye for at least 20 minutes; stabilize an impaled object of the eye; cover both an injured eye and uninjured eye to prevent unnecessary movement; give the patient nothing by mouth; and always transport for evaluation by a physician.

▶ Injuries to the face include injury to the mid-face, jaw, nose, ear, and objects impaled in the cheek. For severe injuries to the face, suspect and treat for cervical spine injury and immediately manage airway, breathing, and circulation problems. Consider advanced life support to provide advanced airway care. An object impaled in the cheek should be stabilized with bulky dressings. If the object has penetrated the cheek all the way and it may obstruct the airway, remove it.

▶ With any blunt or penetrating trauma to the neck, maintain a high index of suspicion for cervical spine injury. Due to the possibility of swelling, crushed airway structures, debris, and clotted blood, maintaining an airway also is extremely important.

TERMS AND CONCEPTS

1. Write the number of each term next to its definition.

    1. aqueous humor
    2. conjunctiva
    3. cornea
    4. iris
    5. pupil
    6. retina
    7. sclera
    8. vitreous humor
    9. lens

    _____ a. Portion of the eye that covers the pupil and the iris
    _____ b. Fluid that fills the anterior chamber of the eye
    _____ c. Clear jelly that fills the large chamber of the eye
    _____ d. Back of the eye
    _____ e. Outer coating of the eye; the white of the eye
    _____ f. Colored portion of the eye that surrounds the pupil

_____ **g.** Thin covering of the inner eyelids and exposed portion of the sclera of the eye

_____ **h.** The dark center of the eye

_____ **i.** The portion of the eye that focuses light on the retina

2. **Label the diagram of the eye with the appropriate terms from the list in item 1.**

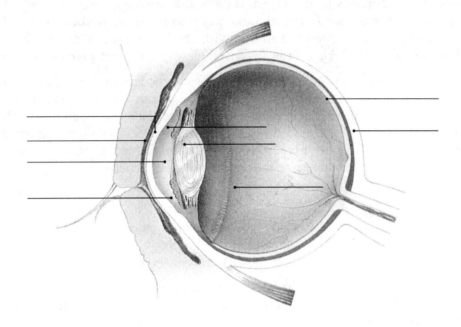

3. **The orbits are**

a. The bony structures that surround the eyes

b. The eyeballs

c. The pupils of the eyes

d. The corneas of the eyes

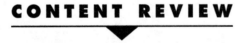

CONTENT REVIEW

1. Briefly explain why you may need to treat the eye-injured patient and family or friends for emotional trauma.

2. During the initial assessment of a patient with facial trauma, establish manual stabilization of the head and neck

a. After assessing the facial trauma

b. On first contact with the patient

c. Following application of oxygen

d. While examining the eye with a penlight

3. Suspect significant damage to the eye if
   a. Vision improves only after blinking
   b. The field of vision increases
   c. There is an injury to the forehead or cheek
   d. There is unusual sensitivity to light

4. Which of the following is considered appropriate when treating an injured eye?
   a. Remove blood clots from the sclera.
   b. Force the eyelids open, if necessary, to examine the pupils.
   c. Have the patient walk to distract him from the pain.
   d. Transport the patient for evaluation by a physician.

5. Only attempt to remove foreign particles that are lodged in the
   a. Conjunctiva
   b. Cornea
   c. Globe
   d. Retina

6. The following items may be acceptable emergency medical care for a lacerated eyelid EXCEPT
   a. Cover with saline soaked sterile gauze.
   b. Apply light pressure from a light dressing.
   c. Cover the uninjured eye with a bandage.
   d. Apply a warm pack to reduce swelling.

7. It is imperative to avoid applying any pressure to a ruptured eyeball, because it may force eye
   contents to leak out.
   a. True
   b. False

8. Begin treatment of a suspected chemical burn of the eye
   a. During the initial assessment
   b. After a rapid trauma assessment
   c. After the focused history and physical exam
   d. During the ongoing assessment

9. To irrigate a chemically burned eye, flush from the inside corner to outside edge for at least
   a. 5 minutes
   b. 10 minutes
   c. 15 minutes
   d. 20 minutes

10. Identify the position in which you would place the patient with an impaled or extruded
    eye injury.
    a. Fowler's position
    b. Lateral recumbent position
    c. Supine position
    d. Prone position

11. All of the following are correct regarding contact lenses EXCEPT
    a. Some patients wear both contact lenses and glasses.
    b. Some patients wear a contact lens in only one eye.
    c. A pen light will help you see a contact lens.
    d. Soft contact lenses show up as shadows over the iris.

12. Which of the following is the correct way to remove a soft contact lens?
    a. Pinch the lens between your thumb and index finger.
    b. Press the lower eyelid under the bottom edge of the lens.
    c. Apply a moistened suction cup.
    d. Slide a fingernail under the edge of the lens and lift.

13. A patient with a painful, deformed, and swollen jaw has dentures that are still intact and in place. It is necessary to remove them immediately.
    a. True
    b. False

14. Your patient is suffering from facial trauma with exposed nerves and tendons. You should
    a. Apply a moist sterile dressing to the injury
    b. Apply a dry sterile dressing to the injury
    c. Do not cover; it may damage the nerves
    d. Cover exposed tissues with an occlusive dressing

15. How would you care for an avulsed tooth resulting from facial trauma?
    a. Scrub it with water, and place it in a saline solution.
    b. Rinse it with saline, and place it in a saline solution.
    c. Scrub it with saline, and place it in dry gauze.
    d. Rinse it with water, and place it in an alcohol solution.

16. An impaled object, which has penetrated the cheek all the way through, is loose. What should you do?
    a. Stabilize it, and be prepared to remove it from the airway.
    b. Stabilize it with bulky dressings, and transport.
    c. Push or pull it out in the same direction in which it entered.
    d. Push or pull it out in the direction opposite to the way it entered.

17. To prevent a patient from swallowing a dressing that is packed between the teeth and cheek, you should
    a. Place a gloved index finger into the mouth to hold the dressing
    b. Have the patient hold onto one end of the dressing
    c. Tape some of the dressing material to the outside of the mouth
    d. Never place dressings into the mouth because they may block the airway

18. Which of the following is the most appropriate for treating a nasal fracture?
    a. Gently pull to align the nose, and transport.
    b. Apply cold compresses, and transport.
    c. Apply a pressure dressing, and transport.
    d. Pack the nostrils, and transport.

19. For clear or bloody fluid draining from the ear
   a. Pack the ear with dressings
   b. Apply pressure dressings
   c. Apply direct pressure
   d. Place a loose dressing across the opening

20. When treating bleeding wounds to the neck, never probe open wounds and always use circumferential bandages.
   a. True
   b. False

CASE STUDY

You and your partner are at the scene of an overturned car. Your patient is a 22-year-old male. He is responsive and supine, with battery acid burns to the eyes and a deep laceration to the left side of the neck that is bleeding heavily. A First Responder will maintain manual stabilization of the head and neck.

1. Should you consider advanced life support backup for this patient? Explain your answer.

2. Which of the following best describes the sequence that should be followed?
   a. Assess the patient, provide emergency care, then transport.
   b. Assess the patient, provide emergency care, and wait for the paramedics.
   c. Provide emergency care for life-threatening injuries first, then assess and treat other injuries, and transport.
   d. Transport immediately, and provide emergency care en route.

3. Which of the following describes the best treatment for this patient's injuries?
   a. Immediately begin flushing the eyes with saline. Simultaneously, place a gloved hand over the neck wound to control bleeding, and administer high flow oxygen.
   b. Immediately begin flushing the eyes with saline. Probe the neck wound to locate and apply pressure to the carotid artery, then administer high flow oxygen.
   c. Immediately stop the profuse bleeding from the neck wound. Then begin flushing the eyes with saline. Administer high flow oxygen as soon as you can.
   d. Once bleeding is under control and you have administered oxygen, check with medical control to find out if you can flush the patient's eyes with saline.

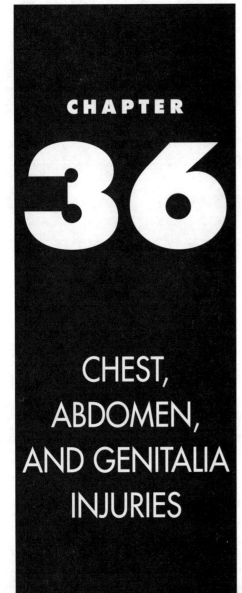

CHAPTER

36

CHEST, ABDOMEN, AND GENITALIA INJURIES

COGNITIVE OBJECTIVES

Numbered objectives are from the United States Department of Transportation 1994 EMT-Basic National Standard Curriculum. Asterisked objectives, if any, pertain to material that is supplemental to the DOT curriculum.

5-2.8 Discuss the emergency medical care considerations for a patient with a penetrating chest injury.

5-2.9 State the emergency medical care considerations for a patient with an open wound to the abdomen.

5-2.10 Differentiate the care of an open wound to the chest from an open wound to the abdomen.

* Review the anatomy of the chest cavity as it pertains to chest injuries.

* Identify signs and symptoms of possible life-threatening chest injuries.

* Describe emergency medical care for life-threatening chest injuries.

* Review the anatomy of the abdomen.

* Recognize the common signs and symptoms of abdominal injuries.

* Describe the emergency medical care for a suspected abdominal injury.

* Describe the emergency medical care for genitalia injuries.

KEY IDEAS

Injuries to the chest and abdomen can be overlooked in the physical assessment because often they are not obvious to the patient or to the EMT. However, injury to vital organs in the chest and abdomen can cause disturbances in respiration, oxygen exchange, and circulation. Rely on the mechanism of injury, a high index of suspicion, and careful physical examination.

▶ Closed chest injuries are the result of blunt trauma to the chest, which can cause extensive damage to ribs and internal organs. An open chest wound is the result of a penetrating injury, which also can cause extensive damage.

▶ Points to remember when assessing the chest injury patient: If blunt trauma to the chest is suspected, establish and maintain in-line spinal stabilization and administer oxygen; quickly expose the chest and examine it; note any sign of respiratory distress; immediately seal any open wound with a gloved hand; if there is paradoxical movement, immediately splint it with your hand. Patients with chest injuries are a high priority; immediate transport with assessment and care continuing en route must be considered.

▶ Emergency care of an open chest injury includes sealing the wound with an occlusive dressing, positioning the patient to ease breathing, and continually assessing respiratory status.

▶ Open wounds to the abdomen include evisceration, in which organs protrude through the skin. Closed abdominal injuries can crush, tear, or rupture a large number of organs, causing severe internal bleeding.

▶ Assessment of abdominal injury includes recognizing that such injury can cause excruciating pain, so much so that other injuries or problems may not be noticed by the patient. A mechanism of injury involving either blunt or penetrating trauma, signs of trauma, early signs and symptoms of shock, shallow rapid respirations, and abdominal pain and rigidity are all significant signs of serious abdominal injury.

▶ Emergency care of both open and closed abdominal injury includes aggressive management of the airway, breathing, and circulation. Early recognition and prompt transport is key. In abdominal evisceration, apply a moist dressing over protruding organs, cover with an occlusive dressing, and add a second dressing over that. Secure the dressings in place with tape, cravats, or a bandage.

▶ While injuries to the genitalia are rarely life threatening, they are typically extremely painful and embarrassing. They may have a number of causes, including sexual assault. Treat such injuries as you would any soft tissue injury.

TERMS AND CONCEPTS

1. **Write the number of each term beside its definition.**

    1. flail segment
    2. paradoxical movement
    3. pneumothorax
    4. sucking chest wound
    5. tension pneumothorax

_____ **a.** A segment of the chest wall that moves inward during inhalation and outward during exhalation

_____ **b.** An open wound to the chest that permits air to enter the thoracic cavity during inhalation

_____ **c.** Two or more consecutive ribs that are fractured in two or more places

_____ **d.** Air in the chest cavity, outside the lungs

_____ **e.** A condition in which the build-up of air and pressure in the thoracic cavity on the injured side is so severe that it begins to shift the lung on that side to the uninjured side, resulting in a compressing of the heart, vessels, and the uninjured lung

CONTENT REVIEW

1. List each of the following terms under the correct heading below.

   aorta   spleen
   heart   stomach
   intestines   superior vena cava
   liver   trachea
   lungs   urinary bladder

Chest Cavity	Abdominal Cavity

2. Briefly explain the difference between an open chest injury and a closed chest injury, and suggest at least one common cause for each.

3. The mechanism of injury suggests an open chest injury. You should quickly expose and examine the patient's chest during which of the following?
   a. Initial assessment
   b. Rapid trauma assessment
   c. Focused history and physical exam
   d. Ongoing assessment

4. Some patients with chest wall injury will breathe with extremely shallow, rapid breaths. What is the probable reason?
   a. The patient is hyperventilating.
   b. It is an attempt to reduce pain.
   c. It is an attempt to relieve hypovolemia.
   d. The patient is hyperglycemic.

5. In subcutaneous emphysema, air is trapped under the skin. When found around the neck and upper chest, what is the usual cause?
   a. Air expelled from the carotid artery
   b. The progressive nature of hypoperfusion
   c. Gravity causing the air to flow upward
   d. Tracheal deviation or jugular distention

6. Which of the following best describes lung sounds produced during a tension pneumothorax?
    a. Absent breath sounds on the uninjured side; decreased breath sounds on the injured side
    b. Absent breath sounds at the lower lobes; decreased breath sounds at the upper lobes
    c. Absent breath sounds on the injured side; decreased breath sounds on the uninjured side
    d. Absent breath sounds at the upper lobes; decreased breath sounds at the lower lobes

7. When there is no spinal injury, place the open chest wound patient
    a. In a semi-Fowler's position
    b. In a left lateral recumbent position
    c. On the uninjured side
    d. On the injured side

8. The spleen is considered to be a hollow organ.
    a. True
    b. False

9. The major complication associated with the laceration or tearing of a solid organ is major bleeding and shock (hypoperfusion).
    a. True
    b. False

10. Often abdominal injuries produce only subtle signs and symptoms. Therefore, you must base your suspicions on
    a. The patient's chief complaint
    b. The patient's sensory response
    c. The mechanism of injury
    d. Bystander information

11. When assessing a patient with abdominal pain, start palpating the abdomen
    a. Without regard to the pain
    b. At the upper right quadrant
    c. Closest to or directly over the pain
    d. Farthest from the pain

12. If no injury to the lower extremities, hips, pelvis, or spine is suspected, place a patient with a closed abdominal injury in a
    a. Lateral recumbent position with both legs flexed
    b. Trendelenburg position with legs flexed at hips
    c. Supine position with legs flexed at knees
    d. Fowler's position with legs straight

13. Identify the dressings that are most appropriate to use with an abdominal evisceration.
    a. Sterile dry paper towels, covered with plastic wrap or aluminum foil
    b. Sterile absorbent cotton soaked in saline and covered with an occlusive dressing
    c. Sterile dressing soaked in saline and covered with plastic wrap and an additional dressing
    d. Sterile dressing soaked in saline and covered by a bulky dressing

14. Identify the best method of transporting an amputated body part.
   a. Wrap it in a dry sterile dressing and place in a plastic bag with ice chips or cubes.
   b. Wrap it in a dry sterile dressing, cover with an occlusive dressing, and place on ice.
   c. Wrap it in a saline-moistened sterile dressing and cover with an occlusive dressing.
   d. Wrap it in a saline-moistened sterile dressing, put in a plastic bag, and place the bag on a cold pack.

15. You are treating a female who has a laceration to her genitalia. Which is the correct way to control the bleeding?
   a. Apply direct pressure, using a moistened sterile compress.
   b. Apply direct pressure, using your gloved hand.
   c. Pack the vagina with a sterile moist dressing.
   d. Place a moist dressing on the laceration and cover with plastic wrap.

CASE STUDY

You and your partner are on the scene of a fall. The injured tree trimmer is lying in the fallen branches. You immediately take in-line spinal stabilization. You introduce yourself and your partner, but the patient can only speak a word or two at a time and must breathe in between. Your partner hears a sucking sound and she quickly exposes the patient's body to find an open chest wound under the left breast and an eviscerated abdomen with protruding bowel. You immediately call for advanced life support backup.

1. Which of the following is the correct IMMEDIATE treatment for the sucking chest wound?
   a. Place an occlusive dressing on the wound during the initial assessment.
   b. Place an occlusive dressing on the wound during the rapid trauma assessment.
   c. Seal the wound with a gloved hand during the initial assessment.
   d. Seal the wound with a gloved hand during the rapid trauma assessment.

2. You apply a dressing to the abdominal evisceration. All of the following are correct regarding dressing the wound EXCEPT
   a. The dressing should be soaked in saline or sterile water.
   b. A moist dressing should be covered by an occlusive dressing.
   c. The dressing should be taped on three sides to allow air to escape.
   d. The dressing should be secured with tape, cravats, or bandages.

Your partner states that it's becoming harder to ventilate the patient. You note cyanosis of the fingertips and quickly look through the examination hole in the cervical spine immobilization collar to visualize the trachea. It appears to be deviated to the right side. Further examination reveals jugular vein distention. You quickly auscultate the lungs and find that breath sounds are absent on the left and decreased on the right.

3. The changes in respiratory status of this patient indicate which possible condition, and what steps should be taken to rectify the problem?
   a. Flail segment with paradoxical movement. Support with pressure from your hand.
   b. Flail segment with paradoxical movement. Roll the patient onto the injured side.
   c. Tension pneumothorax. Transport immediately.
   d. Tension pneumothorax. Lift the corner of the occlusive dressing on the chest wound to allow air to escape.

Numbered objectives are from the United States Department of Transportation 1994 EMT-Basic National Standard Curriculum. Asterisked objectives, if any, pertain to material that is supplemental to the DOT curriculum.

* Describe the general guidelines for emergency care of agricultural injuries and related industrial injuries.

* Identify the mechanisms of injury responsible for the majority of agricultural accidents.

* List the general guidelines for stabilizing and shutting down agricultural equipment and other machinery.

* List the common accidents/mechanisms of injury associated with various types of agricultural machinery, storage devices, and livestock.

* List the general guidelines for industrial rescue.

KEY IDEAS
▼

This chapter focuses on the types of accidents and injuries that you may encounter in agricultural or industrial settings involving heavy machinery and specialized equipment. Such accidents can present unique challenges to the EMT-Basic, so it important to have an understanding of how to approach these situations safely.

▶ Agricultural and industrial accidents often involve unique mechanisms of injury and tremendous kinetic energy resulting in severe trauma. In addition, suffocation, inhalation injuries, and near-drowning are common.

▶ The agricultural and industrial emergency scene is never safe until machinery is stabilized and shut down and any other hazards are controlled. If necessary, wait for fire personnel or specialized hazardous materials teams to control the scene.

▶ Never enter any structure (confined space) without the help of other rescuers, without being tied to a lifeline, and without wearing appropriate protective equipment or a self-contained breathing apparatus.

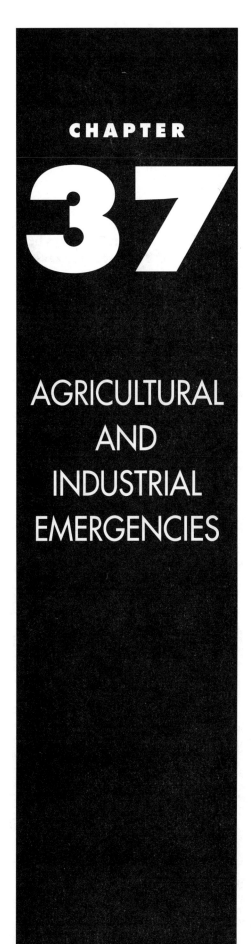

CHAPTER

37

AGRICULTURAL AND INDUSTRIAL EMERGENCIES

CONTENT REVIEW

1. List three hazards that might be found at the scene of an agricultural or industrial accident.

2. You are at the scene of a rollover tractor accident. What is the best approach to this situation?
   a. Due to the potential for severe and extensive traumatic injury, patient extrication and treatment must always be your first priority.
   b. The rescue requires two teams–one to handle the potential fire hazard and one to provide patient extrication and treatment.
   c. Such situations always require a physician on scene because amputation is often necessary to patient rescue.
   d. Due to potential hazards, you should not enter the scene without full "turnout" gear.

3. "Rules" that apply to rescue scenes involving silos or grain tanks include
   a. Extricate the patient immediately to minimize exposure to toxic gases
   b. Anticipate the need for decontamination activities
   c. Never attempt rescue alone or without a lifeline
   d. Use any method available to speed up patient access

4. If your patient was exposed to chemicals or manure during an agricultural accident, your first action should be to
   a. Remove all exposed clothing and flush the patient with copious amounts of water before transport
   b. Control severe bleeding by using direct pressure, unless bleeding is controlled by the pressure of equipment
   c. Administer oxygen by nonrebreather, or initiate positive pressure ventilation if necessary
   d. While maintaining in-line manual spinal stabilization, establish a patent airway using the jaw-thrust maneuver

5. Preserve all avulsed body parts, however mangled their appearance.
   a. True
   b. False

6. Write the number of each mechanism of injury beside its definition.

   1. crush points
   2. pinch points
   3. shear points
   4. stored energy
   5. wrap points

   ____ a. Hazards remain after the machinery is shut down
   ____ b. Aggressive component of machinery moves in a circular motion

230

_____ c. Two objects meet to cause a squeezing or pulling action

_____ d. Two large objects come together to cause a mashing action

_____ e. Two objects move close enough together to cause cutting action

7. All of the following are appropriate ways to stabilize agricultural equipment EXCEPT
   a. Block or chock the vehicle.
   b. Tie it to another vehicle.
   c. Turn off the ignition switch.
   d. Set the parking brake.

8. If the patient is in a life-threatening situation and all other attempts at equipment shutdown have failed, you should
   a. Discharge a fire extinguisher into the air intake
   b. Use the shut-off valve on the bottom of the fuel tank
   c. Clamp the fuel line using vice-grip pliers
   d. Slow the engine down with the throttle

9. In addition to injuries, you should assume that a patient who has been buried in a grain tank is also
   a. Hypovolemic
   b. Hypothermic
   c. Hypoglycemic
   d. Hypoallergenic

10. List three signs of "silo gas" in the environment.

11. Never enter a livestock building or livestock area
    a. Without the owner's permission and guidance
    b. With brightly colored clothing
    c. Until each and every animal is secured
    d. Until the animals have been fed

12. List three guidelines for any industrial rescue.

CASE STUDY

▼

You have arrived on scene at the Wilson farm. John, 16 years old, was accidentally impaled in the abdomen by one of the tines of a forklift and is apparently "pinned" to the wall of the barn. The forklift has been secured and shut down. You find John awake and alert. Your partner initiates in-line manual spinal stabilization. You note that although the tine of the forklift enters the right side of his abdomen, John is moving air adequately. His breathing is rapid, pulse is strong and regular, and skin is warm and slightly diaphoretic. There is very little bleeding coming from the wound. The patient denies any other injuries and has pulses, motion, and sensation in all four extremities.

1. What should you do?

Further assessment reveals that John is merely pushed against the barn wall. The tine does not appear to go all the way through John's abdomen. You also observe that the tine is held in place by two large bolts.

2. Should you remove the tine from John's abdomen?

3. How should you handle the extrication?

John is now immobilized on the long backboard. Reassessment of his pulses, motion, and sensation finds them unchanged from your initial assessment. Baseline vitals: blood pressure 116/78, pulse 90 and regular, respirations 22, with good air exchange. Completing your SAMPLE history, you find that he has no allergies, takes no medications, and has no significant past history. He ate lunch 4 hours ago. John says that he and his brother were "horsing around," and that caused the accident.

4. What should be done now?

MODULE 5 REVIEW
TRAUMA: CHAPTERS 28-37

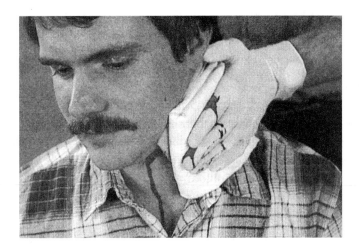

Trauma is an injury or injuries resulting from some outside force, such as a fall, a blow, a motor vehicle collision, a stabbing, or a gunshot. Whether the injury is open (the skin has been broken and, perhaps, an object has penetrated the body) or closed (from a blow that does not break the skin or penetrate the body), the injuries sustained, including injuries to internal organs of the body, may be severe.

Q **Why are mechanism of injury and "index of suspicion" so important?**

A Many injuries cannot be observed. There may be damage to internal organs from a blow that has left only minor marks on the exterior body. In almost any injury, spinal injury should also be suspected, even though the patient may not yet be showing any signs of spinal injury. It is also possible to be distracted by a dramatic-looking injury, such as a deep laceration or a deformed extremity, and be unaware of a far more serious injury that is not visible. Often, the mechanism of injury — how the patient was injured, such as by falling from a height or being struck by a car — is the only clue to hidden injuries the patient may have sustained and how severe these injuries may be. Based on the mechanism of injury, you must maintain a high index of suspicion for injuries that you cannot observe and/or that the patient is unaware of. For example, if the mechanism of injury was one that could cause spinal injury — whether or not the patient shows signs of spinal injury — take in-line manual stabilization of the head and neck on first contact with the patient and maintain it until the patient is secured to a backboard for transport.

Q **What are the chief concerns of the EMT-B at a trauma emergency, in addition to the need for spinal stabilization and immobilization?**

A Airway, airway, and airway! Many mechanisms of injury can cause airway compromise through injury to structures of the airway, broken teeth, dentures, and bone fragments, blood, and secretions. In addition, the injury may cause an altered mental status which can prevent the patient from protecting his airway. Since all other assessments and treatments are of no use if the patient does not have a patent airway, the airway must be the chief concern with any trauma emergency. Also be alert for any signs of inadequate breathing and be prepared to provide positive pressure ventilation with supplemental oxygen if needed.

Q What about bleeding and shock?

A Bleeding is a concern whenever there is trauma. Severe external bleeding must be controlled. You must also be alert for signs of internal bleeding. Whether internal or external, blood loss can cause a life-threatening reduction of perfusion known as shock (hypoperfusion). If shock is suspected, keep the airway open, administer oxygen, keep the patient warm, position with feet elevated, and transport without delay.

Q Are open injuries considered dangerous?

A Yes. Open injuries to the chest and abdomen are always considered life-threatening, as are severe lacerations to the neck. Immediately cover any open injury to the chest or neck with a gloved hand. Then apply dressings, including occlusive dressings. An occlusive dressing to an open chest injury should be taped on only three sides to allow trapped air to escape when the patient exhales, preventing a life-threatening buildup of air in the chest cavity known as tension pneumothorax.

Q What are the major elements of care at a burn emergency?

A Remove clothing and jewelry in the area of the burn, cool the burn with water, apply dressings, keep the patient warm, and transport. Flush a chemical burn with water for at least 20 minutes. If the burn is from a dry chemical, first brush off the chemical before flushing.

Q We have learned that it is important to look for a mechanism of injury or signs of trauma at a medical emergency. Is it also important to assess for signs and symptoms of a medical emergency at the trauma scene?

A Yes. A patient may be suffering from a medical condition as well as from trauma. For example, when a car has gone off the road and the driver is injured, might he have lost control because he was suffering from a medical condition such as a heart attack or diabetic emergency? Or might a medical condition have been brought on or aggravated by the injury? Always keep in mind that the patient may be a trauma patient and a medical patient at the same time.

COGNITIVE OBJECTIVES

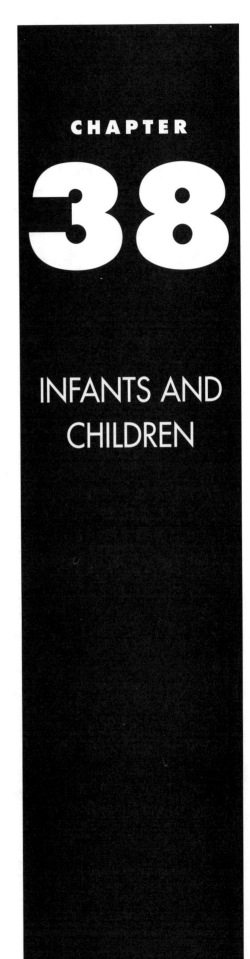

CHAPTER

38

INFANTS AND CHILDREN

Numbered objectives are from the United States Department of Transportation 1994 EMT-Basic National Standard Curriculum. Asterisked objectives, if any, pertain to material that is supplemental to the DOT curriculum.

6-1.1   Identify the developmental considerations for the following age groups:

- infants
- toddlers
- preschool
- school age
- adolescent

6-1.2   Describe the differences in anatomy and physiology of the infant, child, and adult patient.

6-1.3   Differentiate the response of the ill or injured infant or child from that of an adult.

6-1.4   Indicate various causes of respiratory emergencies.

6-1.5   Differentiate between respiratory distress and respiratory failure.

6-1.6   List the steps in the management of foreign body airway obstruction.

6-1.7   Summarize emergency medical care strategies for respiratory distress and respiratory failure.

6-1.8   Identify the signs and symptoms of shock (hypoperfusion) in the infant and child patient.

6-1.9   Describe the method of determining end organ perfusion in the infant and child patient.

6-1.10 State the usual causes of cardiac arrest in infants and children versus adults.

6-1.11 List the common causes of seizures in the infant and child patient.

6-1.12 Describe the management of seizures in the infant and child patient.

6-1.13 Differentiate between the injury patterns in adults, infants, and children.

6-1.14 Discuss the field management of the infant and child trauma patient.

6-1.15 Summarize the indicators of possible child abuse and neglect.

6-1.16 Describe the medical legal responsibilities in suspected child abuse.

6-1.17 Recognize the need for EMT-Basic debriefing following a difficult infant or child transport.

KEY IDEAS

This chapter focuses on the unique assessment and emergency medical management considerations that the EMT-Basic must take into account when providing care to ill or injured infants and children. Most EMS providers find such situations among the most stressful of any emergency call they encounter. A good understanding of the basics about caring for infants and children will go a long way towards increasing your confidence and decreasing your stress.

▶ The ill or injured infant or child is not your only "patient." You must remember that the caregiver will also need your attention.

▶ The developmental classifications of the infant or child patient include neonate, infant, toddler, preschooler, school age, and adolescent. The developmental characteristics related to age will affect your assessment and treatment activities. Management of most infant and child emergencies are identical to the management of the adult patient; however, modifications may need to be made based on anatomical, physiological, and psychological development of the infant or child.

▶ The primary goal in treating any infant or child patient is to anticipate and recognize respiratory problems and to support any function that is compromised or lost.

▶ Capillary refill is an appropriate method of assessment for perfusion in the patient under 6 years of age.

▶ Fever is a common emergency for infants and children and may be due to infection or heat exposure. Sudden infant death syndrome (SIDS) is the leading cause of death among infants from 1 month to 1 year of age. Blunt trauma is the most common injury in children.

▶ Child abuse may take a variety of forms, including physical, emotional, and sexual abuse and neglect.

▶ Infant and child patients with special needs are often cared for at home and may be encountered by EMS personnel as a result of problems with tracheostomies, ventilators, venous access devices, or feeding tubes.

▶ The EMT-Basic can alleviate some of the personal stress of caring for children through advance preparation and by seeking out help when necessary.

TERMS AND CONCEPTS

▼

1. Fill in the chart below. Include at least two characteristics for each stage.

Developmental Stage	Age Group	Characteristics
a. Neonate		
b. Infant		
c. Toddler		
d. Preschooler		
e. School Age		
f. Adolescent		

CONTENT REVIEW

▼

1. Identify a generally helpful method of dealing with caregivers at the scene of an emergency for an infant or child.
   a. The use of technical terms will reassure caregivers that you are qualified to care for their child.
   b. Acknowledge caregivers' concerns and, when appropriate, allow them to assist you in caring for their child.
   c. Immediately remove the child from the scene so that caregivers cannot interfere with your care.
   d. Even if the child is seriously injured, reassure caregivers that "everything will be fine" to help keep them calm.

2. All of the following are characteristics of the infant and young child EXCEPT
   a. The tracheal diameter in a newborn is about the same as an adult's, so vulnerability to inhalation injury is similar.
   b. The tongue is proportionally larger than an adult's, so it is more likely to cause occlusion.
   c. The ribs are more pliable, so pulmonary injury is likely even in the absence of rib fracture.
   d. The head is proportionately larger until about 9 years of age, so pad behind shoulders to maintain neutral alignment.

3. The child's skin surface is large compared to his body mass, thus making him more susceptible to ____.
   a. Hyperventilation
   b. Hyperglycemia
   c. Hypothermia
   d. Hypovolemia

4. Infants and children have faster _____ rates than adults; therefore, they use oxygen from the bloodstream faster than adults do.
   a. Fontanel
   b. Metabolic
   c. Abdominal musculature
   d. Central nervous system

5. The primary goal in treating any infant or child patient is the anticipation and recognition of _____ problems and support of any compromised or lost function.
   a. Central nervous system
   b. Cardiovascular system
   c. Respiratory system
   d. Urinary system

6. List three signs of early respiratory distress in infants and children.

7. Your infant patient is lethargic, has decreased muscle tone, grunting respirations at 80 per minute with obvious use of accessory muscles, and head bobbing. You suspect
   a. Early respiratory distress
   b. Supraclavicular retractions
   c. Decompensated respiratory failure
   d. Cardiopulmonary arrest

8. _____ occurs when the compensatory mechanisms designed to maintain oxygenation of the blood have failed and the body is just moments away from complete cardiopulmonary arrest.
   a. Decompensated respiratory failure
   b. Early cardiopulmonary arrest
   c. Respiratory arrest
   d. Hypotension

9. List three possible causes of rapid breathing in infants and children.

10. Compare the observations you would make in a patient with partial airway obstruction and a patient with complete airway obstruction.

11. If perfusion is adequate, pulses, skin color and temperature, capillary refill, mental status, and
_____ will be normal.
   a. Respiratory effort
   b. Urinary output
   c. Motor function
   d. Intercostal motion

12. Write the numerals 1 to 5 to show the correct order of steps for managing a foreign body airway obstruction in an infant.

____ Support the infant in a prone head-down position on your forearm.

____ Attempt to ventilate; if unsuccessful, repeat sequence.

____ Look in the mouth; if object is visible, sweep it out with your finger.

____ Deliver five sharp back blows between the shoulder blades.

____ Transfer the patient to a supine position, and deliver five chest thrusts using two fingertips.

13. List at least three common causes of seizure in infants and children.

14. Describe the general emergency care procedures for an infant or child who is suffering a seizure.

15. All of the following are included in the emergency medical care of an infant or child with fever EXCEPT
   a. Administer oxygen via nonrebreather mask.
   b. Sponge down the patient with alcohol.
   c. Remove the patient's clothing down to diaper or underwear.
   d. Position the patient on his side.

16. Infants and children compensate for hypoperfusion longer than adults. However, when they do deteriorate because of hypoperfusion, they deteriorate more slowly but more severely than adults.
   a. True
   b. False

17. Describe the emergency medical care of an infant or child with possible shock.

18. In a SIDS emergency, you will provide care for the infant in cardiac arrest as you would for any patient in cardiac arrest.
    a. True
    b. False

19. When obtaining a SAMPLE history in a SIDS emergency, avoid asking the parents and other caregivers any questions. Stick to what you can observe at the scene.
    a. True
    b. False

20. Write the number of each injury pattern next to its most likely emergency situation.

    1. Head and neck injuries

    2. Abdominal and spinal injuries

    3. Head, abdominal, and spinal injuries

    4. Head, chest, and lower extremity injuries

____ a. Young school-age bike rider struck by a car

____ b. Unrestrained infant in a motor vehicle collision

____ c. Young school-age pedestrian struck by a car

____ d. Toddler improperly restrained by seat belt in a motor vehicle collision

21. All of the following are commonly associated with isolated closed head injuries to infants and children EXCEPT
    a. Nausea and vomiting
    b. Respiratory arrest
    c. Scalp and facial injuries
    d. Hypoperfusion

22. You note tire marks on the chest wall of a 5-year-old patient who was struck by a car. However, you feel no deformity to his ribs, so you can safely assume his pliable ribs have protected him from internal injury.
    a. True
    b. False

23. What is the potential danger associated with excessive air in the stomach (gastric insufflation) which may occur as a result of positive pressure ventilation?
    a. Interference with diaphragm movement and lung inflation
    b. Gastric rupture due to excessive air in the stomach
    c. Nausea and projectile vomiting
    d. Gastric regurgitation if the PASG is inflated

24. Just as in the adult trauma patient, the priorities in treating an infant or child trauma patient center around stabilization of the spine, airway management, breathing, and circulatory support.
    a. True
    b. False

25. Infant and child burn patients are at more risk of hypothermia and _____ in part because of their greater skin surface in relation to body mass.
   a. respiratory compromise
   b. fluid loss
   c. altered mental status
   d. scarring

26. List at least five general indications of child abuse.

27. You suspect child abuse. Which of the following statements best describes how you should proceed?
   a. Question neighbors about your suspicions, and flag your prehospital care report by writing "suspected child abuse" on it.
   b. Refuse to leave the scene until the police arrive to arrest the caregivers and restrain them for transport.
   c. Record your objective observations, follow local reporting protocols, and maintain total confidentiality.
   d. Record your objective observations, confront the caregiver, and contact the local child protective services agency.

28. EMT-Bs who are treating infants and children may experience anxiety and stress from lack of experience, fear of failure, or identifying patients with their own children.
   a. True
   b. False

29. In children with tracheostomy tubes, the airway can be easily cleared of mucus by suctioning the tube with a suction catheter that is
   a. One-fourth the diameter of the tube
   b. Half the diameter of the tube
   c. The same diameter as the tube
   d. Twice as large around as the tube

30. You recently ran a call involving a young child who was critically injured. Despite your efforts, she died en route to the hospital. Since then you've been getting anxious every time you're dispatched. Which of the following is most likely to help you?
   a. Request a meeting with the CISD team for everyone involved in the call, since you are probably not alone.
   b. Ignore your anxiety; everyone has tough calls now and then.
   c. Recognize that your anxiety is a sign that you aren't cut out for this kind of work.
   d. Go out with friends for a night on the town to help you forget about everything for awhile.

CASE STUDY

You are dispatched to a women's shelter for "baby not breathing." On arrival, the patient's mother reports that her 5-month-old male infant has had a cold and been fussy for the past 2 days. Today, the child had episodes of coughing that "made him vomit." About 10 minutes ago he appeared to briefly stop breathing, and she called 9-1-1. The infant is lying quietly in his mother's arms. He is awake but lethargic with decreased muscle tone. Eyes appear "glassy." Airway is patent with very rapid, shallow, grunting respirations at 60 per minute. Skin is pale, very warm, and dry. The brachial pulse is strong and regular at 90 per minute. Fontanel appears to be sunken. Capillary refill is greater than 2 seconds. There are no obvious injuries or signs of trauma.

1. How would you categorize this infant's respiratory status?

2. What should you do?

During the SAMPLE history, the mother reports that the patient was born 7 weeks prematurely but has been doing fine. No medications or known allergies. She says that she fed him about 3 hours ago, but he has vomited several times since then. He has not had a wet diaper since this morning. She starts to cry and says it's her fault that the baby is so sick, but she couldn't afford to take him to the doctor when he "caught his cold."

3. How should you deal with the mother's concerns?

MODULE 6 REVIEW
INFANTS AND CHILDREN: CHAPTER 8

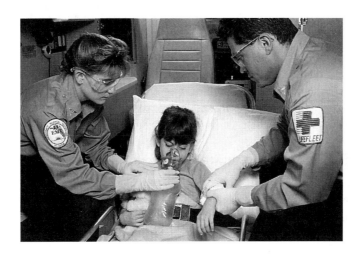

Calls to emergencies involving infants and children are among the most stressful for many EMT-Bs, partly because they are relatively infrequent, partly because many EMTs are not familiar with children, partly because the emotions and reactions of the parents or other caregivers adds to the stress of the event, and partly because the plight of a sick or injured child can be heart-rending.

Q **What are the similarities between emergencies involving infants and children and those involving adults?**

A Infants and children have many of the same medical and trauma problems as adults. They bleed, suffer shock, develop allergies, get stung by insects, and swallow poisonous substances, just as adults do. Most treatments are the same as those for adults.

Q **What are the important differences between adults and infants or children as they may affect emergency care?**

A Some important anatomical differences were discussed in the Airway module. (Children have smaller mouths and noses, relatively larger tongues, softer airway and chest structures, and larger heads that require padding under the shoulders to keep the airway aligned. All of these factors require special alertness to possible airway occlusion.)

Q **Isn't it hard to communicate with children and their parents?**

A It helps to know something about the way children develop. You can also use common sense. You can't ask a baby how he feels, but you can note whether he is alert and crying vigorously or, instead, is lying lethargically and looking ill. Involving the parents or other caregivers can help to keep the adults calm. They can provide information about what is normal for this child and can comfort the child by holding him.

Q **What is the chief concern involving infants or children?**

A *Respiration.* In fact, the primary goal in treating any infant or child is the anticipation and recognition of respiratory problems. With children, respiratory difficulties can rapidly lead to respiratory failure and death.

(Module 6 Review continued)

Q **What are the signs of respiratory distress in the infant or child?**

A Be especially alert for signs of *early* respiratory distress, including a higher-than-normal breathing rate; nasal flaring; retractions of the tissues and muscles above, below, and over the rib cage; audible breathing such as stridor, wheezing, or grunting; or "see-saw" breathing (effort of inspiration draws chest in, forces abdomen out). From early respiratory distress, the child may deteriorate into decompensated respiratory failure (a respiratory rate over 60 per minute, cyanosis, decreased muscle tone, poor peripheral perfusion, and altered mental status), and finally to respiratory arrest (respirations less than 10 per minute or absent, unresponsiveness, slow or absent heart rate, weak or absent peripheral pulses).

Q **What is the emergency care for respiratory distress in the infant or child?**

A If the child is in early respiratory distress and breathing is adequate, provide oxygen and immediate transport. If the child is deteriorating into decompensated respiratory failure or respiratory arrest, establish and maintain a patent airway, suction fluids, and provide positive pressure ventilation with supplemental oxygen. If distress is mild, the child may prefer to sit up. If the child is very ill or unresponsive (without suspected spinal injury), place him on his side to aid drainage from the mouth. If spinal injury is suspected, immobilize him in a supine position with padding beneath the shoulders as needed to keep the airway aligned. Transport without delay.

Q **What are the special concerns regarding trauma in infants and children?**

A A child's relatively larger, heavier head will propel the head forward in a crash, so that head injuries are common. The child's less developed ribs and chest and abdominal walls mean that they may more easily sustain internal injuries without broken ribs or other observable signs of injury. If you observe signs of possible child abuse or neglect, treat the child's injuries as you would ordinarily, do not confront the caregivers, but report your suspicions to the proper authorities according to your state laws or local protocols.

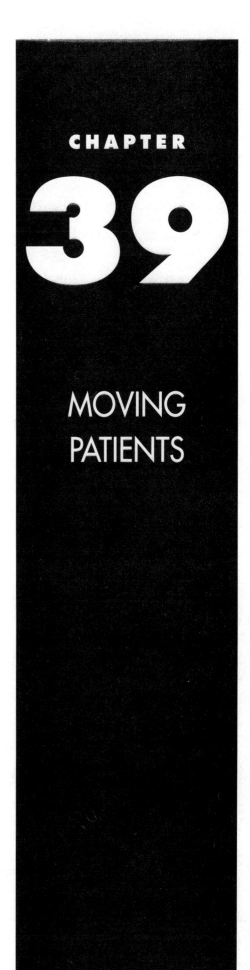

COGNITIVE OBJECTIVES

Numbered objectives are from the United States Department of Transportation 1994 EMT-Basic National Standard Curriculum. Asterisked objectives, if any, pertain to material that is supplemental to the DOT curriculum.

1-6.3   Describe the safe lifting of cots and stretchers.

1-6.10 Discuss the general considerations of moving patients.

1-6.11 State three situations that may require the use of an emergency move.

1-6.12 Identify the following patient carrying devices:

- Wheeled ambulance stretcher
- Portable ambulance stretcher
- Stair chair
- Scoop stretcher
- Long spine board
- Basket stretcher
- Flexible stretcher

KEY IDEAS

Lifting and moving patients is a routine component of the EMT-Basic's responsibilities. You must use a variety of lifting and moving equipment, take a teamwork approach, and use your intelligence and imagination to properly lift and move patients.

▶ There are three categories for moving patients–emergency moves, urgent moves, and nonurgent moves.

▶ Emergency moves should be performed when there is an immediate environmental danger to a patient or the rescuer. These dangers include fire, hazardous materials, inability to gain access to other patients who need life-saving care, and an inability to provide life-saving treatment because of a patient's position.

▶ There are three types of emergency moves–the armpit-forearm drag, the shirt drag, and the blanket drag.

▶ An example of an urgent move is the use of the rapid extrication technique for quick removal of a critical patient from an automobile.

▶ Nonurgent moves include the direct ground lift, extremity lift, direct carry method, and draw sheet method.

▶ Proper packaging of a patient includes selecting and preparing the appropriate carrying device, safely transferring the patient to the device, and moving and carrying the device to the ambulance for loading and unloading.

▶ Patient carrying devices include the wheeled ambulance stretcher, portable stretcher, stair chair, backboard (short and long), scoop stretcher, basket stretcher, and flexible stretcher.

▶ A pregnant woman will feel more comfortable being transported on her left side. This position takes the weight of the baby off the large blood vessels and nerves in the abdomen.

▶ Infants and toddlers can be immobilized and transported in the child's own car seat.

▶ Elderly patients with osteoporosis require extra care to prevent accidental injury from lifting and moving.

▶ Use special care and extra caution when transporting handicapped patients. Strap the patient well and use additional padding as needed.

TERMS AND CONCEPTS

1. **Write the number of each term next to its definition.**

    1. emergency move
    2. nonurgent move
    3. urgent move

_____ a. A move made because there is a threat to life due to the patient's condition and the patient must be moved quickly for transport

_____ b. A move that should be performed when there is immediate danger to the patient or to the rescuer

_____ c. A move made when no immediate threat to life exists

CONTENT REVIEW

1. Which item is NOT a proper lifting and moving technique?
    a. Use teamwork, equipment, and your imagination.
    b. Lift an object as far from your body as possible.
    c. Avoid using back muscles to lift.
    d. Keep ears, shoulders, hips, and feet in alignment.

2. Which situation would require you to make an urgent move?
    a. A patient in a burning building
    b. A patient lying in uncontrolled traffic
    c. A patient who is blocking access to a critically injured patient
    d. A motor vehicle collision patient with a critical head injury

3. To perform _____, insert your hands under the patient's armpits. Then grab the patient's left forearm with your right hand, the right forearm with your left hand, and drag in the direction of the long axis of the body.
   a. The armpit-forearm drag
   b. The drag and pull
   c. The extrication drag
   d. The power-grip technique

4. In which emergency move should you fasten the patient's hands or wrists together and link them to the belt or pants?
   a. The armpit-forearm drag
   b. The blanket drag
   c. The shirt drag
   d. The rapid extrication technique

5. Identify the move. Write the correct caption for each of the following photographs.

A.

B.

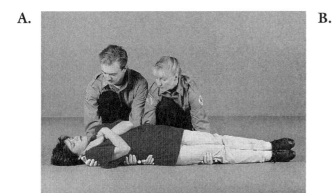

   a. _____
   b. _____

6. Identify the move. Write the correct caption for each of the following photographs.

A.

B.

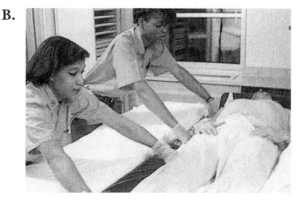

   a. _____
   b. _____

7. The following items are steps in the process of rapid extrication of a patient from an automobile. Number them 1 to 4 to identify the proper sequence.

____ Rotate the patient in several coordinated moves until the patient's back is in the doorway.

____ Place the long backboard next to the patient's buttocks, and lower the patient onto the board.

____ Support the patient's thorax as another rescuer frees the legs from the pedals.

____ Hold in-line stabilization of the head and neck, and apply a cervical-spine immobilization collar.

8. Identify the item that is NOT true about the direct ground lift.
   a. It should be used for heavier patients.
   b. It is not as safe as using a long backboard.
   c. It should be performed by bending at the hips, not at the waist.
   d. The lifting force should be generated from your legs and buttocks.

9. Most wheeled ambulance stretchers are designed to accommodate weights up to
   a. 200 pounds
   b. 300 pounds
   c. 400 pounds
   d. 500 pounds

10. A scoop stretcher
    a. Cannot be used in confined areas
    b. Is designed to carry up to 700 pounds
    c. Is not affected by temperature extremes
    d. Is not recommended for spine-injured patients

11. A stair chair should be used
    a. When the patient has an altered level of consciousness
    b. When the patient has a suspected spinal injury
    c. When a wheeled stretcher cannot traverse narrow corridors
    d. Any time steps are encountered

12. The basket stretcher is also known as a
    a. Stokes basket
    b. Wheeled stretcher
    c. Sholten's basket
    d. Canvas litter

13. Identify the equipment. Write the correct caption for each photograph.

A.

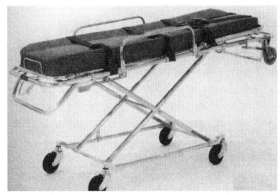

B.

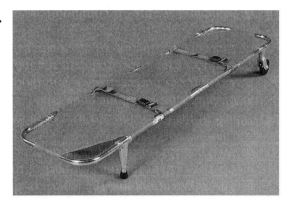

C.

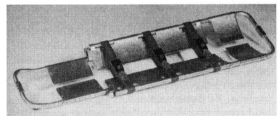

D.

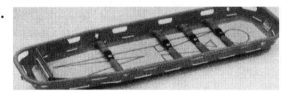

E.

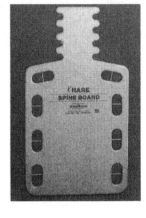

F.

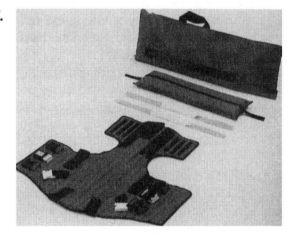

a. _____

b. _____

c. _____

d. _____

e. _____

f. _____

CASE STUDY

▼

You and your partner are dispatched to a call for an elderly patient. A well-dressed man introduces himself as the patient's son and escorts you to the patient. You ask, "Why did you call the ambulance?" He replies, "Mom is in her 60s and lives by herself. She called me today and told me she didn't feel well. I called her doctor and he told me to bring her in. I couldn't take her because she feels dizzy and lightheaded every time she tries to get up." The patient is lying in her bed. Your general impression is that she looks well. Her skin color is pink, respirations are normal, radial pulse is strong and regular. There is no sign of trauma and no obvious bleeding. When you question the patient, she tells you she has been feeling poorly for the past week. She has been unable to eat and has been vomiting for the last few days. She has a history of osteoporosis and high blood pressure.

1. Which method would be preferable for moving this patient onto a wheeled ambulance stretcher?
   a. Extremity lift
   b. Armpit-forearm drag
   c. Shirt drag
   d. Draw sheet method

2. The son suggests that you "walk" the patient to the stretcher. Select the statement that best describes why this would or would not be appropriate.
   a. This would not be appropriate, because the patient is dizzy and lightheaded and may lose her balance.
   b. This would be appropriate if you support her while standing.
   c. This would be appropriate if you position the stretcher next to the bed.
   d. This would be appropriate if both you and your partner support her when she stands.

3. When moving this patient on the wheeled stretcher to the awaiting ambulance, the
   a. EMT at the head pushes the stretcher without assistance
   b. EMT at the head pushes and the EMT at the foot guides
   c. EMT at the head guides and the EMT at the foot pulls
   d. EMT at the head and foot both push, pull, and guide

COGNITIVE OBJECTIVES

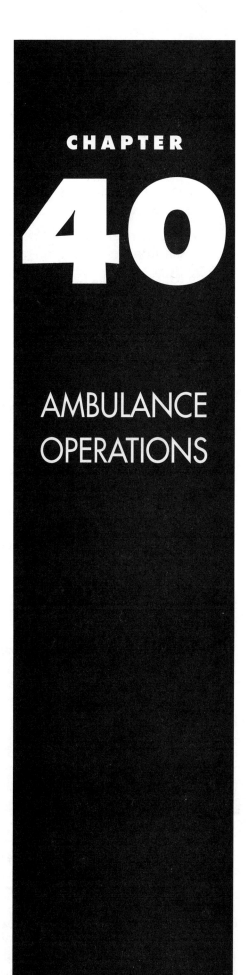

Numbered objectives are from the United States Department of Transportation 1994 EMT-Basic National Standard Curriculum. Asterisked objectives, if any, pertain to material that is supplemental to the DOT curriculum.

7-1.1   Discuss the medical and non-medical equipment needed to respond to a call.

7-1.2   List the phases of an ambulance call.

7-1.3   Describe the general provisions of state laws relating to the operation of the ambulance and privileges in any or all of the following categories:
- Speed
- Warning lights
- Sirens
- Right-of-way
- Parking
- Turning

7-1.4   List contributing factors to unsafe driving conditions.

7-1.5   Describe the considerations that should be given to:
- Request for escorts
- Following an escort vehicle
- Intersections

7-1.6   Discuss "Due Regard for Safety of All Others" while operating an emergency vehicle.

7.1-7   State what information is essential in order to respond to a call.

7-1.8   Discuss various situations that may affect response to a call.

7-1.9   Differentiate between the various methods of moving a patient to the unit based upon injury or illness.

7-1.10 Apply the components of the essential patient information in a written report.

7-1.11 Summarize the importance of preparing the unit for the next response.

7-1.12 Identify what is essential for completion of a call.

7-1.13 Distinguish among the terms "cleansing," "disinfection," "high-level disinfection," and "sterilization."

7-1.14 Describe how to clean or disinfect items following patient care.

KEY IDEAS

As an EMT-Basic, you have the responsibility for getting safely to the scene of an emergency and transporting your patients safely to medical care. This chapter focuses on the safe and effective operation of an ambulance. It also provides information on how to prepare yourself, your equipment, medical supplies, and vehicle for the emergency call.

▶ Operation of an emergency vehicle gives you certain privileges; however at no time is it justified to operate an ambulance in a manner which endangers or jeopardizes anyone else.

▶ Failure to exercise due regard for the safety of others incurs liability for any consequences that may result from your disregard.

▶ Operation of an ambulance requires your familiarity and compliance with the state and local laws and regulations governing all aspects of emergency vehicle operation.

▶ The major phases of an ambulance call include daily pre-run vehicle and equipment preparation, dispatch, en route to the scene, at the scene, en route to the receiving facility, at the receiving facility, en route to the station, and post run.

▶ Infection control procedures play a crucial role in preparing your unit and yourself to return to service.

▶ If your EMS agency interacts with or provides aeromedical emergency service, you must be familiar with landing zone safety considerations and always must comply with them when performing your job.

CONTENT REVIEW

1. List three privileges that are associated with the operation of emergency vehicles.

2. Which of the following demonstrates a FAILURE to exercise "due regard for the safety of others"?
   a. You are en route to the scene of an emergency and cautiously move through a red light, slowing down as you enter the intersection.
   b. En route to an emergency scene, you drive the wrong way down a one-way street without using any warning devices.
   c. You park your vehicle over the crest of a hill on a busy highway, post flares, and direct traffic around your location.
   d. You exceed the speed limit in accordance with state and local regulations while responding to the scene of an emergency.

3. One way to help maintain control of an ambulance is
   a. Accelerate into a curve, decelerate going out
   b. Ensure safe arrival by avoiding alternative routes
   c. Know the "high-traffic" areas and times
   d. Do not get distracted by road safety hazards

4. Select the statement that best describes the appropriate use of escorts.
   a. Since the use of escorts will decrease your response time to the scene of an emergency, they should never be used.
   b. The use of escorts significantly minimizes the dangers associated with emergency driving.
   c. The use of escorts doubles the hazards associated with emergency driving and should only be used as a last resort.
   d. You should make use of escorts even when you are familiar with the area to expedite transport times.

5. Which of the following is NOT a phase of an ambulance call?
   a. Dispatch
   b. Debriefing
   c. Post run
   d. En route to the station

6. List at least three benefits of an emergency vehicle maintenance and inspection schedule.

7. List six points of information you should receive from the dispatcher.

8. En route to the scene, it is a good practice to
   a. Determine and clarify the responsibilities of each team member
   b. Pre-alert medical direction of the nature of the call
   c. Drive as fast as possible to reduce response time
   d. Check on fuel levels to ensure you have enough for the return trip

9. All of the following are basic medical and non-medical supplies and equipment you would find on a properly supplied ambulance EXCEPT
   a. Comprehensive local street maps and personal protective equipment
   b. Patient transfer equipment and basic wound care supplies
   c. "Jaws of Life" and an assortment of hand tools
   d. Airway and oxygenation adjuncts and medications

10. At the scene of a collision, you should park
   a. In front of or behind the collision
   b. On the opposite side of the street or road
   c. As close to the patient(s) as possible
   d. Never park at the scene of a collision

11. Stay a minimum of ___ feet from wreckage or a burning vehicle and ___ feet from hazardous materials spills.
    a. 2000, 100
    b. 100, 2000
    c. 200, 1000
    d. 1000, 200

12. Before moving the ambulance
    a. Make sure the outside compartment doors are secure
    b. Tell the patient where you are taking him
    c. Make sure your patient is settled
    d. All of the above

13. En route to the receiving facility, conduct an ongoing assessment at least every ___ minutes for a stable patient and every ___ minutes for an unstable patient.
    a. 5, 15
    b. 10, 10
    c. 15, 5
    d. 20, 1

14. En route to the receiving facility
    a. Review unit security and check fuel consumption
    b. Do not disturb the driver with patient information
    c. Review patient priorities and check interventions
    d. All of the above

15. A complete oral report should be given to emergency department personnel at the patient's bedside in order to
    a. Ensure proper continuity of care
    b. Expedite the patient's admission into the hospital
    c. Reassess the patient's condition and interventions
    d. Reassure the patient

16. The written prehospital care report
    a. Should never be given to the patient
    b. May substitute for all other reports
    c. Is not necessary if you have given an oral report
    d. Should be left at the emergency department

17. Once you have completed a call, explain what you should do to prepare for a return to service.

18. The word ___ refers to process that kills all microorganisms.
    a. Sterilize
    b. Disinfect
    c. Clean
    d. Wash

19. A formula for making an intermediate-level disinfectant is:
   a. 1:10 solution of household bleach and water
   b. 1:20 solution of household bleach and water
   c. 1:50 solution of household bleach and water
   d. 1:100 solution of household bleach and water

20. Write a number in each blank. Match the level of disinfection or sterilization with the surface or equipment for which it is appropriate.

   1. low-level disinfection

   2. intermediate-level disinfection

   3. high-level disinfection

   4. sterilization

____ a. Reusable instruments that made contact with mucous membranes
____ b. Environmental surfaces with no visible contamination and no suspected TB
____ c. Instruments that are used invasively
____ d. Surfaces that come in contact with intact skin

21. An important guideline to keep in mind when transferring care to or from an aeromedical EMS service is
   a. Make sure the landing area is clear of obstructions
   b. Keep patient and crew clear of the air downwash area
   c. Wear eye and ear protection in the landing zone
   d. All of these

CASE STUDY

You have been dispatched to an "unknown medical emergency involving a school bus" near the intersection of Bruce Road and Fitzgerald Avenue. While your partner verifies the dispatch information and starts the engine of the ambulance, you quickly check the vehicle to make sure all is secure.

1. What should you do en route to prepare for this call?

There are no obvious environmental dangers present at the scene; however, rush hour will begin soon and traffic may pose a problem. The bus is parked at an angle near the shoulder of the road, the engine has been turned off, and all the children have disembarked. They are standing in the field just to the right of the bus. One of the older children has told you, "The bus driver, Mr. Michaels, is in the bus. He is sick and looks really bad." You and your partner have agreed that you will serve as the patient attendant.

2. What should you do first? What should your partner do?

    The police have arrived and taken charge of the children, none of whom were hurt. You have determined that Mr. Michaels is a high priority for transport and have proceeded with patient assessment and emergency care. Then, with the help of your partner, you move Mr. Michaels off the bus onto your stretcher and start him on oxygen via a nonrebreather mask at 15 lpm.

3. What should be done en route to the receiving facility?

GAINING ACCESS AND EXTRICATION

COGNITIVE OBJECTIVES

Numbered objectives are from the United States Department of Transportation 1994 EMT-Basic National Standard Curriculum. Asterisked objectives, if any, pertain to material that is supplemental to the DOT curriculum.

7-2.1   Describe the purpose of extrication.

7-2.2   Discuss the role of the EMT-Basic in extrication.

7-2.3   Identify what equipment for personal safety is required for the EMT-Basic.

7-2.4   Define the fundamental components of extrication.

7-2.5   State the steps that should be taken to protect the patient during extrication.

7-2.6   Evaluate various methods of gaining access to the patient.

7-2.7   Distinguish between simple and complex access.

KEY IDEAS

Your primary role in a rescue situation is gaining access to the patient as quickly as can be safely accomplished in order to perform patient assessment and care. Your two major priorities are to keep yourself and your partner safe and to prevent further harm to the patient.

▶ Proper protective clothing and equipment must be used at every incident in which hazards (such as shattered glass, sharp metal, flammable liquids, battery acid, and body fluids) are present.

▶ If you are first to arrive at the scene, you may be responsible for scene size-up and scene stabilization until police, fire, and other rescue personnel arrive. The most frequent rescue situations are motor vehicle collisions. Related hazards include downed electrical lines and uncontrolled traffic.

▶ After all hazards are addressed and the scene is secure, the vehicles involved must be properly stabilized by specially trained rescue personnel. A vehicle is considered stable when it is in a secured position and can no longer move, rock, or bounce.

▶ Most emergency calls do not present access problems. However, when they do, it is best to call for rescuers who have had specialized training. Residential access includes locating the patient first and evaluating the need for a forced entry based on dispatch information, what you observe at the scene, and your conversation with the patient. In a motor vehicle collision, the access of choice is a door.

▶ The role of the EMT-B in vehicle stabilization and patient extrication is that of patient care provider. Once specialized rescue personnel assure you that a vehicle is stabilized and the scene is safe, you may approach the patient to initiate care. Patient care always precedes removal from the vehicle unless delay would endanger the life of the patient, EMS personnel, or other rescuers.

▶ After gaining access to a patient, provide the same care you would provide to any trauma patient. In addition, you are responsible for assisting the patient through the extrication process and preparing him mentally and physically for disentanglement from the wreckage. Be sure to stabilize and, if possible, immobilize the spine securely before you remove the patient from the vehicle by normal or rapid extrication procedures.

CONTENT REVIEW

1. When should you first begin to plan for access and extrication problems?
   a. When receiving dispatch information
   b. While en route to the incident
   c. While you are approaching the scene
   d. After effectively evaluating the scene

2. Which of the following will present the most frequent rescue problems for an EMT-B?
   a. Water rescue incidents
   b. Motor vehicle collisions
   c. Partial or complete building collapse
   d. Worksite accidents

3. All ambulances should carry _____ to assess the scene from a safe distance.
   a. An air particle sniffer
   b. A cellular telephone
   c. Powerful binoculars
   d. Protective outerwear

4. Identify the most appropriate equipment for personnel involved in the vehicle extrication process.
   a. Full protective turnout gear
   b. Work uniform with helmet
   c. Protective coveralls, helmet, and work gloves
   d. Safety helmet with safety shield

5. When dealing with electrical power lines, which of the following is correct?
   a. Never assume downed lines are electrically alive.
   b. Power lines that are not arcing are considered safe.
   c. Always assume downed lines are electrically alive.
   d. Remove power lines only when wearing rubber gloves.

6. In general, what is the safest method of traffic control at a serious vehicle collision?
   a. Stop all traffic and turn it around.
   b. Stop all traffic and reroute it to different roads.
   c. Slowly guide the vehicles around the scene.
   d. Patiently wait until the scene is cleared.

7. While working a vehicle collision, you notice a small sweater in the rear seat of one of the vehicles. What might this indicate?

8. A vehicle is stable when
   a. Cribbing has been placed front and rear
   b. All four tires are on a flat surface
   c. It can no longer move, rock, or bounce
   d. The engine is off and the parking brake is set

9. The majority of electric current hazards associated with auto collisions can be most simply and quickly eliminated when someone
   a. Disconnects the battery
   b. Pulls the main fuse
   c. Disables the coil wire
   d. Turns off the ignition

10. Briefly explain what steps should be taken to provide patient access in a vehicle collision before turning off or disconnecting the vehhicle's power.

11. If it is necessary to disconnect the car battery, cut or use a wrench
   a. To remove the negative battery cable first
   b. To disconnect the cable on the starter
   c. To disconnect the positive cable first
   d. To lift the battery out of the engine compartment

12. Explain simple access and complex access.
   a. Simple access

   b. Complex access

13. Police are on the scene, and you are about to make forcible entry into a residence for a medical emergency. Which of the following is the quickest, easiest, and least costly method of forcible entry?
    a. Breaking a window
    b. Forcing a door open
    c. Cutting a door lock
    d. Calling a locksmith

14. The patient is pinned inside a vehicle involved in a collision. He is in the driver's seat, facing front. How should you approach him?
    a. From the left side
    b. From the right side
    c. From the front
    d. From directly behind

15. Your patient is pinned inside a vehicle involved in a collision. What is the best way to tell him to unlock the door?
    a. "Unlock the door, but please turn your body at the shoulders."
    b. "Turn your body at the shoulders, then try to unlock the door."
    c. "Try to unlock the door, but don't move your head or neck."
    d. "Without moving your head or neck, try to unlock the door."

16. When using a sharp tool like a screwdriver to break a vehicle window, the tool should be placed ___ of the window.
    a. Against the direct center
    b. Against the upper center
    c. Against a lower corner
    d. Against a upper corner

17. Patient care always precedes removal from the vehicle EXCEPT when
    a. The patient is hysterical and tries to extricate himself
    b. Delaying removal would endanger the patient or rescue personnel
    c. The vehicle extrication will take over an hour
    d. There is minor damage and the patient can be extricated quickly

18. To protect yourself, the patient, and other EMT-Bs from the glass and flying debris that commonly result from disentanglement operations
    a. Cover the patient with your body
    b. Direct the patient to move to the back seat
    c. Share your personal protective equipment with those at the scene
    d. Use blankets, a tarp, or a spine board

19. To help reduce your patient's fears while being extricated, you should
    a. Reassure the patient that you are highly skilled
    b. Explain the activities, noises, and movements
    c. Try to have the patient think of pleasant thoughts
    d. Explain that this is an everyday routine occurrence

20. Stabilize and, if possible, immobilize the spine before you remove the patient from the collision vehicle. Identify the only exception to this rule.

CASE STUDY
▼

You and your partner are working overtime as a standby crew at a local polo match. The last chukker has been completed when you hear a loud screech followed by a terrible crash. You both look toward the highway and see a large luxury car wrapped around a utility pole. Joe quickly advises dispatch of the situation, that the match has ended, and that you will be responding. As you approach the scene, you notice an electrical line that is broken 80 feet from the pole and is lying across the hood of the car. A crowd of bystanders has begun to surround the scene. Joe radios dispatch, advises them of the utility line, and requests the power company. A polo grounds security guard tells you that the power has been shut off by his personnel. You can visualize the patient in the car; the middle-aged man is trying to remove his seat belt.

1. Which of the following is the correct way to secure this scene?
   a. Secure an area that is more than 80 feet in all directions. Do not approach the vehicle. Yell instructions to the patient and advise him to stay in the vehicle.
   b. Secure an area up to 75 feet in all directions in case the power is restored. Approach the vehicle, since the guard advised the power is off, and begin to assess the patient.
   c. There is no reason to secure a perimeter since the power is off; however, you should advise bystanders to keep back so you can work.
   d. Ask bystanders to keep back at least 40 feet (half the distance from the pole). This will keep them clear of danger. Then yell to the patient to stay in the vehicle.

2. Until you are able to gain access, which of the following is the most appropriate way to keep this patient from moving his head and neck?
   a. Instruct the patient to place his hands on either side of his head.
   b. Instruct the patient to close his eyes and try to block out what is happening around him.
   c. Tell the patient to focus and keep his attention on an object directly in front of him.
   d. Have the patient try to lie down across the front seat and remain absolutely still.

3. Briefly explain how you and your partner can decrease the fears that this patient may experience during the noise and confusion that often accompany disentanglement.

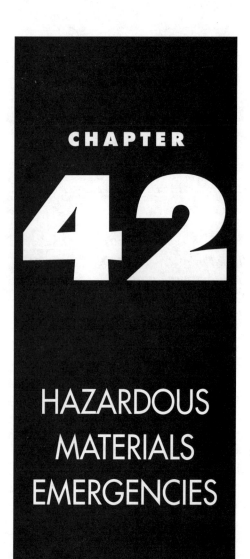

CHAPTER

42

HAZARDOUS
MATERIALS
EMERGENCIES

Numbered objectives are from the United States Department of Transportation 1994 EMT-Basic National Standard Curriculum. Asterisked objectives, if any, pertain to material that is supplemental to the DOT curriculum.

7-3.1 Explain the EMT-Basic's role during a call involving hazardous materials.

7-3.2 Describe what the EMT-Basic should do if there is reason to believe that there is a hazard at the scene.

7-3.3 Describe the actions that an EMT-Basic should take to ensure bystander safety.

7-3.4 State the role the EMT-Basic should perform until appropriately trained personnel arrive at the scene of a hazardous materials situation.

7-3.5 Break down the steps to approaching a hazardous situation.

7-3.6 Discuss the various environmental hazards that affect EMS.

7-3.11 Describe basic concepts of incident management.

7-3.12 Explain the methods for preventing contamination of self, equipment, and facilities.

KEY IDEAS

Hazardous materials spills and incidents are increasing in frequency. The EMT-Basic's role in such emergencies is to recognize that a hazardous material emergency exists and to secure the scene until trained rescuers arrive. This chapter reviews recognition and EMS management of hazardous materials emergencies. Personal safety of the EMT-Basic is emphasized.

▶ The principle dangers from hazardous materials are toxicity, flammability, and reactivity.

▶ The amount of injury caused by a hazardous material depends upon the dose, concentration, and amount of time the patient is exposed.

▶ The primary concerns in any hazardous materials emergency are rescuer safety, public safety, and patient safety.

▶ The U.S. Department of Transportation's regulations require hazardous materials packages and containers to be marked and accompanied by shipping papers.

▶ Resources for hazardous materials identification and management include state and local agencies, state and local hazardous materials teams, the U.S. Department of Transportation's *Hazardous Materials: Emergency Response Guidebook*, and CHEMTREC (1-800-424-9300).

▶ Avoid contact with any unidentified material, regardless of the level of protection offered by your clothing and equipment.

▶ The most essential part of hazardous materials rescue is pre-incident planning. Plan for the worst possible scenario and tailor the plan to the individual community. As part of your plan, predesignate an incident command officer, establish a clear chain of command and a system of communications, and predesignate receiving facilities.

▶ An early priority at the scene of any hazardous material emergency is to establish safety zones in which rescue operations may be carried out. These zones are the hot (contaminated) zone, warm (control) zone, and the cold (safe) zones.

▶ Do not enter the hazardous materials area unless you are trained at least to the hazardous materials technician level and are trained in the use of SCBA (self-contained breathing apparatus). If you have had no training, radio immediately for help. While you are waiting for help to arrive, protect yourself and bystanders by keeping uphill, upwind, and away from danger.

TERMS AND CONCEPTS

1. **Write the number of the correct term next to each definition.**

   1. warm zone
   2. cold zone
   3. safety zone
   4. hot zone

   _____ **a.** Area surrounding an accident involving hazardous materials, designated for specific rescue operations

   _____ **b.** Area adjacent to the warm zone in a hazardous materials emergency; normal triage, treatment, and stabilization are performed here; also called safe zone

   _____ **c.** Area where contamination is actually present; it generally is the area that is immediately adjacent to the accident site and where contamination can still occur; also called contamination zone

   _____ **d.** Area that is established surrounding or immediately adjacent to the hot zone, the purpose of which is to prevent the spread of contamination; also called control zone

CONTENT REVIEW

1. The primary concern in any hazardous materials emergency is
   a. Preservation of property
   b. Rescuer, public, and patient safety
   c. Rapid control and removal of the hazard
   d. Locating placards and shipping papers

2. The amount of damage caused by exposure to hazardous materials depends upon
   a. Dose, concentration, time exposed
   b. Dose, expiration date, time exposed
   c. Dose, route of exposure, time exposed
   d. Dose, whether internal or external, time exposed

3. A hazardous materials warning label required by the U.S. Department of Transportation is usually
   a. A circle with a triangle in the center
   b. Two concentric circles
   c. A four-sided diamond shape
   d. A triangle with the point down

4. In the internationally recognized NFPA 704 Hazardous Materials Identification System, a blue diamond indicates a
   a. Health hazard
   b. Fire hazard
   c. Reactivity hazard
   d. Protective equipment required

5. An important resource available to rescuers 24 hours per day is a public service division of the Chemical Manufacturer's Association. It is referred to as
   a. Chemical Transportation Emergency Center (CHEMTREC)
   b. Chemical Transportation Awareness Program (CHEMAWARE)
   c. Chemical Emergency Response Guide (CHEMERG)
   d. Chemical Manufacturer's Association Center (CHEMMAC)

6. List at least three visual clues that can indicate the probable presence of a hazardous material.

7. Never just assume that the area surrounding a spill or leak is dangerous.
   a. True
   b. False

8. If you have the four-digit identification number of the hazardous material, you can find complete emergency instructions in a book published by the U.S. Department of Transportation. What is the title of this important resource?

9. OSHA (Occupational Safety and Health Administration) and the EPA (Environmental Protection Agency) have developed regulations meant to enhance the safety of rescuers. List the four levels of training OSHA and the EPA identify as necessary for dealing with hazardous materials emergencies.

10. Smoke from a hazardous materials fire
    a. Has been rendered harmless by the fire
    b. Poses no concern to health and safety
    c. Presents an environmental hazard
    d. Has only short-term health effects

11. Avoid contact with any unidentified material, regardless of the level of protection offered by your clothing and equipment.
    a. True
    b. False

12. There are three general priorities in a hazardous materials emergency in an order that never changes. Indicate that order by writing 1, 2, and 3.
    ____ a. Decontaminate clothing, equipment, and the vehicle.
    ____ b. Protect the safety of all rescuers and victims.
    ____ c. Provide patient care.

13. Your duty is to risk your life and/or your health in a hazardous materials emergency, even if the only threat is to the environment.
    a. True
    b. False

14. Prior to air transport of a contaminated patient be sure to
    a. Establish a landing zone within the hot zone
    b. Decontaminate the patient fully
    c. Contact the patient's family
    d. Contact the receiving facility

15. If you have no training to handle a hazardous materials emergency, radio immediately for help and
    a. Keep downhill, downwind, and away from the danger
    b. Keep downhill, upwind, and away from the danger
    c. Keep uphill, upwind, and away from the danger
    d. Keep uphill, downwind, and away from the danger

16. List six steps you should take in the personal care of your body when you are accidentally exposed to hazardous materials.

CASE STUDY 1

You have responded to a call for an overturned tractor-trailer on a remote stretch of highway. From a distance you observe green smoke escaping from the back of the trailer. A man, standing about 100 yards away, waves you down. You pull over and watch him walk up to you. The man is about 45 years old and looks well. He has a normal gait and does not appear to be injured. You ask him "Why did you call the ambulance?" He says, "I don't know who called you. I called the police. Hey, I was alone, I fell asleep, I ran off the road. I bounced around inside the truck, and then I was crawling out of it." While talking to the patient, you use your binoculars and spot an orange panel on the back of the truck. You take out your Guidebook to look up the ID number and determine that the number refers to chlorine gas.

1. What is your next BEST action to take?
   a. Enter the truck cab and search for shipping papers.
   b. Approach from downwind to survey the scene.
   c. Enter the truck cab and search for additional victims.
   d. Quickly request additional assistance.

2. After taking the action above, what is your next BEST action?
   a. Call CHEMTREC for hazard control information.
   b. Enter the trailer and begin decontamination procedures.
   c. Keep uphill, upwind, and protect yourself and the patient.
   d. Crack open the trailer doors to vent and prevent build-up of fumes.

CASE STUDY 2

You have responded to a hazardous materials accident. The patient is being decontaminated. You arrive on scene and report to the staging area. Shortly after, you are called to the cold zone to transport the patient.

1. You are accidentally splashed with contamination from an anxious and fatigued rescuer. Contamination can occur most easily in what areas of your body?
   a. Lower legs and feet
   b. Lower arms and hands
   c. Under the arms and in the groin
   d. Back

2. How should you decontaminate yourself?
   a. Wash with green soap and plenty of running water, irrigating skin for at least 20 minutes.
   b. Use high pressure hoses to wash and irrigate skin for at least 20 minutes.
   c. Use baking soda to neutralize the contaminant, then stand under running water for at least 20 minutes.
   d. Blot your skin with towels for at least 20 minutes, and dispose of the towels in a sealed biohazard container.

3. What precautions should be undertaken prior to transport of the decontaminated patient?
   a. Treat the patient's major and minor injuries in the hot zone before moving.
   b. Cover exposed areas of the vehicle with plastic sheeting.
   c. Transport the patient's clothing with the patient and leave it at the hospital.
   d. Transport with the patient any contaminated patient care equipment used in the hot zone.

CASE STUDY 3

You have responded to a call for a "man down" at a local fertilizer distributor. You arrive on scene and observe smoke billowing from the building. A bystander is preparing to enter the building to put the fire out with a garden hose.

1. What should you do?
   a. You should remove the bystander, evacuate the area, and contact dispatch.
   b. You, the bystander, and your partner should enter to put out the fire.
   c. You should contact dispatch while your partner puts out the fire.
   d. You should contact dispatch and remain near the building to direct fire fighters.

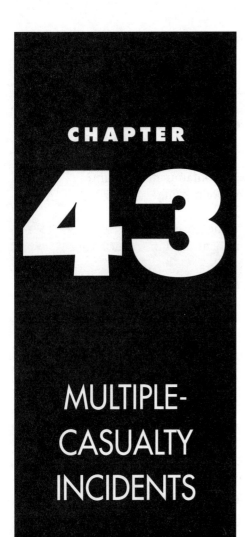

CHAPTER

43

MULTIPLE-
CASUALTY
INCIDENTS

COGNITIVE OBJECTIVES

Numbered objectives are from the United States Department of Transportation 1994 EMT-Basic National Standard Curriculum. Asterisked objectives, if any, pertain to material that is supplemental to the DOT curriculum.

7-3.7   Describe the criteria for a multiple-casualty situation.

7-3.8   Evaluate the role of the EMT-Basic in the multiple-casualty situation.

7-3.9   Summarize the components of basic triage.

7-3.10 Define the role of the EMT-Basic in a disaster operation.

7-3.11 Describe the basic concepts of incident management.

7-3.13 Review the local mass casualty incident plan.

*Outline the ways to get help in a multiple-casualty incident.

*Describe various approaches for reducing rescue personnel stress during an MCI or disaster.

KEY IDEAS

A multiple-casualty incident (MCI) can occur without warning at any time or place. This chapter reviews fundamental management techniques for MCIs. Review local community plans for specific MCI procedures.

▶ A multiple-casualty incident (MCI) is an event that places excessive demands on personnel and equipment.

▶ In any MCI, call for plenty of help as quickly as possible.

▶ An incident management system is a written plan to help control, direct, and coordinate emergency personnel and equipment in the event of an MCI. In a unified command system, decisions are made in collaboration by representatives of EMS, fire, and law enforcement agencies. In a single command system, one agency is given the authority to manage all emergency response resources.

▶ The EMS incident manager is the senior EMT who is first to arrive at the scene of an MCI or may be a predesignated officer. The EMS incident manager may or may not also be the incident manager, in charge of EMS and all other emergency response resources at the scene of an MCI.

▶ The incident manager establishes seven sectors that are managed by sector officers. These include mobile command, supply, extrication, triage, treatment, staging, and transportation sectors.

▶ The communications center should be provided the following information as soon as possible by the incident manager: name of agency calling, type of incident, location of incident, approximate number of patients, additional EMS personnel and/or equipment/supplies needed, and any additional emergency agencies or expert response required.

▶ EMT-Bs responding to the scene should first report to the mobile command sector for instructions.

▶ Triage is a system used for sorting patients to determine the order in which they will receive care. Triage is performed in the triage sector. If you are assigned to the triage sector, perform a quick initial assessment of all patients. The initial treatments are limited to airway and bleeding control until all patients have been triaged.

▶ Typically, there are three or four triage priority levels. Level 1 (High Priority) are patients who require immediate transport, Level 2 (Second Priority) patients who will survive even if care is somewhat delayed, and Level 3 (Low Priority) those who do not require or will not benefit from prompt care. A four-level system uses Priority 0 to identify the dead or fatally injured.

▶ Typical patient identification systems use colors to signify priorities of care: High = red, Second = yellow, Low = green, Priority 0 = gray or black.

▶ To reduce stress on yourself and other rescue personnel who are involved in an MCI, rest at regular intervals. Be aware of your exact assignment. Several workers should watch for signs of physical exhaustion and stress in other rescuers. Plenty of food and drinks should be provided, and workers should be encouraged to talk among themselves.

TERMS AND CONCEPTS

1. Write the number of the correct term next to each definition.

　　1. treatment sector

　　2. disaster

　　3. triage

　　4. multiple-casualty incident (MCI)

　　5. mobile command center

　　6. extrication sector

　　7. EMS incident manager

　　8. transportation sector

　　9. incident manager

　10. triage sector

　11. incident management system

　12. supply sector

　13. staging sector

_____ **a.** Monitors, inventories, and directs available ambulances to the treatment sector at the request of the transportation officer

_____ **b.** An event that places excessive demands on EMS personnel and equipment

_____ **c.** The senior EMT who is the first to arrive at a multiple-casualty scene or a predesignated officer; responsible for seeing that the multiple-casualty incident is responded to in a controlled and orderly way and that all responsibilities are carried out

_____ **d.** Responsible for prioritizing patients for emergency medical care and transport

_____ **e.** The headquarters for the incident manger; the EMS command post — coordinates the MCI response activities of all sectors

_____ **f.** The person in charge of the incident management system at an MCI; also called the incident commander

_____ **g.** A sudden catastrophic event that overwhelms natural order and causes great loss of property and/or life

_____ **h.** Responsible for inventory and distribution of the medical materials and equipment necessary to render care

_____ **i.** Responsible for freeing patients from wreckage and managing them at the accident site

_____ **j.** The process of sorting patients to determine the order in which they will receive care or transport

_____ **k.** A written plan to help control, direct, and coordinate emergency personnel at the scene of an MCI

_____ **l.** Responsible for collecting and treating patients in a centralized treatment area

_____ **m.** Coordinates patient transportation with the triage and staging sectors and its officer communicates with the hospitals involved

CONTENT REVIEW

1. This system works best when the MCI involves more that one emergency response agency.
   a. Multiple command system
   b. Unified command system
   c. Single command system
   d. Disaster command system

2. The incident manager (commander) should be stationed in a command center located
   a. Near the supply sector
   b. Near the area where patients are extricated
   c. Near or at the staging sector for the MCI
   d. Near the area where patients will be loaded for transport

3. The senior EMT who arrives first at the scene of an MCI or disaster
   a. Assumes EMS incident manager until relieved
   b. Assumes command of the staging sector
   c. Assumes command of the transport sector
   d. Assumes command of the treatment sector

4. Each sector officer
   a. Coordinates all aspects of the incident
   b. Works without the control of the incident manager
   c. Wears a highly visible reflective vest
   d. Determines transport priorities for all patients to the hospital(s)

5. The goals of triage include
   a. To assess and assign a priority to each patient
   b. To provide comprehensive treatment to each patient
   c. To perform a detailed physical exam on each patient
   d. To transport all patients as rapidly as possible

6. To perform a rapid triage of multiple patients you should
   a. Check for an airway only
   b. Check for airway and pulse only
   c. Check for bleeding only
   d. Perform a quick initial assessment

7. Patients who are transported first in a three-level priority triage system are
   a. Priority 1
   b. Priority 2
   c. Priority 3
   d. Priority 0

8. Cardiac arrest patients are generally assigned to what priority when there are limited numbers of rescuers on scene?
   a. High priority
   b. Second priority
   c. Low priority
   d. These patient are moved and transported rapidly, so they are not assigned a priority.

9. A typical patient tagging system uses colors to triage and identify patients. Red would be used to signify a
   a. High priority patient
   b. Second priority patient
   c. Low priority patient
   d. Priority 0 or fourth level

10. Patients should be organized in the treatment area according to
   a. Approximate age
   b. Order they were brought to the treatment area
   c. Kind of injury or condition
   d. Triage or priority level

11. Which of the following will help to reduce stress on rescuers during an MCI incident?
   a. Have rescuers work in 8-to-10-hour shifts and then perform less stressful tasks.
   b. Give a motivating talk to any rescuer who becomes hysterical.
   c. Provide plenty of nourishing food and drinks.
   d. Encourage rescue workers not to talk among themselves.

CASE STUDY

▼

You have been dispatched to the scene of a bus-train collision. You are the senior EMT-B on the vehicle and you are the closest responding unit to the scene. Your partner quickly pulls out the local "Disaster Response Packet" and reviews the MCI plan. You arrive on scene and observe a large commercial bus that has been struck by a train. The bus has been pushed at least 50 yards from the crossing. There is extensive damage to the bus. There are at least 10 bystanders who are next to the bus waving at you to hurry. Several patients have been removed from the bus and are being treated by bystanders. A law enforcement officer grabs you by the arm as you exit the vehicle and tells you, "You had better get some help out here! There are at least 40 people injured. There are people lying all over the place. Tell 'em to hurry!"

1. What is your BEST first action to take?
    a. Establish a mobile command sector.
    b. Request additional help and assistance.
    c. Have the walking wounded patients walk to the treatment area.
    d. Triage all patients to determine the total number of injured patients.

2. Who should initially assume the role of EMS incident manager?
    a. The Law Enforcement officer
    b. First-arriving fire service personnel
    c. You, as the senior EMT on the scene
    d. No one. Wait for the designated EMS MCI incident manager to arrive on the scene.

3. The EMS incident manager should work closely with fire and law enforcement to
    a. Begin the transport of the walking wounded
    b. Communicate with the media
    c. Position arriving rescue vehicles
    d. Move the obviously dead patients to the morgue holding area

4. Triage the following patients from this bus accident as High Priority (H), Second Priority (S), or Low Priority (L).

    _____ a. A patient with a large leg wound that is bleeding severely

    _____ b. A patient who is unresponsive to verbal or painful stimuli

    _____ c. A patient complaining of back pain who is unable to feel or move his legs

    _____ d. A patient with several lacerations and minor bleeding

    _____ e. A patient with breathing difficulty

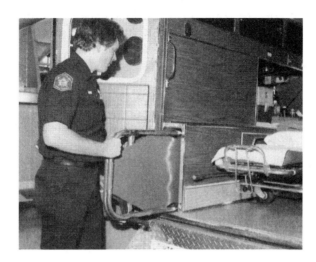

Previous modules have dealt with the assessment and emergency care of patients. In the operations module, you have been learning primarily about the daily nuts-and-bolts nonmedical aspects of your job as an EMT-Basic — as well as approaches to some special situations such as gaining access and the management of hazardous materials emergencies and multiple-casualty incidents.

Q What are the major aspects of ambulance operation?

A For the EMT-Basic who will drive the ambulance, development of safe and effective driving skills and knowledge of the special laws regulating operation of emergency vehicles are essential. All members of the crew must participate in the necessary chores of making sure that the unit is operational, that the ambulance is fully supplied at all times, and that the unit is properly cleaned and disinfected before notifying dispatch that you are clear for the next call. Specific tasks must be performed during each of the eight phases of an ambulance call: pre-run preparation, dispatch, en route to the scene, at the scene, en route to the receiving facility, at the receiving facility, en route to the station, and post run.

Q What is the primary role of the EMT-Basic during a rescue operation?

A If you are not a trained member of a rescue crew, you must call for expert assistance and wait until they have secured the scene, for example, by stabilizing a collision vehicle. Your role as an EMT-B is to gain access to the patient or patients as quickly as can be safely accomplished in order to perform patient assessment and care, even as the rescue operation proceeds. Your major priorities at the rescue scene are to keep yourself and your partner safe and to prevent further harm to your patient.

Q What is the role of the EMT-B at a hazardous materials emergency?

A The EMT-B is not required to deal with hazardous materials. You should be able to identify the possibility of a hazardous material accident from a safe distance, call for the assistance of a specialized hazardous materials team, and protect yourself and bystanders by keeping uphill, upwind, and away from the danger. Patients will be removed from the accident site and decontaminated by those equipped to do so. However, even after decontamination, there may still be some contamination present on patients or equipment. Exercise caution and take measures to protect your equipment and vehicle from contamination. Prior to transport, cover all benches, floor, and other exposed areas of your unit with thick plastic sheeting secured with duct tape. Leave all contaminated clothing and equipment at the scene. Following the incident, wash your unit and equipment, your clothing, and yourself thoroughly. Seek medical help immediately if you develop symptoms of illness following a hazardous material incident.

Q   What is the role of the EMT-B at a multiple-casualty incident?

A   Emergency care at a multiple-casualty incident will be conducted according to a preset disaster response plan. Most jurisdictions use some version of the incident management system. Under this system, the senior EMT who arrives first becomes the EMS incident manager until relieved by a more senior or predesignated person. Under a unified system, management of the disaster is coordinated by predesignated representatives of EMS, fire, and police services. In an incident command system, the following sectors are usually established at the scene of the multiple-casualty incident: mobile command sector, supply sector, extrication sector, triage sector, treatment sector, staging sector, and transportation sector. Patients are generally triaged under a three- or four-level priority system in which Priority 1 patients are those whose survival requires treatment or transport without delay and Priority 3 and 4 patients are those who do not require or will not benefit from prompt care. As an EMT-B arriving at a multiple-casualty scene, unless you are the first and senior EMT to arrive and must take command, you will be assigned to a sector and a task for which you will ideally have practiced and prepared in advance of the emergency.

Numbered objectives are from the United States Department of Transportation 1994 EMT-Basic National Standard Curriculum. Asterisked objectives, if any, pertain to material that is supplemental to the DOT curriculum.

8-1.1 Identify and describe the airway anatomy in the infant, child, and the adult.

8-1.2 Differentiate between the anatomy in the infant, child, and the adult.

8-1.3 Explain the pathophysiology of airway compromise.

8-1.4 Describe the proper use of airway adjuncts.

8-1.5 Review the use of oxygen therapy in airway management.

8-1.6 Describe the indications, contraindications, and techniques for insertion of nasal gastric tubes.

8-1.7 Describe how to perform the Sellick maneuver (cricoid pressure).

8-1.8 Describe the indications for advanced airway management.

8-1.9 List the equipment required for orotracheal intubation.

8-1.10 Describe the proper use of the curved blade for orotracheal intubation.

8-1.11 Describe the proper use of the straight blade for orotracheal intubation.

8-1.12 State the reasons for and proper use of the stylet in orotracheal intubation.

8-1.13 Describe the methods of choosing the appropriate size endotracheal tube in an adult patient.

8-1.14 State the formula for sizing the infant or child endotracheal tube.

8-1.15 List complications associated with advanced airway management.

8-1.16 Define the various alternative methods for sizing the infant and child endotracheal tube.

8-1.17 Describe the skill of orotracheal intubation in the adult patient.

8-1.18 Describe the skill of orotracheal intubation in the infant and child patient.

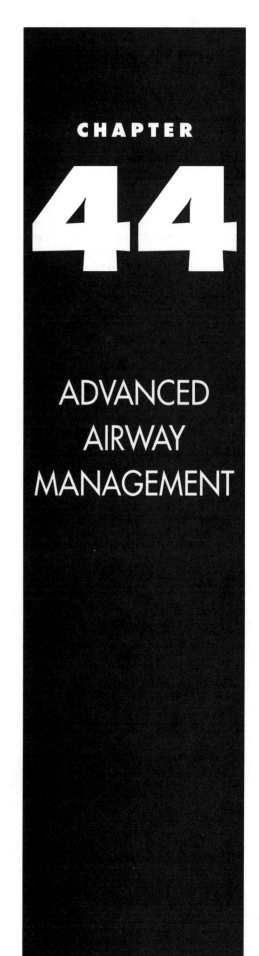

CHAPTER

44

ADVANCED AIRWAY MANAGEMENT

8-1.19 Describe the skill of confirming endotracheal tube placement in the adult, infant, and child patient.

8-1.20 State the consequence of and the need to recognize unintentional esophageal intubation.

8-1.21 Describe the skill of securing the endotracheal tube in the adult, infant, and child patient.

KEY IDEAS
▼

In some situations, manual maneuvers and basic airway adjuncts are inadequate to maintain or even to establish an airway. In these situations, the use of advanced airway adjuncts is necessary. For this reason, some EMS jurisdictions and medical directors now require EMT-Bs to become proficient in advanced airway management skills. These skills are difficult to master and require a high degree of accuracy; performed correctly, however, they offer a real opportunity to save lives.

▶ It is important to know the anatomy of the upper airway, especially the landmark structures that differentiate the opening of the larynx from the opening of the esophagus, to avoid accidental insertion of the endotracheal tube into the esophagus – a dangerous and possibly fatal error.

▶ It is important to understand how the right and left mainstem bronchi branch from the trachea at the level of the carina, the right mainstem bronchus at a much lesser angle than the left. If the endotracheal tube is advanced too far, it is likely to enter the right mainstem bronchus so that air is entering only the right lung, causing inadequate oxygenation.

▶ It is critical to master the techniques of confirming correct placement of the endotracheal tube by watching for chest rise and fall and auscultating the lungs and the epigastrium.

▶ It is critical to understand differences in airway anatomy of infants and children as compared to adults. An infant's larger head will cause the supine infant's head to tilt forward, constricting the airway; padding must be placed under the infant's shoulders to keep the airway aligned. The infant or young child's tongue is larger in proportion to the mouth and can not only cause obstruction by falling back into the airway but can also interfere with visualization of anatomical structures during intubation. The infant and child airway is narrowest at the level of the cricoid cartilage, so that a tube that passes easily through the vocal cords may be too large to pass through the cricoid ring; tubes a half-size larger and smaller than the size you estimate must be available to deal with such problems. Infant and child airway structures are softer; pressure on the cricoid and overextension of the neck during intubation can constrict the airway. Airway structures are shorter in infants and children, making intubation of the mainstem bronchus more likely.

▶ Before advanced airway techniques are initiated, basic airway techniques including manual opening of the airway, hyperventilation of the patient, and oropharyngeal suctioning must be performed.

▶ Indications for the use of endotracheal intubation include the following: the EMT-B is unable to ventilate the apneic patient with standard methods such as mouth-to-mask or bag-valve-mask ventilation; the patient cannot protect his own airway (is unresponsive to any stimulus or has no cough or gag reflex).

▶ Because the EMT-B must get very close to the patient's open mouth and contact with the patient's secretions, vomitus, and blood is unavoidable, body substance isolation including gloves, eye protection, and mask are essential during advanced airway procedures.

► The equipment used in endotracheal intubation includes the laryngoscope (used to lift the epiglottis and provide a light source for visualization of the vocal cords and glottic opening); the endotracheal tube; a stylet to stiffen the tube during insertion; a water-soluble lubricant; a 10 cc syringe to inflate the cuff at the distal end of the tube and create an airtight seal; a securing device to prevent the tube, once correctly positioned, from slipping inward or pulling outward; suctioning equipment, including a large-bore rigid catheter for clearing the oropharynx and a flexible French catheter for endoctracheal suctioning; towels or padding to raise the head or shoulders as needed for airway alignment; and a stethoscope for auscultation of the lungs and epigastrium to confirm tube placement. Special sizes of equipment must be used for infants and children. For best displacement of the tongue and visualization of the glottic opening, a straight blade is preferred in infants and children up to 8 years of age; a curved blade could be used for children 8 years and older. Uncuffed tubes are used in children under 8 years of age because the narrow cricoid ring seals the airway.

► Sellick's maneuver, also called cricoid pressure, is pressure applied over the cricoid cartilage to close off the esophagus (cutting off airflow into the stomach and helping to prevent vomiting of stomach contents) and to slightly move the glottic structures into a better position for visualization.

► Some of the more common complications of endotracheal intubation include the following: hypertension (elevated blood pressure), tachycardia (increased heart rate), and arrhythmias (irregular heart rhythms); in infants and children and some adults bradycardia (decreased heart rate) and hypotension (depressed blood pressure) may be seen; trauma to the lips, tongue, gums, teeth, and airway; inadequate oxygenation and hypoxia from prolonged (longer than 30 seconds) attempts at intubation during which the patient is receiving no oxygen; right mainstem bronchial intubation; misplacement of the endotracheal tube in the esophagus; vomiting from stimulation of the gag reflex; deflation of the cuff, causing air leakage; laryngospasm caused by stimulation of the epiglottis or vocal cords; and accidental extubation or self-extubation if the patient becomes responsive enough to pull out the tube.

► Nasogastric intubation (insertion of a flexible tube through the nose into the stomach) may be required in infants and children to relieve gastric distention that is preventing effective ventilation or when the patient is unresponsive and at risk of vomiting stomach contents.

► Contraindications to use of the nasogastric (NG) tube are as follows: An NG tube should not be inserted in a patient who has suffered major facial, head, or spinal trauma. Consult medical direction about oral insertion in such patients. An NG tube should not be inserted in a patient suspected of suffering an airway disease, which can cause spasms or exacerbate swelling to the point of occluding the airway. An NG tube should not be inserted in a patient who has ingested some caustic substances or hydrocarbons. Consult medical direction.

► Possible complications of nasogastric intubation include: tracheal intubation; nasal trauma; stimulation of the gag reflex causing vomiting; curling or kinking of the tube; perforation of the esophagus; and (rarely) passage of the tube into the cranium through a basilar skull fracture.

► Orotracheal suctioning (suctioning of the trachea to the level of the carina, as differentiated from oropharyngeal suctioning of the mouth and pharynx) can be performed by inserting a soft catheter through the endotracheal tube to remove heavy secretions that might block the airway. Possible complications include hypoxia (which can be prevented by aggressive hyperventilation of the patient before and after suctioning and applying suction for no more than 15 seconds at a time); cardiac arrhythmias or abnormal (fast or slow) heart rates resulting from stimulation of the airway or from hypoxia; coughing (which can increase pressure inside the skull and decrease blood flow to the brain, very dangerous in the case of head injury or stroke); damage to the mucosa caused by the catheter; and bronchospasm if the catheter is inserted beyond the carina into the bronchi.

TERMS AND CONCEPTS

▼

1. **Write the correct term next to each definition.**

   1. carina
   2. cricoid cartilage
   3. cuneiforms
   4. epiglottis
   5. extubation
   6. glottic opening

   7. laryngoscopy
   8. Murphy eye
   9. thyroid cartilage
   10. trachea
   11. vallecula

   _____ a. The procedure of using a laryngoscope to lift the epiglottis to visualize the vocal cords and glottic opening

   _____ b. A tubular structure that extends from the lower portion of the larynx to the bronchi

   _____ c. The bulky shield-like structure that forms the anterior surface of the larynx

   _____ d. The point of bifurcation at about the level of the fifth thoracic vertebra where the trachea splits into the right and left mainstem bronchi

   _____ e. The removal of a tube, such as an endotracheal tube

   _____ f. The space between the vocal cords

   _____ g. Elongated cartilage attached to the posterior arytenoids

   _____ h. A firm and complete circular ring located below the thyroid cartilage and attached to the first ring of the trachea

   _____ i. A leaf-shaped cartilaginous structure that covers the opening of the larynx during swallowing

   _____ j. A depression located between the base of the tongue and the epiglottis

   _____ k. A small hole opposite the bevel at the distal end of an endotracheal tube

CONTENT REVIEW

1. Fill in each term, naming the epiglottis and nearby structures, on the appropriate line.

epiglottis
glossoepiglottic ligament
tongue
vallecula

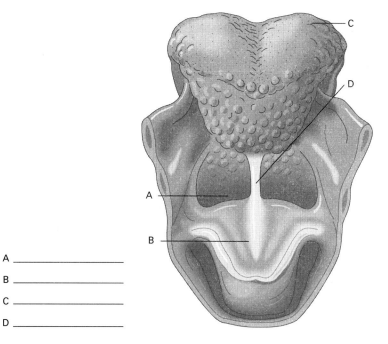

A _____

B _____

C _____

D _____

2. Fill in each term, naming the glottis and associated structures, on the appropriate line.

aryepiglottic fold
corniculate cartilage
cuneiform cartilage
epiglottis
false vocal cords
glottis
true vocal cords

A _____

B _____

C _____

D _____

E _____

F _____

G _____

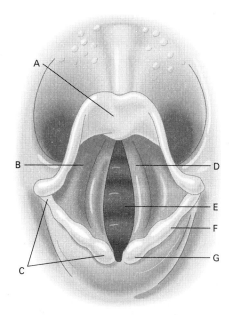

3. Which of the following explains why it is easier to misplace an endotracheal tube into the right mainstem bronchus?
   a. The left bronchioles branch from the trachea at a greater angle than the right.
   b. The right bronchioles branch from the trachea at a greater angle than the left.
   c. The left mainstem bronchus branches from the trachea at a lesser angle.
   d. The right mainstem bronchus branches from the trachea at a lesser angle.

4. To keep the airway aligned and assure airflow with the infant or small child you should
   a. Place a small folded towel under the shoulders
   b. Place padding under the back of the head (occiput)
   c. Place a small folded towel or padding under the feet
   d. With patient lying prone, place padding under the head

5. Briefly explain what may happen in most situations when basic airway management steps are not taken prior to advanced airway management.

6. When you hear gurgling sounds during ventilations, which of the following is correct?
   a. Gurgling indicates that the patient has a stoma, and this is a normal sound heard.
   b. Gurgling indicates a narrowing of the airway, and a bronchodilator is needed.
   c. Gurgling indicates an obstructed airway, and back blows are needed immediately.
   d. Gurgling indicates liquid in the airway, and suction is needed immediately.

7. List four advantages of endotracheal intubation.

8. Briefly list the indications for endotracheal intubation.

9. Which of the following is the most appropriate way to determine if a patient has lost the gag reflex?
   a. You are able to insert your index finger into the back of the throat without incident.
   b. You are able to insert an oropharyngeal airway without incident.
   c. You are able to insert a hard suction catheter without incident.
   d. You are able to insert the endotracheal tube into the oropharnx without incident.

10. Which of the following body substance isolation devices should be worn when performing endotracheal intubation?
    a. Gloves
    b. Mask
    c. Eye protection
    d. All of these

11. On the curved laryngoscope blade, the broad surface and tall flange are used to
    a. Spread the teeth to keep the mouth open
    b. Lift the vallecula
    c. Lift the epiglottis
    d. Hold the tongue out of the way

12. The curved laryngoscope blade lifts the epiglottis by
    a. Pressing on the corniculate cartilage to lift the epiglottis indirectly
    b. Pressing on the glossoepiglottic ligament to lift the epiglottis indirectly
    c. Placing the tip under the epiglottis to lift it directly
    d. Displacing the aryepiglottic fold to lift the epiglottis directly

13. If the laryngoscope light is not working or is not bright and white, briefly explain what should be checked to rectify the problem.

14. In an emergency, which size endotracheal tube will fit either an adult male or and adult female?
    a. 7.0 mm i.d.
    b. 7.5 mm i.d.
    c. 8.0 mm i.d.
    d. 9.0 mm i.d.

15. Fill in each term, naming a part of the endotracheal tube, on the correct line.

15 mm adapter

bevel

centimeter marker

cuff

inflation port

Murpy eye

pilot balloon

A _____

B _____

C _____

D _____

E _____

F _____

G _____

16. What is the purpose of the Murphy eye on the endotracheal tube?
    a. Permits airflow in the case of tube obstruction
    b. Permits easy access for suctioning the trachea
    c. Permits attachment of securing device
    d. Protects the stylet tip from injuring the trachea

17. Which of the following is true of a properly placed endotracheal tube?
    a. Distal tip of tube is in the esophagus, midway between the carina and vocal cords
    b. Distal tip of tube is in the trachea, midway between the carina and vocal cords
    c. Proximal tip of tube is in the trachea, with the distal tip extending past the carina
    d. Proximal tip of tube is in the trachea, midway between the carina and vocal cords

18. All of the following are correct regarding the use of the stylet EXCEPT
    a. Lubricate the stylet with a water-soluble jelly.
    b. Place the stylet in the tube and bend into hockey stick shape.
    c. Extend the tip of the stylet past the Murphy eye of the tube.
    d. Hold the tube securely when removing the stylet.

19. When checking an endotracheal tube prior to insertion, you should inject _____ of air into the cuff to ensure that it is working properly.
    a. 5 cc
    b. 10 cc
    c. 15 cc
    d. 20 cc

20. Briefly describe the purpose of the cuff on the endotracheal tube.

21. Briefly describe how to perform the Sellick's maneuver and how it aids in intubation.

22. Which of the following is the correct sequence for inserting the laryngoscope?
    a. Hold scope in left hand, insert into left corner of mouth, sweep tongue to right.
    b. Hold scope in left hand, insert into right corner of mouth, sweep tongue to left.
    c. Hold scope in right hand, insert into left corner of mouth, sweep tongue to left.
    d. Hold scope in right hand, insert into right corner of mouth, sweep tongue to right.

23. Briefly describe the three anatomical characteristics or landmarks that identify the glottic opening.

24. Briefly describe how to confirm correct endotracheal tube placement.

25. Which of the following are possible complications of endotracheal intubation in an adult?

1. bradycardia
2. heart dysrhythmia
3. hypertension
4. hypotension
5. tachycardia

    a. 4 and 5

    b. 1, 2, and 4

    c. 2, 3, and 5

    d. 1, 2, 3, 4, and 5

26. All of the following are indications for orotracheal intubation in infants and children EXCEPT
    a. Prolonged positive pressure ventilation is required.
    b. The patient is responsive and in severe respiratory distress.
    c. The patient is apneic and in respiratory arrest.
    d. Bag-valve mask and mouth-to-mask ventilations are inadequate.

27. All of the following statements are true regarding the straight laryngoscope blade EXCEPT
    a. The straight blade is preferred in infants because it displaces the tongue better for visualization.
    b. The straight blade directly lifts the epiglottis, exposing the vocal cords.
    c. Straight blades come in sizes 0 to 4, sizes 0 to 2 usually being used for infants and children.
    d. The straight blade is placed into the vallecula to put pressure on the glossoepiglottic ligament to lift the epiglottis.

28. Which of the following is appropriate for selecting endotracheal tube size in the infant and child?
    a. Refer to a sizing chart or commercially available resuscitation tape.
    b. Use this formula: Tube size = (12 + patient's age in years) ÷ 2.
    c. Match the child's thumb with the outside diameter of the tube.
    d. Any of these

29. All of the following can cause inadequate lung expansion or tidal volume following orotracheal intubation EXCEPT
    a. A deactivated pop-off valve on the BVM
    b. Using too small a tube so that air leaks around it
    c. The tube has become blocked with secretions.
    d. The tube has become kinked and limits the flow.

30. Briefly list two indications for nasogastric intubation in infants and children.

31. Briefly list the contraindications for nasogastric intubation in infants and children.

32. Which of the following is the correct way to measure for a nasogastric tube?
   a. Measure from angle of jaw, around the ear extending downward, until the distal end is past the xiphoid process.
   b. Measure from tip of nose, around the ear extending downward, until the distal end is past the xiphoid process.
   c. Measure from the corner of mouth, around the ear extending downward, until the distal end is past the xiphoid process.
   d. None of the above is correct.

33. Briefly explain the five possible complications of orotracheal suctioning.

CASE STUDY

It's a beautiful summer afternoon in the coastal community you work. You and your part-ner, Jill, are relaxing at your EMS station when the radio alerting system sounds: "Unit 5, respond to a report of a boat accident at Inlet State Park. Park rangers are reporting a middle-aged male not breathing." You and Jill request paramedic back-up, but you antici-pate that your unit will arrive before the back-up. As you arrive on scene, you find a crowd surrounding the patient. Park rangers are performing rescue breathing with a pocket mask. One of the rangers advises you that the patient fell out of the boat and then the boat crashed onto the rocks. Jill reports that the patient has a strong pulse but is unresponsive to painful stimulus and apneic. You ask the park ranger to hold in-line stabilization of the patient's neck since he fell from a moving boat.

1. What procedures should you immediately undertake for this patient?
   a. Measure an endotracheal tube, prepare the laryngoscope, and visualize the glottic opening.
   b. Perform a jaw thrust, insert an oropharyngeal airway, and hyperventilate with a bag-valve mask.
   c. Have the park rangers continue artificial ventilation with the pocket mask until paramedic back-up arrives.
   d. Describe the patient's condition to medical direction and then proceed according to on-line orders.

2. Is advanced airway management indicated in this case? Briefly explain your answer.

While ventilating the patient you note a gurgling sound in the upper airway. You inspect the oropharnx and find that it is full of sea water.

3. Which of the following is the most appropriate treatment for this condition?
a. Turn the patient's head to the side to allow the water to drain.
b. Do nothing; sea water will not injure the patient's oropharynx.
c. Immediately suction the sea water with a rigid catheter.
d. Immediately suction the sea water with a soft catheter.

At this point, you and Jill decide to initiate endotracheal intubation. As you prepare the appropriate equipment, Jill is hyperventilating the patient.

4. Which of the following is the most appropriate rate at which to hyperventilate this patient?
a. 12 breath per minute for up to 1 minute prior to intubating
b. 16 breaths per minute for at least 1 minute prior to intubating
c. 20 breaths per minute for at least 2 minutes prior to intubating
d. 24 breaths per minute for at least 1 minute prior to intubating

Jill ceases ventilations so that you can attempt to intubate the patient. You immediately initiate visualization of the patient's glottic opening. Jill silently counts to herself and will advise you when the patient needs to be ventilated again.

5. Briefly explain how you and Jill would work together to achieve maximum visualization of the glottic opening.

6. Jill will notify you that the patient needs to be ventilated after silently counting to
a. 15 seconds
b. 30 seconds
c. 45 seconds
d. 60 seconds

After identifying the glottic opening and being careful not to lose sight of it, you watch as you guide the endotracheal tube through the opening. You remove the laryngoscope from the patient's mouth and carefully remove the stylet from the tube. You then inflate the cuff. Jill attaches the bag-valve device to the endotracheal tube and begins to ventilate so that you can confirm tube placement. The chest rises and falls during ventilations, and there are no gurgling sounds in the epigastrium. However, when you auscultate the lung fields, the left side is silent while there are normal breath sounds on the right.

7. Approximately how far beyond the vocal cords should you place the proximal end of the cuff on this patient?
   a. $1/2$ inch to 1 inch past the vocal cords
   b. 1 inch to $1^1/_2$ inches past the vocal cords
   c. $1^1/_2$ inches to 2 inches past the cords
   d. $1/_2$ inch to 2 inches past the vocal cords

8. Which of the following best describes the cause of the unequal lung sounds and the action that should be taken?
   a. The tube is past the carina and in the left mainstem bronchus. Deflate the cuff and pull back enough to restore lung sounds on the right side. When equal sounds are restored, reinflate the cuff.
   b. The tube is past the carina and in the right mainstem bronchus. Deflate the cuff and pull back enough to restore lung sounds on the left side. When equal sounds are restored, reinflate the cuff.
   c. The tube has not been properly secured in place and has been pulled out of the trachea. Hyperventilate the patient, reinsert the tube, secure in place, and reassess for correct placement.
   d. The tube has been misplaced in the esophagus. Remove the tube, hyperventilate the patient, insert the tube into the trachea, secure in place, and reassess for correct placement.

After correcting the problem with the unequal lung sounds you place an end-tidal carbon dioxide detector on the endotracheal tube. The paramedic back-up team has arrived, and you proceed to give them a complete assessment and report. The senior paramedic, Lieutenant Wilson, assesses the lung sounds and advises that there is good chest rise and fall, no sounds are heard over the epigastrium, and breath sounds and present and equal in both lungs. The patient responds to treatment and is released from the hospital a few days later. You and Jill are justified in feeling that you have saved the man's life by performing basic and advanced airway management procedures efficiently and correctly.

MODULE 8 REVIEW
ADVANCED AIRWAY MANAGEMENT:
CHAPTER 44

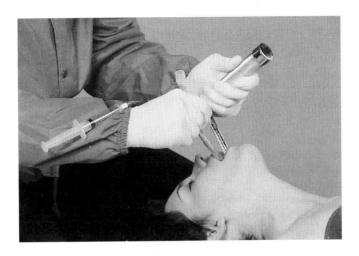

In the past, performance of advanced airway procedures was reserved for ALS personnel. However, it is the EMT-Basic who is usually first on the scene, and the ability of the EMT-B to perform advanced airway procedures before ALS assistance arrives may, in some situations, make the difference between life and death for the patient. For this reason, although advanced airway skills are difficult to master and maintain, some jurisdictions, at the discretion of the medical director, may now require that EMT-Bs receive advanced airway management training. If you are assigned to such a jurisdiction, this module will be required. If not, you may skip this module or you may want to study it as additional background.

Q **At the discretion of the medical director, and if trained to perform them, what advanced airway procedures may be performed by EMT-Bs?**

A Orotracheal intubation, nasogastric intubation in infants and children, and orotracheal suctioning.

Q **What is orotracheal intubation and when is it performed?**

A Orotracheal intubation is the insertion of a tube through the mouth and along the oropharynx and larynx, directly into the trachea. (Because the tube goes into the trachea, it is called an endotracheal tube.) The advantages of orotracheal intubation include isolation and complete control of the airway, to prevent aspiration of vomitus and other substances. Not every patient requires endotracheal intubation. It should be attempted only after basic airway techniques (such as the head-tilt, chin-lift maneuver, suctioning, and insertion of an airway adjunct such as an oropharyngeal airway) and normal ventilation methods (such as mouth-to-mask or bag-valve-mask ventilation) have been attempted. Orotracheal intubation should then be attempted if ventilation by ordinary methods is ineffective and if the patient cannot protect his own airway (is unresponsive to any stimuli and has no gag or cough reflex). Extreme care must be taken to confirm that the tube is correctly placed in the trachea. Mistaken placement of the tube in the esophagus or advancement of the tube into the right mainstem bronchus can
cause severe hypoxia and death.

(Module 8 Review continued)

Q   What is nasogastric intubation and when is it performed?

A   Nasogastric intubation is performed by the EMT-B primarily to relieve gastric distention in infants and children. (It is far easier to mistakenly force air into the esophagus in an infant or child than in an adult. If distention is severe, it will force the diaphragm upward against the lungs and prevent adequate ventilation.) A flexible tube is measured from the tip of the nose, around the ear, to below the xiphoid process. The lubricated tube is inserted through a nostril and into the esophagus. The tube is then attached to low suction to aspirate gastric contents. A nasogastric (NG) tube should not be inserted in a patient who has suffered major facial, head, or spinal trauma nor in a patient with suspected airway disease.

Q   What is orotracheal suctioning and when is it performed?

A   Orotracheal suctioning is peformed by inserting a soft suction catheter through an already-inserted endotracheal tube to clear secretions. The tube can be advanced down the endotracheal tube to the level of the carina (the point where the right and left mainstem bronchi branch off from the trachea). There are two main indications for orotracheal suctioning: obvious secretions in the endotracheal tube, and poor compliance or increased resistance when ventilating through the endotracheal tube, which may indicate a blockage in the tube. Because the patient cannot receive oxygen during orotracheal suctioning, aggressive hyperventilation for 2 minutes before and after suctioning is required and suction must be limited to 15 seconds or less in order to prevent hypoxia.

1. Which department of the United States government was charged with developing an Emergency Medical Services (EMS) system and upgrading prehospital emergency care?
   a. Department of Assessment Standards
   b. Department of Technical Assistance
   c. Department of Labor and Employment
   d. Department of Transportation (DOT)

2. The process of ensuring scene safety is BEST described by which of the following statements?
   a. Ensuring scene safety is accomplished upon arrival on scene.
   b. Ensuring scene safety is dynamic and ongoing.
   c. Ensuring scene safety begins with patient contact.
   d. Ensuring scene safety is continued until patient contact.

3. You are dispatched to a rock climber injured on a very steep hillside. Knowing that you are not trained in this type of rescue, you should
   a. Wait for a trained rescue crew
   b. Climb down to the patient
   c. Secure the patient with ropes
   d. From below, climb up to the patient

4. You are dispatched to a residence where all of the family members, including the dog, are experiencing the same signs and symptoms. What should you suspect?
   a. The dog has infected the family.
   b. The patients have the flu.
   c. The patients have become hysterical.
   d. The environment is toxic.

5. A simple way to gain consent from the adult patient is to
   a. Advise the patient that you are going to transport him/her to the hospital
   b. Ask the patient, "Is it all right for me to help you?"
   c. Ask the patient, "What happened today?"
   d. Ask the patient's family for permission to treat the patient

6. A life-threatening condition that is found during the initial assessment
   a. Should be treated once the initial assessment is completed
   b. Should be treated once the patient priorities are established
   c. Should be treated immediately as it is found
   d. Should be treated after assessing the circulation

7. Inadequate breathing should be suspected in an unresponsive patient with a respiratory rate of
   a. Less than 10 or greater than 22 per minute
   b. Less than 8 or greater than 24 per minute
   c. Less than 10 or greater than 20 per minute
   d. Less than 4 or greater than 20 per minute

8. The focused history and physical exam is performed to
   a. Identify any additional injuries or conditions that may also be life threatening
   b. Rapidly make the initial identification of life-threatening conditions
   c. Identify potential hazards that may be present on the scene
   d. Identify the total number of patients ill or injured

Course Review Self Test

9. A trauma patient with a mid-facial fracture, unequal pupils, and a deteriorating mental status requires
   a. Rapid transport without spinal immobilization
   b. Hyperventilation at 24-30 per minute with supplemental oxygen
   c. Placement of a nasopharyngeal airway and hyperventilation at 24-30 per minute
   d. Spinal immobilization and rapid transport only

10. The "S" in the SAMPLE history represents
    a. Signs and symptoms
    b. Symptoms and severity
    c. Signs and setting
    d. Setting and scenario

11. The chest of the medical patient should be auscultated at the
    a. Third intercostal space at the midclavicular line and fifth intercostal space at the midaxillary line
    b. First intercostal space at the midclavicular line and sixth intercostal space at the midaxillary line
    c. Second intercostal space at the midclavicular line and fourth intercostal space at the midaxillary line
    d. Sixth intercostal space at the midclavicular line and sixth intercostal space at the midaxillary line

12. The detailed physical exam is
    a. Always conducted on every patient
    b. Most often performed on scene prior to patient transport on the critical patient
    c. Performed to rapidly identify life threats
    d. Performed following the focused history and physical exam and after life-threatening injuries are controlled

13. A pupil that is large in size and not responding to light should be referred to as
    a. Dilated and glazed
    b. Fixed and dilated
    c. Fixed and constricted
    d. A consensual reflex

14. The purpose of the ongoing assessment is to
    a. Determine potential scene hazards
    b. Determine patient changes and assess treatments
    c. Establish priorities of patient management
    d. Evaluate system effectiveness

15. Vital signs in the unstable patient should be reassessed every _____ minutes.
    a. 2
    b. 3
    c. 5
    d. 15

16. A situation in which a drug should NOT be administered is
    a. A side effect
    b. A therapeutic effect
    c. An indication
    d. A contraindication

17. There are many different routes by which medications may be administered. Which of the following describes the correct route for administration of nitroglycerin spray?
    a. Oral
    b. Sublingual
    c. Inhalation
    d. Intramuscular

18. When you must lift a patient you should
    a. Keep your back in an unlocked position
    b. Keep your back in a locked-in position
    c. Lean backward from the waist and bend knees
    d. Lean forward from the waist and lock knees

19. When pulling an object you should keep the load
    a. Between your shoulders and hips and close to your body
    b. Between your shoulders and waist and away from your body
    c. Above the shoulders and avoid bending at the waist if possible
    d. Below the waist and avoid bending at the waist when possible

20. In which of the following circumstances should you perform an emergency move?
    a. The patient is unresponsive but is breathing and has a pulse.
    b. It is necessary to gain access to a patient who needs spinal immobilization.
    c. The patient is responsive but has an obvious head injury.
    d. It is necessary to gain access to other patients who display immediate life threats.

21. From the following, when would you NOT want to use the stair chair?
    a. The corridors and stairway are narrow.
    b. The patient has an injury to the chest.
    c. The patient weighs more than 200 pounds.
    d. The patient has an altered mental status.

22. To help take the weight of the fetus off the large blood vessels and nerves, a woman in advanced pregnancy should be placed in which position?
    a. On her left side
    b. On her right side
    c. Supine
    d. Prone

23. Each 3-month period of the approximately 9-month pregnancy is referred to as a
    a. Trimester
    b. Trigeminal
    c. Stage
    d. Period

24. The third stage of labor is the period during which
    a. Complete cervical dilation occurs
    b. The placenta is expelled
    c. The infant moves through the birth canal
    d. The amniotic sac ruptures

25. The organ that contains the developing infant is called the
    a. Perineum
    b. Cervix
    c. Placenta
    d. Uterus

26. Delivery of the infant can be expected within a few minutes if
    a. Contractions are less than 5 minutes apart and last from 15 to 20 seconds
    b. Contractions are less than 4 minutes apart and last from 15 to 25 seconds
    c. Contractions are less than 3 minutes apart and last from 20 to 25 seconds
    d. Contractions are less than 2 minutes apart and last from 30 to 90 seconds

27. When suctioning the infant's airway
    a. Suction the nose first then the mouth
    b. Suction the mouth first then the nose
    c. The nose and mouth are typically clear and do not need suction
    d. Suction either the nose or the mouth first

28. A newborn infant has bluish discoloration of the skin but has spontaneous breathing and an adequate heart rate. Select the most appropriate treatment.
    a. Begin CPR.
    b. Provide ventilations by bag-valve mask with supplemental oxygen.
    c. Provide free-flow oxygen by the "blow-by" method.
    d. Insert a nasogastric tube to decompress the stomach.

29. An anatomical difference between the airway of infants and children and the airway of adults is that in the infant's or child's airway
   a. The tongue is smaller and takes up less space in the pharynx
   b. The nose and mouth are larger
   c. The epiglottis is more U-shaped and can protrude into the pharynx
   d. The trachea is wider, harder, and less flexible

30. A "patent airway" is
   a. Partially obstructed by food or vomitus
   b. An airway that is open
   c. Also called an oropharyngeal airway
   d. Completely obstructed by the tongue

31. The oropharyngeal airway
   a. Is available in adult sizes only
   b. Passes through and extends below the larynx to hold the tongue in position
   c. Can be used on responsive patients
   d. Is rotated 180 degrees after the tip is positioned at the back of the soft palate

32. The nasopharyngeal airway
   a. Is available in one size
   b. Is more likely to stimulate vomiting than an oropharyngeal airway
   c. Can enter the esophagus if improperly measured
   d. Does not require lubrication prior to placement

33. The depth of a patient's breathing may also be referred to as
   a. Chest ventilation
   b. Tidal volume
   c. Total volume
   d. Breathing capacity

34. Excessively rapid breathing is referred to as
   a. Tachypnea
   b. Hyperpnea
   c. Dyspnea
   d. Bradypnea

35. The preferred method for performing artificial ventilation is
   a. Mouth-to-mask
   b. Bag-valve mask
   c. Flow-restricted, oxygen-powered ventilation device
   d. Automatic transport ventilator

36. The preferred method for ventilation of a patient using the bag-valve mask device requires that
   a. One EMT-B should ventilate the patient
   b. The EMT-B who ventilates should be positioned at the patient's side
   c. The pop-off valve should be activated
   d. Two EMT-Bs should ventilate the patient

37. The flow-restricted, oxygen-powered ventilation device provides
   a. A flow rate of more than 50 lpm of 60 percent oxygen
   b. Easy operation, requiring little or no training
   c. 100 percent oxygen with each ventilation
   d. Positive pressure ventilation for the adult or child patient

38. A full oxygen cylinder will generally read
   a. 1,000 PSI
   b. 1,500 PSI
   c. 1,750 PSI
   d. 2,000 PSI

39. The safe use of oxygen includes
   a. Use of oil or grease on the regulator and fittings
   b. Keeping cylinders secured when in transit
   c. Use of a valve that has been modified from another gas cylinder
   d. Storing cylinders below 200°F

40. The preferred method for the delivery of oxygen in the prehospital setting is with a
    a. Nasal cannula
    b. Simple face mask
    c. Nonrebreather mask
    d. Partial rebreather mask

41. Which of the following signs and symptoms is associated with a patient who is suffering an altered mental status with a history of diabetes controlled by medication?
    a. Slow heart rate
    b. Combativeness
    c. Warm, dry skin
    d. Calmness

42. Before oral glucose may be administered, what criteria must first be met, in addition to an on-line or off-line order from medical direction?
    a. Unresponsiveness, history of diabetes controlled by diet, ability to swallow
    b. Altered mental status, history of diabetes controlled by medication, ability to swallow
    c. Unresponsiveness, history of diabetes controlled by injections, present gag reflex
    d. Open airway, history of diabetes controlled by exercise, present gag reflex

43. When assessing pulse quality, the term "thready" refers to
    a. Strong, irregular pulse
    b. Strong, regular pulse
    c. Weak, rapid pulse
    d. Weak, irregular pulse

44. To gather the most effective information during the history-taking, you should
    a. Ask open-ended questions
    b. Ask yes-or-no questions
    c. Question a family member
    d. Ask challenging questions

45. Which of the following sets of vital signs is considered normal for a 42-year-old male?
    a. Pulse 82, blood pressure 154/72, breathing rate 24
    b. Pulse 98, blood pressure 146/92, breathing rate 18
    c. Pulse 78, blood pressure 142/68, breathing rate 12
    d. Pulse 58, blood pressure 122/54, breathing rate 10

46. Which of the following is a meeting that may precede a CISD (critical incident stress debriefing) to allow the rescuers to vent their emotions and get information before the larger group meeting?
    a. Defusing
    b. Critiquing
    c. Teaching
    d. Debriefing

47. Which of the following is the single most important way you can prevent the spread of infection?
    a. Wearing gloves
    b. Wearing a mask
    c. Hand washing
    d. Clean equipment

48. When might it be appropriate to apply a surgical mask to the patient?
    a. When blood may be splashed into the patient's face
    b. When you suspect an airborne infectious disease
    c. When the patient is suspected of having AIDS
    d. When transporting more than one patient at a time

49. Dark red blood that flows steadily from a wound usually indicates a severed or damaged
    a. Artery
    b. Vein
    c. Capillary
    d. Arteriole

50. Your patient has a large laceration to the forearm. After you have applied direct pressure and elevation, the wound continues to bleed profusely. You should
   a. Compress the popliteal pressure point
   b. Compress the femoral pressure point
   c. Compress the brachial pressure point
   d. Compress the carotid pressure point

51. Which of the following is a sign or symptom of shock?
   a. Constricted pupils
   b. Absent peripheral pulses
   c. Red, warm, dry skin
   d. Slow deep breathing

52. A child from 1 year to 3 years of age is referred to as
   a. A neonate
   b. An infant
   c. A toddler
   d. A preschooler

53. The primary goal in treating any infant or child patient is
   a. To recognize and treat respiratory problems
   b. To provide rapid transport to the hospital
   c. To reduce pain and suffering
   d. To provide spinal immobilization when required

54. An indication of respiratory arrest in the infant or child patient is
   a. Regular respirations
   b. Respiratory rate less than 10 per minute
   c. Hyperactive patient
   d. Strong peripheral pulses and an elevated heart rate

55. The best indication of a complete airway obstruction in the infant or child patient is
   a. Crying or talking
   b. Stridor upon inspiration
   c. Pale, cool, clammy skin
   d. Ineffective or absent cough

56. The normal ranges of respirations in the infant and the child are, respectively,
   a. 25-50 and 15-30
   b. 30-40 and 20-25
   c. 40-50 and 15-20
   d. 30-40 and 12-20

57. A sign of hypoperfusion in the infant or child patient is
   a. Warm, pink, dry skin
   b. Rapid, bounding pulse
   c. Capillary refill under 2 seconds
   d. Absence of tears when crying

58. SIDS (sudden infant death syndrome) has a peak incidence at around ____ of age.
   a. 2 weeks
   b. 1 month
   c. 4 months
   d. 1 year

59. Gastrostomy tubes in the child are used to provide
   a. Long term drainage of cerebrospinal fluid
   b. Long term feeding directly to the stomach
   c. Long term intravenous access
   d. Long term airway access

60. You are the triage officer on an MCI (multiple-casualty incident). As you triage the patients, your treatment should be limited to
    a. Airway management and protection of the spine
    b. Airway management and severe bleeding control
    c. Oxygen therapy and management of hemorrhages
    d. Spine immobilization and severe bleeding control

61. In the three-priority system of triage tagging, which of the following injuries would indicate a Priority 2 patient?
    a. Airway and breathing difficulties
    b. Multiple bone or joint injuries
    c. Decreased mental status
    d. Diabetic or cardiac emergencies

62. A patient is found in severe respiratory distress, sitting upright and leaning slightly forward, supporting himself with his arms. This position is called a
    a. Trendelenburg position
    b Tripod position
    c Distress position
    d. Bronchospasm position

63. A cough that produces mucus is known as a
    a. Diminished cough
    b. Productive cough
    c. Paradoxical cough
    d. Wet cough

64. Cyanosis is
    a. An early sign of hypoperfusion
    b. An early sign of breathing difficulty
    c. A late sign of breathing difficulty
    d. A late sign of altered mental status

65. An infant with cyanosis, an altered mental status, and a slow heart rate should be provided
    a. Positive pressure ventilation with supplemental oxygen
    b. Oxygen via simple face mask
    c. Oxygen via nonrebreather mask
    d. Oxygen via the "blow by" method

66. Which of the following is an "S" question in the OPQRST questions used to evaluate a patient with respiratory distress?
    a. "When did the difficulty in breathing start?"
    b. "Does lying flat make the breathing more difficult?"
    c. "How bad is this breathing difficulty on a scale of 1 to 10?"
    d. "What were you doing when the breathing difficulty started?"

67. A patient with difficulty in breathing is considered a
    a. High priority patient
    b. Low priority patient
    c. Medium priority patient
    d. A patient not assigned to a priority

68. A loose flap of skin and soft tissue that has been torn loose or pulled completely off is known as an
    a. Articulation
    b. Amputation
    c. Avulsion
    d. Abrasion

69. You are treating a patient who has an abdominal injury with exposed organs. Which treatment is most appropriate?
    a. Apply sterile gauze moistened with sterile water, then an occlusive dressing.
    b. Apply an occlusive dressing, then sterile gauze moistened with sterile water.
    c. Apply a dry sterile cotton dressing; then use direct pressure to help control bleeding.
    d. Apply a dry gauze dressing to control bleeding, then cover with an occlusive dressing.

70. Which is the best way to transport an amputated body part?
    a. Place the body part in a plastic bag; label the bag; immediately place the bag on ice.
    b. Immediately immerse the body part in a bag of ice water; label the bag; transport.
    c. Wrap the body part in dry sterile dressing; place in a plastic bag; label the bag; keep the part cool.
    d. Do not delay to wrap or label the part; transport the part and the patient at once.

71. Which of the following is an early sign or symptom of neurologic deficit that is commonly found in the patient suffering a nontraumatic brain injury?
    a. Paralysis to both legs
    b. Bilateral numbness to hands
    c. Stiff neck
    d. Loss of vision in one eye

72. Which of the following is the most appropriate means of administering oxygen to the nontraumatic-brain-injured patient who is unresponsive and breathing inadequately?
    a. Nasal cannula with a flow of 4-6 lpm
    b. Nonrebreather mask with a flow of 15 lpm
    c. Positive pressure ventilation at 12 per minute
    d. Positive pressure ventilation at 24 per minute

73. Implied consent applies to which of the following?
    a. The patient adamantly refuses treatment, then becomes unresponsive.
    b. The patient is of legal age and able to make rational decisions.
    c. The parent or legal guardian has consented to treatment and transport.
    d. The patient consents orally or by a nod or an affirming gesture.

74. By law, which of the following constitutes negligence?
    a. While off duty, you pass the scene and make no attempt to call for help.
    b. You stop providing care without ensuring that equivalent or better care will be provided.
    c. You provide emergency care to a patient without his consent.
    d. Your care deviates from the accepted standard and results in further injury to the patient.

75. Which chamber of the heart receives oxygen-rich blood from the lungs?
    a. Left ventricle
    b. Right ventricle
    c. Left atrium
    d. Right atrium

76. Which of the following is the most appropriate emergency medical treatment for a responsive patient suffering from a cardiac emergency?
    a. Administer oxygen at 10 lpm via nonrebreather mask and consider calling for ALS backup.
    b. Administer oxygen at 15 lpm via nonrebreather mask and consider calling for ALS backup.
    c. Administer oxygen at 10 lpm via nasal cannula and consider calling for ALS backup.
    d. Administer oxygen at 6 lpm via nasal cannula and consider calling for ALS backup.

77. Which of the following statements is FALSE regarding nitroglycerin?
    a. It dilates the coronary arteries, increasing the blood flow to the heart.
    b. A second dose can be administered 2 minutes after the first dose.
    c. The patient's systolic blood pressure must be above 100 mmHg.
    d. Nitroglycerin is contraindicated in patients suffering from a head injury.

78. When using the AED, the decision to transport the patient to the emergency facility should occur after which of the following conditions is met?
    a. A total of six shocks have been delivered by the AED.
    b. The AED has given two consecutive no shock messages.
    c. The patient regains a pulse and then slips back into cardiac arrest.
    d. The patient has been shocked four times and remains pulseless.

79. Which of the following statements is FALSE regarding the AED?
    a. Before depressing the shock button, you should say, "Clear the patient."
    b. Before delivering shocks in the ambulance, stop and turn the motor off.
    c. The AED cannot be used on a patient who has an implanted pacemaker.
    d. Shocking a patient who is wearing a nitroglycerin patch may cause a fire.

80. You are treating a patient who has partial thickness burns that encircle the right arm and cover the anterior trunk. What is the total BSA burned and the severity?
   a. 36%; critical burns
   b. 27%; critical burns
   c. 36%; moderate burns
   d. 27%; moderate burns

81. You are treating a patient with dry lime burns on both legs. Which is the appropriate treatment?
   a. Remove clothing; do not attempt to brush the chemical off; flush for 20 minutes while transporting.
   b. Remove clothing; brush the chemical off; flush for 20 minutes while transporting.
   c. Brush the chemical off; remove clothing; flush for 20 minutes; then transport.
   d. Remove clothing; do not attempt to brush the chemical off; flush for 20 minutes; then transport.

82. When dealing with a patient suffering from a behavioral emergency, which of the following statements to the patient would be most appropriate?
   a. "You have nothing to worry about; everything will be better before long."
   b. "Trust me; things will be all right after we go to the hospital and see the doctor."
   c. "I'm sensitive to your problems and I'm sure you can be cured."
   d. "Even with all of your problems, you seem to have people who care about you."

83. Which of the following restraints are considered humane and may be used when restraining a patient who may be a danger to you or himself?
   a. Metal police handcuffs
   b. Soft leather restraints
   c. Disposable flex cuffs
   d. Wide adhesive tape

84. When an error is made while writing the prehospital care report, how should you correct the mistake?
   a. Use a commercially available correction fluid.
   b. Erase the mistake, then write over the error.
   c. Draw a single line through the error and initial it.
   d. Completely blacken out the mistake and initial it.

85. Your patient is adamantly refusing treatment and transport to a medical facility. The patient is also refusing to sign a refusal-of-care form. You should
   a. Have the police respond to the scene and force the patient to sign the form
   b. Advise the patient that if the form is not signed he will have to be transported
   c. Have someone else sign the form, verifying that the patient refused to sign
   d. If the patient refuses to sign the form, there is nothing you can do. Clear the scene.

86. According to the National Fire Protection Association (NFPA), a diamond-shaped symbol identifies potentially dangerous cargo. Which color and number represent an extreme health hazard?
   a. Red diamond with the number 1 inside the triangle
   b. Red diamond with the number 4 inside the triangle
   c. Blue diamond with the number 1 inside the triangle
   d. Blue diamond with the number 4 inside the triangle

87. At a hazardous material scene, the zone where contamination is actually present or that is immediately adjacent to the accident site and where contamination can still occur is the
   a. Safety zone
   b. Hot zone
   c. Warm zone
   d. Cold zone

88. While you are waiting for specially trained personnel to arrive to handle a hazardous material scene, you should protect yourself and bystanders by
   a. Keeping downhill and upwind from the scene
   b. Keeping uphill and downwind from the scene
   c. Keeping downhill and downwind from the scene
   d. Keeping uphill and upwind from the scene

89. This division of the nervous system influences the activities of skeletal muscles and movements throughout the body.
   a. Automatic nervous system
   b. Voluntary nervous system
   c. Autonomic nervous system
   d. Involuntary nervous system

90. A spinal injury resulting from hanging would be caused by which of the following mechanisms of spine injury?
   a. Flexion
   b. Extension
   c. Lateral bending
   d. Distraction

91. Manual stabilization of the potentially spine-injured patient's neck should
   a. Not be released until the cervical spine immobilization collar is applied
   b. Be released if the patient complains of discomfort
   c. Not be released until the patient is securely immobilized to a backboard
   d. Be released if the patient's level of responsiveness deteriorates

92. A patient who is walking around at a collision scene
   a. Does not have a spinal injury
   b. Should never be immobilized
   c. May have a spinal injury
   d. Should always be immobilized

93. Paralysis to all four extremities is called
   a. Quadriplegia
   b. Paraplegia
   c. Biplegia
   d. Hemiplegia

94. Your patient has ingested a poisonous plant and will only respond to painful stimuli. In which position should you place the patient?
   a. On his side
   b. On his back
   c. Sitting up
   d. Feet elevated

95. After administering activated charcoal to a 6-year-old patient who has ingested all of her mother's blood pressure medicine, the patient vomits. You should now
   a. Contact medical direction to authorize one repeat dose of 10 grams
   b. Contact medical direction to authorize one repeat dose of 25 grams
   c. Contact medical direction to authorize one repeat dose of 60 grams
   d. NOT contact medical direction, repeating the dose is contraindicated

96. When treating a patient who has inhaled a poisonous gas, your FIRST treatment priority is to
   a. Administer high-flow oxygen
   b. Place the patient on his side
   c. Start positive pressure ventilation
   d. Move the patient out of the toxic environment

97. Your patient has been involved in a farm accident. All conventional methods of shutting down the tractor have failed. Which of these methods of shutting off the engine may be used but may cause engine damage?
   a. Pulling the air shut-off lever instead of using the key
   b. Discharging a 20-pound CO_2 extinguisher into the air intake
   c. Closing the fuel valve at the bottom of the fuel tank
   d. Clamping the fuel line by using a pair of vise-grip pliers

98. Which of the following best describes silo gas?
   a. Carbon dioxide, rotten-egg-like smell, lighter than air, can kill within hours
   b. Carbon monoxide, gasoline-like smell, lighter than air, can kill within minutes
   c. Methane gas, vodka-like odor, heavier than air, can kill within hours
   d. Oxides of nitrogen, bleach-like odor, heavier than air, can kill within minutes

99. The term that means "toward the center of the body" is
   a. Superior
   b. Medial
   c. Dorsal
   d. Lateral

100. The term that refers to the center of each of the collarbones is
   a. Midclavicular
   b. Distal
   c. Midanterior
   d. Midaxillary

101. In this body position the patient is lying on the back with the head elevated at a 45-degree to 60-degree angle.
   a. Supine position
   b. Lateral recumbent position
   c. Fowler's position
   d. Trendelenburg position

102. Which heart valve is located between the left atrium and the left ventricle?
   a. Mitral valve
   b. Aortic valve
   c. Pulmonary valve
   d. Tricuspid valve

103. This organ is solid, is located in the left upper quadrant of the abdominal cavity, and aids in the production of red blood cells and the filtration of blood.
   a. Gallbladder
   b. Spleen
   c. Ileum
   d. Duodenum

104. The five vertebrae that form the lower back and are located between the sacral and the thoracic spine form the
   a. Iliac spine
   b. Humeral spine
   c. Cervical spine
   d. Lumbar spine

105. When the amount of heat the body produces or gains exceeds the amount the body loses the result is
   a. Heat stroke
   b. Hyperthermia
   c. Heat cramps
   d. Hypothermia

106. Fixed dilated pupils, coma, slow respirations, and possible cardiac arrest occur in hypothermia at what core body temperature?
   a 68-82° F
   b 82-86° F
   c. 86-90° F
   d. 90-95° F

107. The earliest stage of hypothermia is
   a. Decreased vital signs
   b. Decreased level of responsiveness
   c. Apathy
   d. Shivering

108. A hyperthermic patient with moist, pale skin that is normal-to-cool in temperature should be
   a. Placed in a bath filled with ice water
   b. Moved to a cool environment
   c. Placed in a supine position with the head elevated
   d. Given fluids if unresponsive

109. A patient has been stung by a bee. Which of the following methods is the best way to remove the stinger?
    a. Use tweezers.
    b. Use your fingers.
    c. Use forceps.
    d. Gently scrape it.

110. You are treating a patient who has been struck in the head with a baseball bat. Which of the following is the correct way to treat the bleeding from the right ear?
    a. Cover the ear with a sterile gauze dressing; then apply a pressure dressing.
    b. Cover the ear with a sterile gauze dressing; then apply an occlusive dressing.
    c. Cover the ear with a sterile gauze dressing; do not try to stop the bleeding.
    d. Cover the ear with a sterile gauze dressing; then apply direct pressure.

111. Your patient responds to painful stimuli by extending both arms down to his sides and extending his legs, then arching his back. Which best describes this response?
    a. Lowest level of purposeful response, known as decorticate posturing
    b. Lowest level of nonpurposeful response, known as decerebrate posturing
    c. Second lowest level of nonpurposeful response, known as decorticate posturing
    d. Second lowest level of purposeful response, known as decerebrate posturing

112. Which of the following signs and symptoms best describes those that would be found in a patient who is suffering from an abdominal aortic aneurysm?
    a. Sudden onset of tearing pain felt in the chest and left arm; pale cool skin
    b. Abdominal pain with pale skin above the chest and normal color below
    c. Constant, severe abdominal pain and a pulsating abdominal mass
    d. Sudden onset of intermittent abdominal pain that radiates to the neck

113. Which is the correct way of performing the physical assessment of a patient with acute abdominal pain?
    a. Have the patient first point to the area that is most painful; then palpate each quadrant, beginning with the area farthest from the pain.
    b. Palpate the lower two quadrants first; next palpate the upper two quadrants; then have the patient point to the area that is most painful.
    c. Have the patient first point to the area that is most painful; palpate that area first, moving toward the less painful areas.
    d. Palpate all four quadrants to find the area that is most painful.

114. What is the main purpose for assessing the elderly patient's mental status?
    a. To determine the degree of senility
    b. To determine if circulation is adequate
    c. To determine if a stroke has occurred
    d. To protect the airway and breathing

115. Which of the following is NOT true regarding an altered mental status in an elderly patient?
    a. An altered mental status may be caused by chronic condition such as Alzheimer's disease.
    b. An altered mental status may result from the use of drugs and medications.
    c. An altered mental status may be the result of the acute onset of an emergency such as a stroke.
    d. An altered mental status is normal and to be expected in an elderly patient.

116. Nearly one-third of all elderly victims of heart attack never experience pain. This is widely known as
    a. An atypical heart attack
    b. A painless heart attack
    c. A false heart attack
    d. A silent heart attack

117. The quickest way to eliminate the majority of electrical current hazards associated with a motor vehicle crash is to
    a. Disconnect the battery
    b. Disconnect the coil wire
    c. Turn off vehicle ignition
    d. Disconnect the main fuse

118. Which of the following is most likely to help prevent a motor vehicle crash victim from moving his head before you are able to gain access and immobilize him?
    a. From the patient's side, call out to him and ask him not to move.
    b. Approach the patient from the driver's side and hold his head.
    c. Have the patient focus on an object directly in front of him.
    d. Have the patient focus on you and instruct him not to move.

119. In a vehicle collision, the up-and-over or the down-and-under pathway commonly occurs with a
    a. Lateral impact
    b. Rear end impact
    c. Rollover
    d. Frontal impact

120. A "whiplash" injury is commonly caused by a
    a. Lateral impact
    b. Rear end impact
    c. Rollover
    d. Frontal impact

121. Which of the following is the most common mechanism of injury?
    a. Motor vehicle collisions
    b. Motorcycle collisions
    c. Gunshot wounds
    d. Falls

122. Penetrating injuries are classified as
    a. Hollow, solid, and mixed
    b. Open, closed, and mixed
    c. Low, medium, and high velocity
    d. Partial, complete, and closed

123. This is called "pathway expansion" and is caused by a pressure wave resulting from the kinetic energy of the bullet.
    a. Cavitation
    b. Profile
    c. Drag
    d. Trajectory

124. The three phases of an explosion that cause specific injury patterns are the
    a. First, second, and third phase
    b. Initial, medial, and final phase
    c. Preliminary, general, and specific phase
    d. Primary, secondary, and tertiary phase

125. You are treating a patient with an injured forearm and no other apparent or suspected injuries. There is no distal pulse, and the extremity appears cyanotic. Which of the following is correct?
    a. Immobilize the extremity immediately following the focused history; then transport.
    b. Immobilize the extremity immediately following the initial assessment; then transport.
    c. Following the initial assessment, immediately transport; immobilize while en route.
    d. Following the focused history, immediately transport; immobilize while en route.

126. Which of the following describes the correct way to immobilize long bone injuries?
    a. Immobilize the joint above the injury.
    b. Immobilize the joint below the injury.
    c. Immobilize the joints above and below the injury.
    d. Immobilize the injured long bone only, not the joints.

127. The traction splint should not be used in which of the following circumstances?
    a. When the pelvis has also been injured
    b. When the injury is within 3 inches of the hip
    c. When the injury is to the middle of the thigh
    d. When the injury is within 6 inches of the ankle

128. After receiving an on-line order from medical direction, you should
    a. Tell medical direction that you have received the order
    b. Repeat the order back to medical direction, word for word
    c. Have medical direction repeat the order at least twice
    d. Write the order on a notepad

129. To establish effective face-to-face communication with people in an emergency situation, you should convey all of the following qualities EXCEPT
    a. Callousness
    b. Competence
    c. Confidence
    d. Compassion

130. When trying to rescue a responsive patient who is struggling near the shore of a lake, which order of rescuing the patient is preferred?
    1. Swim to the patient by using a flotation device.
    2. Reach to the patient by holding out an object.
    3. Throw a weighted polypropylene rope to the patient.
    4. Row a boat to the patient if one is immediately available.

    a. 3, 2, 1, 4
    b. 2, 3, 4, 1
    c. 3, 2, 4, 1
    d. 2, 4, 3, 1

131. You are treating a suspected spine-injured swimmer who is in the water. Which of the following is correct?
    a. Slide the backboard under the patient while in the water; secure the torso, then the head.
    b. Apply a cervical spine immobilization collar, then slide the backboard under the patient and secure the torso and legs.
    c. Support the patient's head; move him to shore; then place him onto the backboard.
    d. Apply a cervical spine immobilization collar; move the patient to shore; then secure him to the backboard.

132. When operating an emergency vehicle, you must exercise "due regard for the safety of others." Which statement is true regarding this concept?
    a. You will not be held responsible for your actions if your emergency lights and siren are operating.
    b. Even under the special laws that apply in cases of true emergency, you can be held liable if you do not exercise reasonable care for the safety of others.
    c. You will not be held responsible for your actions if you exceed the speed limit by no more than 10 miles per hour over the posted speed limit.
    d. You must slow down only at red lights or stop signs.

133. Which of the following is NOT true of an excellent ambulance operator?
    a. Holds the wheel at the nine o'clock and three o'clock positions
    b. Is familiar with how the ambulance accelerates and decelerates
    c. Recognizes and responds to changes in weather and road conditions
    d. Drives as fast as possible to get the patient to the hospital without delay

134. The first major phase of an ambulance call is the
    a. Arrival at scene
    b. Dispatch
    c. Equipment preparation
    d. Post run

135. A daytime landing area for a small helicopter requires an area
    a. 30 x 30 feet
    b. 40 x 40 feet
    c. 50 x 50 feet
    d. 60 x 60 feet

136. The four corners of a helicopter landing area should be marked. A fifth device should be positioned where?
    a. On the approach side of the landing area
    b. At the location of the patient
    c. On the upwind side of the landing area
    d. At the location of the ambulance

137. Which of the following is the most common cause of seizures?
    a. Diabetes
    b. Stroke
    c. Head injury
    d. Epilepsy

138. Which condition below is a dire medical emergency that requires aggressive airway management?
    a. Postictal state
    b. Status epilepticus
    c. Tonic-clonic seizure
    d. Grand mal seizure

139. Which of the following drugs is considered to be a central nervous system depressant?
    a. Alcohol
    b. Cocaine
    c. LSD
    d. Ephedrine

140. In which of the following overdose cases (in which the drug taken is known) would you NOT use the talk-down technique?
    a. PCP
    b. LSD
    c. Heroin
    d. Cocaine

141. The patient with an eye injury should be asked to follow your finger as you move it left and right, up and down, to evaluate all of the following EXCEPT
    a. Pain on movement
    b. Paralysis of gaze
    c. Accommodation to light
    d. Abnormal gaze

142. Removal of foreign particle from the eye should not generally be attempted in the field. If required, you should attempt removal of a particle only if
    a. It is lodged on the conjunctiva
    b. It is lodged on the globe
    c. It is lodged on the cornea
    d. It is lodged on the iris

143. An injury to the globe of the eye should be treated with
    a. Patches applied lightly to both eyes
    b. A firm compress applied to both eyes
    c. Firm hand pressure to the globe of the injured eye
    d. Direct pressure to the globes of both eyes

144. When a patient has suffered an injury to the face, which of the following BEST states the other areas or structures to which compromise or injury should be suspected?
    a. The airway, spine, and skull
    b. The airway and spine
    c. The spine and skull
    d. The airway and skull

145. Which of the following is the correct way to dress and bandage a bleeding neck wound?
    a. An occlusive dressing covered by a regular dressing and a circumferential bandage
    b. A bulky dressing covered by an occlusive dressing and a circumferential bandage
    c. An occlusive dressing covered by a regular dressing and a figure-eight bandage
    d. A regular dressing covered by an occlusive dressing and a self-adhesive bandage

146. When administering an epinephrine auto-injector to a patient who is experiencing a severe allergic reaction, which injection site is correct?
    a. Any of the large arm veins
    b. Right or left buttocks
    c. Lateral portion of the thigh
    d. Deltoid or shoulder muscle

147. Which of the following key categories of signs and symptoms specifically indicates a severe allergic reaction (anaphylaxis) and indicates immediate intervention and administration of epinephrine?
    a. Itchy, watery eyes with a slow heart rate
    b. Intense itching, increased blood pressure
    c. Respiratory compromise and shock (hypoperfusion)
    d. Hives with a warm tingling feeling to hands

148. Your patient has been stabbed in the chest. You quickly expose the chest and find an open wound to the anterior chest. Which of the following is your correct FIRST action?
    a. Perform a focused history and physical exam.
    b. Perform a rapid trauma assessment.
    c. Seal the wound with a nonocclusive dressing.
    d. Seal the wound with a gloved hand.

149. Which of the following is an EARLY sign or symptom that indicates a complication associated with the sealed chest wound and a developing tension pneumothorax?
    a. A breathing rate that is faster than normal
    b. A heart rate that is slower than normal
    c. High blood pressure with a widening pulse pressure
    d. Tracheal deviation away from the injured side

150. You are treating a patient with an abdominal injury but no suspected spinal injury. Which is the best position in which to place the patient?
    a. On the left side with the legs straight
    b. Supine with the legs flexed at the knees
    c. Fowler's position with the legs flexed
    d. Trendelenburg position with legs straight

OPTIONAL: ADVANCED AIRWAY MANAGEMENT

151. Before any advanced airway techniques are attempted, it is necessary to do all of the following EXCEPT
    a. Open the airway with a manual maneuver such as the jaw thrust or the head-tilt, chin-lift.
    b. Suction the oropharynx to remove secretions, blood, vomitus, or other substances.
    c. Suction the trachea to remove secretions, blood, vomitus, or other substances.
    d. Insert a mechanical airway adjunct such as an oropharyngeal or nasopharyngeal airway.

152. In orotracheal intubation, the tube should be inserted
    a. Through the nose and into the esophagus
    b. Through the mouth and into the trachea
    c. Through the mouth and into the esophagus
    d. Through the nose and into the larynx

153. Equipment used for orotracheal intubation includes all of the following EXCEPT
    a. Laryngoscope
    b. Stylet
    c. Nasogastric tube
    d. 10 cc syringe

154. In orotracheal intubation, the epiglottis must be lifted in order to
    a. Provide visualization of the vocal cords and glottic opening
    b. Prevent aspiration of blood, secretions, and vomitus
    c. Open the esophageal structures
    d. Move the tongue aside

155. In orotracheal intubation, the
    a. Straight blade is inserted into the vallecula to lift the epiglottis directly
    b. Curved blade is fitted under the epiglottis to spread the glottic opening directly
    c. Straight blade is inserted between the vocal cords to separate them directly
    d. Curved blade is inserted into the vallecula to lift the epiglottis indirectly

156. During Sellick's maneuver, pressure is applied
    a. To the stomach, to relieve gastric distention
    b. To the larynx, to prevent regurgitation and aspiration
    c. To the cricoid cartilage, to push the glottic structures into the visual field
    d. To the 10 cc syringe, to inflate the distal cuff

157. To assess for correct placement of an endotracheal tube, use all of the following procedures EXCEPT
    a. Auscultate over the epigastrium.
    b. Watch for chest rise and fall during ventilation.
    c. Auscultate breath sounds in both lungs.
    d. Palpate all four thoracic quadrants.

158. Endotracheal tubes in infants and children under age 8 are typically
    a. Uncuffed because the narrow cricoid ring seals the trachea
    b. Measured from the tip of the nose, around the ear, to the xiphoid process
    c. Not used because of the danger of severe gastric distention
    d. One-half size larger than the diameter of the patient's thumb

159. A CONTRAINDICATION for the insertion of a nasogastric tube in an infant or child is
    a. You are unable to provide effective positive pressure ventilation due to gastric distention
    b. The patient is unresponsive and at risk of vomiting gastric contents
    c. Ingested poisons need to be diluted
    d. The patient has suffered major facial trauma

160. In orotracheal suctioning
    a. A rigid catheter is used to suction the oropharynx
    b. A soft catheter is used to suction to the level of the carina
    c. A soft catheter is used to suction to the level of the larynx
    d. A rigid catheter is used to suction to the level of the xiphoid process

The National Registry of Emergency Medical Technicians is an organization founded in 1970, one of whose goals is to establish nationwide professional standards for EMTs. Many state EMS systems use examinations developed by the National Registry to establish certification of EMTs.

The National Registry has prepared a certification examination correlated to the 1994 Department of Transportation Emergency Medical Technician-Basic: National Standard Curriculum. The examination includes both a written portion and a practical portion that consists of a series of performance-based skill stations.

To assist students in preparing for the skill stations that are part of the EMT-Basic examination, as well as to establish guidelines and parameters for those who will evaluate students' performance at the skill stations, the National Registry has developed a series of skill sheets. Each skill sheet contains a set of directions, the skill criteria, and the critical criteria that if not met by the student results in immediate failure of the station.

In studying for the National Registry examination, these skill sheets should be used in conjunction with the material presented in the textbook and not as the sole means of learning the individual skills. The skill sheets will aid you in organizing the steps necessary to perform each skill and in identifying the criteria that will be used to evaluate your performance. You can use these sheets to evaluate your own performance when practicing these skills and preparing for your practical skills evaluation.

Note: Three skill sheets regarding advanced airway management are included. The use of these skills will vary based on your medical director, training program, and local protocol.

National Registry Skill Sheets

ORGANIZATION OF THE NATIONAL REGISTRY EXAMINATION

The practical examination consists of six stations, five mandatory stations and one random basic skill station, consisting of both skill-based and scenario-based testing. The random skill station is conducted so the candidate is totally unaware of the skill to be tested until he or she arrives at the test site.

The candidate will be tested individually in each station and will be expected to direct the actions of any assistant EMTs who may be present in the station. The candidate should pass or fail the examination based solely on his or her actions and decisions.

The following is a list of the stations and their established time limits. The maximum time is determined by the number and difficulty of tasks to be completed.

Station 1:	Patient Assessment/Management — Trauma	10 min
Station 2:	Patient Assessment/Management — Medical	10 min
Station 3:	Cardiac Arrest Management/AED	15 min
Station 4:	Bag-Valve Mask — Apneic Patient	10 min
Station 5:	Spinal Immobilization Station:	
	Spinal Immobilization — Supine Patient	10 min
	Spinal Immobilization — Seated Patient	10 min
Station 6:	Random Basic Skill Verification:	
	Long Bone Injury	5 min
	Joint Injury	5 min
	Traction Splint	10 min
	Bleeding Control/Shock Management	10 min
	Upper Airway Adjuncts and Suction	5 min
	Mouth-to-Mask with Supplemental Oxygen	5 min
	Supplemental Oxygen Administration	5 min

INSTRUCTIONS TO THE CANDIDATE:
PATIENT ASSESSMENT/MANAGEMENT — TRAUMA

This station is designed to test your ability to perform a patient assessment of a victim of multi-system trauma and voice-treat all conditions and injuries discovered. You must conduct your assessment as you would in the field, including communicating with your patient. You may remove the patient's clothing down to shorts or swimsuit if you feel it is necessary. As you conduct your assessment, you should state everything you are assessing. Clinical information not obtainable by visual or physical inspection, for example blood pressure, will be given to you after you demonstrate how you would normally gain that information. You may assume that you have two EMTs working with you and that they are correctly carrying out the verbal treatments you indicate. You have (10) ten minutes to complete this skill station. Do you have any questions?

INSTRUCTIONS TO THE CANDIDATE:
PATIENT ASSESSMENT/MANAGEMENT — MEDICAL

This station is designed to test your ability to perform a patient assessment of a victim with a chief complaint of a medical nature and voice-treat all conditions and injuries discovered. You must conduct your assessment as you would in the field, including communicating with your patient. As you conduct your assessment, you should state everything you are assessing. Clinical information not obtainable by visual or physical inspection, for example, blood pressure, will be given to you after you demonstrate how you would normally gain that information. You may assume that you have two EMTs working with you and that they are correctly carrying out the verbal treatments you indicate. You have (10) ten minutes to complete this skill station. Do you have any questions?

INSTRUCTIONS TO THE CANDIDATE:
CARDIAC ARREST MANAGEMENT

This station is designed to test your ability to manage a pre-hospital cardiac arrest by integrating CPR skills, defibrillation, airway adjuncts, and patient/scene management skills. There will be an EMT assistant in this station. The EMT assistant will only do as you instruct him. As you arrive on the scene you will encounter a patient in cardiac arrest. A first responder will be present performing single rescuer CPR. You must immediately establish control of the scene and begin resuscitation of the patient with an automated external defibrillator. At the appropriate time, you must control the airway and ventilate the victim using adjunctive equipment. You may not delegate this action to the EMT assistant. You may use any of the supplies available in this room. You have (15) fifteen minutes to complete this skill station. Do you have any questions?

INSTRUCTIONS TO THE CANDIDATE:
AIRWAY, OXYGEN, VENTILATION SKILLS
BAG-VALVE MASK APNEIC PATIENT WITH PULSE

This station is designed to test your ability to ventilate a patient using a bag-valve mask. As you enter the station you will find an apneic patient with a palpable central pulse. There are no bystanders and artificial ventilation has not been initiated. The only patient intervention required is airway management and ventilatory support using a bag-valve mask. You must initially ventilate the patient for a minimum of 30 seconds. You will be evaluated on the appropriateness of ventilator volumes. I will inform you that a second rescuer has arrived and will instruct you that you must control the airway and the mask seal while the second rescuer provides ventilation. You may use only the equipment available in this room. Do you have any questions?

INSTRUCTIONS TO THE CANDIDATE:
SPINAL IMMOBILIZATION — SUPINE PATIENT

This station is designed to test your ability to provide spinal immobilization on a patient using a long spine immobilization device. You arrive on the scene with an EMT assistant. The assistant EMT has completed the scene size-up as well as the initial and focused assessments. As you begin the station there are no airway, breathing, or circulatory problems. You are required to treat the specific, isolated problem of an unstable spine using a long spine immobilization device. When moving the patient to the device, you should use the help of the assistant EMT and the evaluator. The assistant EMT should control the head and cervical spine of the patient while you and the evaluator move the patient to the immobilization device. You are responsible for the direction and subsequent action of the EMT assistant. You may use any equipment available in this room. You have (10) ten minutes to complete this procedure. Do you have any questions?

INSTRUCTIONS TO THE CANDIDATE:
SPINAL IMMOBILIZATION SKILLS — SEATED PATIENT

This station is designed to test your ability to provide spinal immobilization on a patient using a half spine immobilization device. You arrive on the scene with an EMT assistant. The assistant EMT has completed the scene size-up, initial and focused assessments. As you begin the station, there are no airway, breathing, or circulatory problems. You are required to treat the specific, isolated problem of an unstable spine using a half spine immobilization device. Continued assessment of airway, breathing, and central circulation is not necessary. You are responsible for the direction and subsequent actions of the EMT assistant.

Transferring the patient to the long spine board should be accomplished verbally. You may use any equipment available in this room. You have (10) ten minutes to complete this procedure. Do you have any questions?

INSTRUCTIONS TO THE CANDIDATE:
IMMOBILIZATION SKILLS — LONG BONE

This station is designed to test your ability to properly immobilize a closed, non-angulated long bone injury. You are required to treat only the specific, isolated injury. The scene size-up and initial assessment have been completed and during the focused assessment a closed, non-angulated injury of the _____ (radius, ulna, tibia, fibula) was detected. Ongoing assessment of the patient's airway, breathing, and central circulation is not necessary. You may use any equipment available in this room. You have (5) five minutes to complete this procedure. Do you have any questions?

INSTRUCTIONS TO THE CANDIDATE:
IMMOBILIZATION SKILLS — JOINT INJURY

This station is designed to test your ability to properly immobilize a non-complicated shoulder injury. You are required to treat only the specific, isolated injury. The scene size-up and initial assessment have been accomplished on the victim and during the focused assessment a shoulder injury was detected. Ongoing assessment of the patient's airway, breathing, and central circulation is not necessary. You may use any equipment available in this room. You have (5) five minutes to complete this procedure. Do you have any questions?

INSTRUCTIONS TO THE CANDIDATE: IMMOBILIZATION SKILLS — TRACTION SPLINTING

This station is designed to test your ability to properly immobilize a mid-shaft femur injury with a traction splint. You will have an EMT assistant to help you in the application of the device by applying manual traction when directed to do so. You are required to treat only the specific, isolated injury. The scene size-up and initial assessment have been accomplished on the victim and during the focused assessment a mid-shaft femur deformity was detected. Ongoing assessment of the patient's airway, breathing, and central circulation is not necessary. You may use any equipment available in this room. You have (10) ten minutes to complete this procedure. Do you have any questions?

INSTRUCTIONS TO THE CANDIDATE: BLEEDING CONTROL/SHOCK MANAGEMENT

This station is designed to test your ability to control hemorrhage. This is a scenario-based testing station. As you progress through the scenario, you will be offered various signs and symptoms appropriate for the patient's condition. You will be required to manage the patient based on these signs and symptoms. A scenario will be read aloud to you and you will be given an opportunity to ask clarifying questions about the scenario; however, you will not receive answers to any questions about the actual steps of the procedures to be performed. You may use any of the supplies and equipment available in this room. You have (10) ten minutes to complete this skill station. Do you have any questions?

INSTRUCTIONS TO THE CANDIDATE: AIRWAY, OXYGEN, VENTILATION SKILLS UPPER AIRWAY ADJUNCTS AND SUCTION

This station is designed to test your ability to properly measure, insert, and remove an oropharyngeal and a nasopharyngeal airway as well as suction a patient's upper airway. This is an isolated skills test comprised of three separate skills. You may use any equipment available in this room. Do you have any questions?

INSTRUCTIONS TO THE CANDIDATE:
AIRWAY, OXYGEN, VENTILATION SKILLS
MOUTH-TO-MASK WITH SUPPLEMENTAL OXYGEN

This station is designed to test your ability to ventilate a patient with supplemental oxygen using a mouth-to-mask technique. This is an isolated skills test. You may assume that mouth-to-mouth ventilation is in progress and that the patient has a central pulse. The only patient management required is ventilator support using a mouth-to-mask technique with supplemental oxygen. You must ventilate the patient for at least 30 seconds. You will be evaluated on the appropriateness of ventilatory volumes. You may use any equipment available in this room. Do you have any questions?

INSTRUCTIONS TO THE CANDIDATE:
AIRWAY, OXYGEN, VENTILATION SKILLS
SUPPLEMENTAL OXYGEN ADMINISTRATION

This station is designed to test your ability to correctly assemble the equipment needed to administer supplemental oxygen in the pre-hospital setting. This is an isolated skills test. You will be required to assemble an oxygen tank and regulator and administer oxygen to a patient using a nonrebreather mask. At this point you will be instructed to discontinue oxygen administration by the nonrebreather mask because the patient cannot tolerate the mask and start oxygen administration using a nasal cannula. Once you have initiated oxygen administration using a nasal cannula, you will be instructed to discontinue oxygen administration completely. You may use only the equipment available in this room. Do you have any questions?

PATIENT ASSESSMENT/MANAGEMENT
TRAUMA

		Points Possible	Points Awarded
Takes or verbalizes body substance isolation precautions		1	
SCENE SIZE-UP			
Determines the scene is safe		1	
Determines the mechanism of injury		1	
Determines the number of patients		1	
Requests additional help if necessary		1	
Considers stabilization of spine		1	
INITIAL ASSESSMENT			
Verbalizes general impression of patient		1	
Determines responsiveness		1	
Determines chief complaint/apparent life threats		1	
Assesses airway and breathing	Assessment	1	
	Initiates appropriate oxygen therapy	1	
	Assures adequate ventilation	1	
	Injury management	1	
Assesses Circulation	Assesses for and controls major bleeding	1	
	Assesses pulse	1	
	Assesses skin (color, temperature and condition)	1	
Identifies priority patients/makes transport decision		1	
FOCUSED HISTORY AND PHYSICAL EXAM/RAPID TRAUMA ASSESSMENT			
Selects appropriate assessment (focused or rapid assessment)		1	
Obtains or directs assistant to obtain baseline vital signs		1	
Obtains SAMPLE history		1	
DETAILED PHYSICAL EXAMINATION			
Assesses the head	Inspects and palpates the scalp and ears	1	
	Assesses the eyes	1	
	Assesses the facial area including oral and nasal area	1	
Assesses the neck	Inspects and palpates the neck	1	
	Assesses for JVD	1	
	Assesses for tracheal deviation	1	
Assesses the chest	Inspects	1	
	Palpates	1	
	Auscultates the chest	1	
Assesses the abdomen/pelvis	Assesses the abdomen	1	
	Assesses the pelvis	1	
	Verbalizes assessment of genitalia/perineum as needed	1	
Assesses the extremities	1 point for each extremity includes inspection, palpation, and assessment of pulses, sensory and motor activities	4	
Assesses the posterior	Assesses thorax	1	
	Assesses lumbar	1	
Manages secondary injuries and wounds appropriately **1 point for appropriate management of secondary injury/wound**		1	
Verbalizes reassessment of the vital signs		1	
	TOTAL:	40	

CRITICAL CRITERIA

___ Did not take or verbalize body substance isolation precautions
___ Did not assess for spinal protection
___ Did not provide for spinal protection when indicated
___ Did not provide high concentration of oxygen
___ Did not find or manage problems associated with airway, breathing, hemorrhage or shock (hypoperfusion)
___ Did not differentiate patient's needing transportation versus continued on scene assessment
___ Does other detailed physical examination before assessing airway, breathing and circulation
___ Did not transport patient within ten (10) minute time limit

PATIENT ASSESSMENT/MANAGEMENT
MEDICAL

	Points Possible	Points Awarded
Takes or verbalizes body substance isolation precautions	1	
SCENE SIZE-UP		
Determines the scene is safe	1	
Determines the mechanism of injury/nature of illness	1	
Determines the number of patients	1	
Requests additional help if necessary	1	
Considers stabilization of spine	1	
INITIAL ASSESSMENT		
Verbalizes general impression of patient	1	
Determines responsiveness/level of consciousness	1	
Determines chief complaint/apparent life threats	1	

Assesses airway and breathing	Assessment	1	
	Initiates appropriate oxygen therapy	1	
	Assures adequate ventilation	1	
Assesses Circulation	Assesses/controls major bleeding	1	
	Assesses pulse	1	
	Assesses skin (color, temperature and condition)	1	
Identifies priority patients/makes transport decision		1	

FOCUSED HISTORY AND PHYSICAL EXAM/RAPID ASSESSMENT

Signs and Symptoms (Assess history of present illness)	4	

Respiratory	Cardiac	Altered Mental Status	Allergic Reaction	Poisoning/ Overdose	Environmental Emergency	Obstetrics	Behavioral
•Onset? •Provokes? •Quality? •Radiates? •Severity? •Time? •Interventions?	•Onset? •Provokes? •Quality? •Radiates? •Severity? •Time? •Interventions?	•Description of the episode •Onset? •Duration? •Associated symptoms? •Evidence of trauma? •Interventions? •Seizures? •Fever?	•History of allergies? •What were you exposed to? •How were you exposed? •Effects? •Progression? •Interventions?	•Substance? •When did you ingest/become exposed? •How much did you ingest? •Over what time period? •Interventions? •Estimated weight? •Effects?	•Source? •Environment? •Duration? •Loss of consciousness? •Effects - General or local?	•Are you pregnant? •How long have you been pregnant? •Pain or contractions? •Bleeding or discharge? •Do you feel the need to push? •Last menstrual period? •Crowning?	•How do you feel? •Determine suicidal tendencies •Is the patient a threat to self or others? •Is there a medical problem? •Interventions?

Allergies	1	
Medications	1	
Past medical history	1	
Last Meal	1	
Events leading to present illness (rule out trauma)	1	
Performs focused physical examination Assesses affected body part/system or, if indicated, completes rapid assessment	1	
VITALS (Obtains baseline vital signs)	1	
INTERVENTIONS Obtains medical direction or verbalizes standing order for medication interventions and verbalizes proper additional intervention/treatment	1	
TRANSPORT (Re-evaluates transport decision)	1	
Verbalizes the consideration for completing a detailed physical examination	1	
ONGOING ASSESSMENT (verbalized)		
Repeats initial assessment	1	
Repeats vital signs	1	
Repeats focused assessment regarding patient complaint or injuries	1	
Checks interventions	1	
CRITICAL CRITERIA TOTAL:	34	

___ Did not take or verbalize body substance isolation precautions if necessary
___ Did not determine scene safety
___ Did not obtain medical direction or verbalize standing orders for medication interventions
___ Did not provide high concentration of oxygen
___ Did not evaluate and find conditions of airway, breathing, circulation
___ Did not find or manage problems associated with airway, breathing, hemorrhage or shock (hypoperfusion)
___ Did not differentiate patient's needing transportation versus continued assessment at the scene
___ Does detailed or focused history/physical examination before assessing airway, breathing and circulation
___ Did not ask questions about the present illness
___ Administered a dangerous or inappropriate intervention

CARDIAC ARREST MANAGEMENT/AED

	Points Possible	Points Awarded
ASSESSMENT		
Takes or verbalizes body substances isolation precautions	1	
Briefly questions rescuer about events	1	
Directs rescuer to stop CPR	1	
Verifies absence of spontaneous pulse *(skill station examiner states "no pulse")*	1	
Turns on defibrillator power	1	
Attaches automated defibrillator to patient	1	
Ensures all individuals are standing clear of the patient	1	
Initiates analysis of rhythm	1	
Delivers shock (up to three successive shocks)	1	
Verifies absence of spontaneous pulse *(skill station examiner states "no pulse")*	1	
TRANSITION		
Directs resumption of CPR	1	
Gathers additional information on arrest event	1	
Confirms effectiveness of CPR (ventilation and compressions)	1	
INTEGRATION		
Directs insertion of a simple airway adjunct (oropharyngeal/nasopharyngeal)	1	
Directs ventilation of patient	1	
Assures high concentration of oxygen connected to the ventilatory adjunct	1	
Assures CPR continues without unnecessary/prolonged interruption	1	
Re-evaluates patient/CPR in approximately one minute	1	
Repeats defibrillator sequence	1	
TRANSPORTATION		
Verbalizes transportation of patient	1	
TOTAL:	20	

CRITICAL CRITERIA

___ Did not take or verbalize body substance isolation precautions
___ Did not evaluate the need for immediate use of the AED
___ Did not direct initiation/resumption of ventilation/compressions at appropriate times
___ Did not assure all individuals were clear of patient before delivering each shock
___ Did not operate the AED properly (inability to deliver shock)

BAG-VALVE-MASK
APNEIC PATIENT

	Points Possible	Points Awarded
Takes or verbalizes body substance isolation precautions	1	
Voices opening the airway	1	
Voices inserting an airway adjunct	1	
Selects appropriate size mask	1	
Creates a proper mask-to-face seal	1	
Ventilates patient at no less than 800 ml volume **(The examiner must witness for at least 30 seconds)**	1	
Connects reservoir and oxygen	1	
Adjust liter flow to 15 liters/minute or greater	1	
The examiner indicates the arrival of second EMT. The second EMT is instructed to ventilate the patient while the candidate controls the mask and the airway.		
Voices re-opening the airway	1	
Creates a proper mask-to-face seal	1	
Instructs assistant to resume ventilation at proper volume per breath **(The examiner must witness for at least 30 seconds)**	1	
TOTAL:	11	

CRITICAL CRITERIA

___ Did not take or verbalize body substance isolation precautions
___ Did not immediately ventilate the patient
___ Interrupted ventilations for more than **20** seconds
___ Did not provide high concentration of oxygen
___ Did not provide or direct assistant to provide proper volume/breath
    (more than 2 ventilations per minute are below 800 ml)
___ Did not allow adequate exhalation

SPINAL IMMOBILIZATION
SUPINE PATIENT

	Points Possible	Points Awarded
Takes or verbalizes body substance isolation precautions	1	
Directs assistant to place/maintain head in neutral in-line position	1	
Directs assistant to maintain manual immobilization of the head	1	
Assesses motor, sensory, and distal circulation in extremities	1	
Applies appropriate size extrication collar	1	
Positions the immobilization device appropriately	1	
Directs movement of the patient onto device without compromising the integrity of the spine	1	
Applies padding to voids between the torso and the boards as necessary	1	
Immobilizes the patient's torso to the device	1	
Evaluates the pads behind the patient's head as necessary	1	
Immobilizes the patient's head to the device	1	
Secures the patient's legs to the device	1	
Secures the patient's arms to the device	1	
Reassesses motor, sensory, and distal circulation in extremities	1	
TOTAL:	14	

CRITICAL CRITERIA

___ Did not immediately direct or take manual immobilization of the head
___ Releases or orders release of manual immobilization before it was maintained mechanically
___ Patient manipulated or moved excessively, causing potential spinal compromise
___ Patient moves excessively up, down, left, or right on the device.
___ Head immobilization allows for excessive movement
___ Upon completion of immobilization, head is not in the neutral in-line position
___ Did not reassess motor, sensory, and distal circulation after immobilization to the device
___ Immobilized head to the board before securing torso

SPINAL IMMOBILIZATION
SEATED PATIENT

	Points Possible	Points Awarded
Takes or verbalizes body substance isolation precautions	1	
Directs assistant to place/maintain head in neutral in-line position	1	
Directs assistant to maintain manual immobilization of the head	1	
Reassesses motor, sensory, and distal circulation in extremities	1	
Applies appropriate size extrication collar	1	
Positions the immobilization device behind the patient	1	
Secures the device to the patient's torso	1	
Evaluates torso fixation and adjusts as necessary	1	
Evaluates and pads behind the patient's head as necessary	1	
Secures the patient's head to the device	1	
Verbalizes moving the patient to a long board	1	
Reassesses motor, sensory, and distal circulation in extremities	1	
TOTAL:	12	

CRITICAL CRITERIA

___ Did not immediately direct or take manual immobilization of the head
___ Releases or orders release of manual immobilization before it was maintained mechanically
___ Patient manipulated or moved excessively, causing potential spinal compromise
___ Device moves excessively up, down, left, or right on patient's torso.
___ Head immobilization allows for excessive movement
___ Torso fixation inhibits chest rise, resulting in respiratory compromise
___ Upon completion of immobilization, head is not in the neutral position
___ Did not reassess motor, sensory, and distal circulation after voicing immobilization
    to the long board
___ Immobilized head to the board before securing the torso

IMMOBILIZATION SKILLS
LONG BONE

	Points Possible	Points Awarded
Takes or verbalizes body substance isolation precautions	1	
Directs application of manual stabilization	1	
Assesses motor, sensory, and distal circulation	1	
NOTE: The examiner acknowledges present and normal		
Measures splint	1	
Applies splint	1	
Immobilizes the joint above the injury site	1	
Immobilizes the joint below the injury site	1	
Secures the entire injured extremity	1	
Immobilizes hand/foot in the position of function	1	
Reassesses motor, sensory, and distal circulation	1	
NOTE: The examiner acknowledges present and normal		
TOTAL:	10	

CRITICAL CRITERIA

___ Grossly moves injured extremity
___ Did not immobilize adjacent joints
___ Did not assess motor, sensory, and distal circulation before and after splinting

IMMOBILIZATION SKILLS
JOINT INJURY

	Points Possible	Points Awarded
Takes or verbalizes body substance isolation precautions	1	
Directs application of manual stabilization of the injury	1	
Assesses motor, sensory, and distal circulation	1	
NOTE: The examiner acknowledges present and normal		
Selects proper splinting material	1	
Immobilizes the site of the injury	1	
Immobilizes bone above injured joint	1	
Immobilizes bone below injured joint	1	
Reassesses motor, sensory, and distal circulation	1	
NOTE: The examiner acknowledges present and normal		
TOTAL:	8	

CRITICAL CRITERIA

___ Did not support the joint so that the joint did not bear distal weight

___ Did not immobilize bone above and below injured joint

___ Did not reassess motor, sensory amd distal circulation before and after splinting

IMMOBILIZATION SKILLS
TRACTION SPLINTING

	Points Possible	Points Awarded
Takes or verbalizes body substance isolation precautions	1	
Directs application of manual stabilization of the injured leg	1	
Directs the application of manual traction	1	
Assesses motor, sensory, and distal circulation	1	
NOTE: The examiner acknowledges present and normal.		
Prepares/adjusts splint to the proper length	1	
Positions the splint at the injured leg	1	
Applies the proximal securing device (e.g., ischial strap)	1	
Applies the distal securing device (e.g., ankle hitch)	1	
Applies mechanical traction	1	
Positions/secures the support straps	1	
Re-evaluates the proximal/distal securing devices	1	
Reassesses motor, sensory, and distal circulation	1	
NOTE: The examiner acknowledges present and normal		
NOTE: The examiner must ask candidate how he/she would prepare the patient for transportation.		
Verbalizes securing the torso to the long board to immobilize the hip	1	
Verbalizes securing the splint to the long board to prevent movement of the splint	1	
TOTAL:	14	

CRITICAL CRITERIA:

___ Loss of traction at any point after it is assumed
___ Did not reassess motor, sensory, and distal circulation before and after splinting
___ The foot is excessively rotated or extended after splinting
___ Did not secure the ischial strap before taking traction
___ Final immobilization failed to support the femur or prevent rotation of the injured leg
___ Secures leg to splint before applying mechanical traction

NOTE: If the Sager splint or Kendrick Traction Device is used without elevating the patient's leg, application of manual traction is not necessary. The candidate should be awarded 1 point as if manual traction were applied.

NOTE: If the leg is elevated at all, manual traction must be applied before elevating the leg. The ankle hitch may be applied before elevating the leg and used to provide manual traction.

	Points Possible	Points Awarded
Takes or verbalizes body substance isolation precautions	1	
Applies direct pressure to the wound	1	
Elevates the extremity	1	
NOTE: The examiner must now inform the candidate that the wound continues to bleed.		
Applies an additional dressing to the wound	1	
NOTE: The examiner must now inform the candidate that the wound still continues to bleed. The second dressing does not control the bleeding.		
Locates and applies pressure to appropriate arterial pressure point	1	
NOTE: The examiner must now inform the candidate that the bleeding is controlled.		
Bandages the wound	1	
NOTE: The examiner must now inform the candidate that the patient is showing signs and symptoms indicative of hypoperfusion.		
Properly positions the patient	1	
Applies high concentration oxygen	1	
Initiates steps to prevent heat loss from the patient	1	
Indicates need for immediate transportation	1	
TOTAL:	10	

CRITICAL CRITERIA

___ Did not take or verbalize body substance isolation precautions
___ Did not apply high concentration of oxygen
___ Applies tourniquet before attempting other methods of bleeding control
___ Did not control hemorrhage in a timely manner
___ Did not indicate a need for immediate transportation

AIRWAY, OXYGEN, AND VENTILATION SKILLS
UPPER AIRWAY ADJUNCTS AND SUCTION

OROPHARYNGEAL AIRWAY

	Points Possible	Points Awarded
Takes or verbalizes body substance isolation precautions	1	
Selects appropriate size airway	1	
Measures airway	1	
Inserts airway without pushing the tongue posteriorly	1	
NOTE: The examiner must advise the candidate that the patient is gagging and becoming conscious.		
Removes oropharyngeal airway	1	

SUCTION

NOTE: The examiner must advise the candidate to suction the patient's oropharynx/nasopharynx		
Turns on/prepares suction device	1	
Assures presence of mechanical suction	1	
Inserts suction tip without suction	1	
Applies suction to the oropharynx/nasopharynx	1	

NASOPHARYNGEAL AIRWAY

NOTE: The examiner must advise the candidate to insert a nasopharyngeal airway.		
Selects appropriate airway	1	
Measures airway	1	
Verbalizes lubrication of the nasal airway	1	
Fully inserts the airway with the bevel facing toward the septum	1	
TOTAL:	13	

CRITICAL CRITERIA

___ Did not take or verbalize body substance isolation precautions
___ Did not obtain a patent airway with the oropharyngeal airway
___ Did not obtain a patent airway with the nasopharyngeal airway
___ Did not demonstrate an acceptable suction technique
___ Inserts any adjunct in a manner dangerous to the patient

NATIONAL REGISTRY SKILL SHEETS   **323**

MOUTH-TO-MASK WITH SUPPLEMENTAL OXYGEN

	Points Possible	Points Awarded
Takes or verbalizes body substance isolation precautions	1	
Connects one-way valve to mask	1	
Opens patient's airway or confirms patient's airway is open (manually or with adjunct)	1	
Establishes and maintains a proper mask to face seal	1	
Ventilates the patient at the proper volume and rate (800–1200 ml per breath/10–20 breaths per minute)	1	
Connects mask to high concentration oxygen	1	
Adjusts flow rate to 15 liters/minute or greater	1	
Continues ventilation at proper volume and rate (800–1200 ml per breath/10–20 breaths per minute)	1	
NOTE: The examiner must witness ventilations for at least 30 seconds.		
TOTAL:	8	

CRITICAL CRITERIA

___ Did not take or verbalize body substance isolation precautions

___ Did not adjust liter flow to 15 L/min or greater

___ Did not provide proper volume per breath
  (more than 2 ventilations per minute are below 800 ml)

___ Did not ventilate the patient at 10-20 breaths per minute

___ Did not allow for complete exhalation

OXYGEN ADMINISTRATION

	Points Possible	Points Awarded
Takes or verbalizes body substance isolation precautions	1	
Assembles regulator to tank	1	
Opens tank	1	
Checks for leaks	1	
Checks tank pressure	1	
Attaches non-rebreather mask	1	
Prefills reservoir	1	
Adjusts liter flow to 12 liters/minute or greater	1	
Applies and adjusts mask to the patient's face	1	
NOTE: The examiner must advise the candidate that the patient is not tolerating the non-rebreather mask. Medical direction has ordered you to apply a nasal cannula to the patient.		
Attaches nasal cannula to oxygen	1	
Adjusts liter flow up to 6 liters/minute or less	1	
Applies nasal cannula to the patient	1	
NOTE: The examiner must advise the candidate to discontinue oxygen therapy.		
Removes the nasal cannula	1	
Shuts off the regulator	1	
Relieves the pressure within the regulator	1	
TOTAL:	15	

CRITICAL CRITERIA

___ Did not take or verbalize body substance isolation precautions
___ Did not assemble the tank and regulator without leaks
___ Did not prefill the reservoir bag
___ Did not adjust the device to the correct liter flow for the non-rebreather mask
     (12 L/min or greater)
___ Did not adjust the device to the correct liter flow for the nasal cannula (up to 6 L/min)

VENTILATORY MANAGEMENT
ENDOTRACHEAL INTUBATION

NOTE: If a candidate elects to initially ventilate with a BVM attached to a reservoir and oxygen, full credit must be awarded for steps denoted by "**" if the first ventilation is delivered within the initial 30 seconds

	Points Possible	Points Awarded
Takes or verbalizes body substance isolation precautions	1	
Opens airway manually	1	
Elevates tongue and inserts simple airway adjunct (oropharyngeal or nasopharyngeal airway)	1	
NOTE: The examiner now informs the candidate no gag reflect is present and the patient accepts the adjunct.		
**Ventilates the patient immediately using a BVM device unattached to oxygen	1	
**Hyperventilates the patient with room air	1	
Note: The examiner now informs the candidate that ventilation is being performed without difficulty.		
Attaches the oxygen reservoir to the BVM	1	
Attaches BVM to high-flow oxygen	1	
Ventilates the patient at the proper volume and rate (800–1200 ml per breath/10–20 breaths per minute)	1	
NOTE: After 30 seconds, the examiner auscultates and reports breath sounds are present and equal bilaterally and medical control has ordered intubation. The examiner must now take over ventilation.		
Directs assistant to hyperventilate patient	1	
Identifies/selects proper equipment for intubation	1	
Checks equipment — Checks for cuff leaks	1	
Checks equipment — Checks laryngoscope operation and bulb tightness	1	
NOTE: The examiner must remove the OPA and move out of the way when the candidate is prepared to intubate.		
Positions the head properly	1	
Inserts the laryngoscope blade while displacing the tongue	1	
Elevates the mandible with the laryngoscope	1	
Introduces the ET tube and advances it to the proper depth	1	
Inflates the cuff to the proper pressure	1	
Disconnects the syringe from the cuff inlet port	1	
Directs ventilation of the patient	1	
Confirms proper placement by auscultation bilaterally and over the epigastrium	1	
NOTE: The examiner must ask, "If you had proper placement, what would you expect to hear?"		
Secures the ET tube (*may be verbalized*)	1	
TOTAL:	21	

CRITICAL CRITERIA

___ Did not take or verbalize body substance isolation precautions
___ Did not initiate ventilations within 30 seconds after applying gloves or interrupts ventilations for greater than 30 seconds at any time
___ Did not voice or provide high oxygen concentrations (15 L/min or greater)
___ Did not ventilate patient at a rate of at least 10/minute
___ Did not provide adequate volume per breath (maximum of 2 errors/minute permissible)
___ Did not hyperventilate the patient prior to intubation
___ Did not successfully intubate within 3 attempts
___ Used the patient's teeth as a fulcrum
___ Did not assure proper tube placement by auscultation bilaterally and over the epigastrium
___ If used, the stylette extended beyond the end of the ET tube
___ Inserts any adjunct in a manner that would be dangerous to the patient
___ Did not disconnect syringe from cuff inlet port

		Points Possible	Points Awarded
Continues body substance isolation precautions		1	
Confirms the patient is being properly ventilated with high percentage oxygen		1	
Directs assistant to hyperventilate the patient		1	
Checks/prepares airway device		1	
Lubricates distal tip of the device (*may be verbalized*)		1	
Removes the oropharyngeal airway		1	
Positions the head properly		1	
Performs a tongue-jaw lift		1	
Inserts airway device to proper depth		1	
COMBI-TUBE	PTL		
Inflates pharyngeal cuff and removes syringe	Secures strap	1	
Inflates distal cuff and removes syringe	Blows into tube #1 to inflate both cuffs	1	
Ventilates through proper first lumen		1	
Confirms placement by observing chest rise and auscultating over the epigastrium and bilaterally over the chest		1	
NOTE: The examiner states: "You do not see rise and fall of the chest and hear sounds only over the epigastrium."			
Ventilates through the alternate lumen		1	
Confirms placement by observing chest rise and auscultating over the epigastrium and bilaterally over the chest		1	
NOTE: The examiner confirms adequate chest rise, bilateral breath sounds, and absent sounds over the epigastrium.			
Secures tube at appropriate step in sequence		1	
	TOTAL:	16	

CRITICAL CRITERIA

___ Did not take or verbalize body substance isolation precautions.
___ Interrupts ventilation for greater than 30 seconds.
___ Did not direct hyperventilation of the patient prior to placement of the device.
___ Did not assure proper placement of the device.
___ Did not successfully ventilate patient.
___ Did not provide high flow oxygen (15 L/min or greater).
___ Inserts any adjunct in a manner that would be dangerous to the patient.

VENTILATORY MANAGEMENT
ESOPHAGEAL OBTURATOR AIRWAY INSERTION FOLLOWING
AN UNSUCCESSFUL ENDOTRACHEAL INTUBATION ATTEMPT

	Points Possible	Points Awarded
Continues body substance isolation precautions	1	
Confirms the patient is being properly ventilated	1	
Directs assistant to hyperventilate the patient	1	
Identifies/selects proper equipment	1	
Assembles airway	1	
Tests cuff	1	
Inflates mask	1	
Lubricates tube (*may be verbalized*)	1	
Removes the oropharyngeal airway	1	
Positions head properly with neck in the neutral or slightly flexed position	1	
Grasps and elevates tongue and mandible	1	
Inserts and elevates tongue and mandible	1	
Inserts tube in the same direction as the curvature of the pharynx	1	
Advances tube until the mask is sealed against the face	1	
Ventilates the patient while maintaining a tight mask seal	1	
Confirms placement by observing chest rise and auscultating over the epigastrium and bilaterally over the chest	1	
NOTE: The examiner confirms adequate chest rise, bilateral breath sounds and absent sounds over the epigastrium.		
Inflates the cuff to the proper pressure	1	
Disconnects the syringe	1	
Continues ventilation of the patient	1	
TOTAL:	18	

CRITICAL CRITERIA

___ Did not take or verbalize body substance isolation precautions.
___ Interrupts ventilation for more than 30 seconds
___ Did not direct hyperventilation of the patient prior to placement of the device.
___ Did not assure proper placement of the device
___ Did not successfully ventilate the patient
___ Did not provide high flow oxygen (15 L/min or greater)
___ Inserts any adjunct in a manner that would be dangerous to the patient

328   NATIONAL REGISTRY SKILL SHEETS

The number(s) following each question refer to the textbook page(s) where the answer can be found or supported.

CHAPTER 1 — INTRODUCTION TO EMERGENCY MEDICAL CARE

Terms and Concepts

1. a. 4 b. 5 c. 1 d. 6 e. 3 f. 2 *(pp. 3-5)*

Content Review

1. **b.** The other items are EMT-I or EMT-P skills. *(pp. 4-5)*
2. **a.** YOUR safety first and always; then other rescuers/bystander safety. When the scene is secure you may then provide care for the patient. *(pp. 5-6)*
3. **c.** All the items listed are potential hazards. Be especially aware of the hazards from traffic at nighttime scenes. *(p. 6)*
4. At nighttime traffic scenes: **a.** Wear reflective clothing; **b.** Provide adequate lighting *(p. 6)*
5. **b.** This will result in much discussion. The best answer, given the situation described, is to move or retreat to an area where you can observe the scene and await the arrival of law enforcement. You should not approach until law enforcement tells you the scene is safe. *(p. 6)*
6. **b.** Quality improvement. *(pp. 9-10)*
7. **b.** Latex or other disposable gloves, eye protection, mask, and gown are the most commonly used equipment worn to protect against infectious diseases. Disposable gloves and eye protection are the most commonly worn. If the potential for splash of body fluid exists then the mask and cover gown would be added. Leather gloves, turnout gear, helmets or hard hats, and boots would be worn at an accident scene. Self contained breathing apparatus is used mainly by hazardous materials teams when toxic fumes are present. *(p. 6)*
8. The medical director is: **a.** Legally responsible for clinical and patient care aspects; **b.** Responsible for overseeing quality improvement for the EMS System *(p. 9)*
9. **b.** The EMT-B functions as an agent of the system medical director. *(p. 9)*
10. Be honest in your rankings. Ask a friend to rank you on these items; then compare the results. Nobody's perfect but you must recognize your limitations so you can improve. *(pp. 8-9)*
11. **d.** Patient advocacy includes actions such as collecting patient valuables (if time permits), protecting patients from onlookers, and honoring the patient's requests (as possible). *(pp. 7-8)*
12. **c.** Agencies commonly accessed by 9-1-1 include law enforcement, fire services, and EMS. *(pp. 3-4)*

Case Study

1. **d.** Law enforcement has the primary responsibility for traffic control. At this scene, the car was just over the crest of a hill. This could create a potential hazard to rescuers while working this scene. If law enforcement is not on scene when you arrive you (or others) will need to control traffic until they arrive.
2. **a.** The fire department has the primary responsibility for extrication and hazard control at this scene. The fire/rescue department, if properly trained, may need to secure downed power lines in emergency situations when the power company is not on scene. Otherwise the power company would deal with electrical hazards.
3. **b.** EMS/ambulance service has the primary responsibility for patient care and transport. In many areas the fire service also provides EMS.
4. **d.** Do what you can, when you can for the patient. Patient advocacy requires doing what is in the patient's best interest.
5. **d.** Prehospital care reports and feedback from crews and patients all provide information that contributes to quality improvement.

Chapters Answer Key

6. **d.** Traffic is certainly a hazard given that the accident occurred on a steep hill at night. The danger of fire is a possibility at any vehicle accident and the vehicle could have been in an unstable position. Downed power lines could also be a potential hazard.

CHAPTER 2 — THE WELL-BEING OF THE EMT-BASIC

Terms and Concepts
1. **a.** 1 **b.** 3 **c.** 2 **d.** 5 **e.** 4 *(p. 28)*

Content Review
1. Denial, depression. The five emotional stages associated with death and dying are: denial, anger, bargaining, depression, acceptance. *(p. 14)*
2. Answers may include any three of the following: Maintain the patient's dignity. Show respect for the patient. Communicate with the patient. Allow family members to express themselves. Listen empathetically. Do not give false assurances. Use a gentle tone. Let the patient know that everything that can be done will be done. Use a reassuring touch. Do what you can to comfort the family. [If done, these should not delay treatment or transport.] *(pp. 14-15)*
3. **d.** All of these are signs of stress. *(p. 15)*
4. Defusing. *(p. 18)*
5. Pathogens *(p. 18)*
6. **a.** Handwashing *(p. 20)*
7. Specialized teams (experts) *(p. 25)*
8. **a.** 5 **b.** 2 **c.** 3 **d.** 1 **e.** 4. Identify hazards with binoculars and guidebook, await scene control by hazmat team, put on necessary protective clothing, and then (and only then) provide patient assessment and emergency care. *(p. 23)*
9. **a.** Call for police assistance before entering a potentially violent scene. *(pp. 25-26)*
10. **b.** Avoid disturbing a crime scene, but remember that your priority as an EMT-B is patient care. *(pp. 25-26)*

Case Study
1. Your patient seems to be exhibiting the acceptance stage of emotional response to death and dying.
2. Honor the patient's request for privacy and allow him time alone with his wife. Reassure him that you'll be only a short distance away if he should want anything.
3. Your signs and symptoms indicate that you are suffering from critical incident stress. You should request that a critical incident stress debriefing be conducted for all of the rescuers who were involved in this call. It is very understandable to have a significant emotional reaction to an incident like this, and other rescuers may be having similar reactions.

CHAPTER 3 — MEDICAL, LEGAL, AND ETHICAL ISSUES

Terms and Concepts
1. **a.** 4 **b.** 6 **c.** 5 **d.** 2 **e.** 3 **f.** 1 *(p. 38)*

Content Review
1. **b.** Federal laws *(p. 31)*
2. **d.** Battery *(p. 32)*

3. **c.** Good Samaritan law *(p. 31)*
4. **a.** Standard of care *(p. 31)*
5. **b.** The patient's expressed or implied consent *(pp. 32-33)*
6. **a.** Implied consent. (It is not minor consent, which must be given by a parent or guardian.) *(p. 34)*
7. **c.** 1 and 2 (To refuse care, a patient must be mentally competent and informed. He is not legally required to sign a release, although the EMT-B should attempt to get a signed and witnessed release for the legal protection of the EMT-B and the EMS system.) *(p. 34)*
8. **c.** Both a and b. (Shaking the head, pushing away, or any other indication that care is not welcome — before or after care is begun — constitutes valid refusal if the patient is a competent adult.) *(p. 34)*
9. **b.** Abandonment *(p. 35)*)
10. **a.** Patient information may not be given to an off-duty EMT-B or any other person without a legitimate need for the information. (The other 3 choices name circumstances in which confidential information may be released.) *(pp. 35-36)*

Case Study 1
1. **b.** 2 and 3. (The patient seemed mentally competent but gave signs of not understanding the information and appeared to sign the release without reading it. The feelings of the other EMT-B are not a priority.)
2. **d.** (The other choices should be pursued only when all efforts to persuade the patient have failed.)

Case Study 2
1. **a.** Y **b.** Y **c.** Y **d.** Y (This situation meets all four criteria for a successful negligence suit.)

CHAPTER 4 — THE HUMAN BODY

Terms and Concepts
1. **a.** transverse line **b.** posterior **c.** prone **d.** superior **e.** normal anatomical position **f.** midaxillary **g.** inferior **h.** lateral **i.** anterior **j.** distal **k.** midline *(pp. 68-70)*

Content Review
1. **c.** The patient's right *(p. 42)*
2. **a.** midline **b.** proximal **c.** distal **d.** medial **e.** lateral **f.** palmar **g.** plantar **h.** anterior **i.** posterior **j.** superior **k.** midaxillary **l.** inferior *(pp. 42, 44)*
3. **a.** Bilateral refers to right and left; the femur is the thigh bone. *(pp. 42, 46)*
4. **a.** Posterior means "toward the back." *(p. 42)*
5. **c.** Lateral means "toward or on the side"; recumbent means "lying down." *(p. 40)*
6. **d.** Thoracic spine *(p. 46)*
7. **a.** Cervical spine (the neck) *(p. 46)*
8. **d.** Ball and socket joints *(p. 49, 50)*
9. **c.** Voluntary muscles can be consciously controlled; involuntary muscle movements are automatic. *(p. 50)*

10. **b.** The unresponsive patient may not be able to protect his airway, partly because the epiglottis fails to close over the trachea. *(p. 52)*

11. **b.** The thoracic cavity increases, creating lower pressure inside the chest than in the atmosphere, causing air to flow into the lungs. *(p. 52)*

12. **b.** The infant or child's tongue takes up proportionately *more* space in the smaller mouth. *(pp. 52-53)*

13. **d.** Use of accessory muscles (e.g., muscles of the neck, above the clavicles, below the ribs) to aid in breathing is a sign that normal breathing mechanisms are not functioning adequately. The other choices are signs of adequate breathing. *(p. 55)*

14. **a.** cranium **b.** zygomatic bone **c.** maxilla **d.** cervical vertebra **e.** sternum **f.** xiphoid process **g.** iliac crest **h.** ilium **i.** pelvic girdle **j.** greater trochanter **k.** symphysis pubis **l.** frontal bone **m.** parietal bone **n.** occipital bone **o.** temporal bone **p.** mandible **q.** clavicle **r.** scapula **s.** ribs **t.** humerus **u.** elbow **v.** ulna **w.** radius **x.** sacrum **y.** coccyx **z.** carpals **aa.** metacarpals **bb.** phalanges **cc.** femur **dd.** patella **ee.** tibia **ff.** fibula **gg.** tarsals **hh.** metatarsals **ii.** calcaneus *(pp. 45-49)*

15. **a.** Gas exchange takes place between capillaries and alveoli and between capillaries and the body's cells. *(pp. 54-55)*

16. **d.** (1) atria (2) ventricles *(p. 58)*

17. **d.** The white blood cells *(p. 59)*

18. **c.** The carotid (in the neck) is a central pulse. The radial (wrist), brachial (upper arm), and tibial (ankle) are considered peripheral pulses (away from the center). *(p. 59)*

19. **d.** Perfusion ("Hypo" in hypoperfusion means "low" – so hypoperfusion is low, or inadequate, perfusion.) *(p. 59)*

20. **a.** Brain and spinal cord *(pp. 59-60)*

21. **b.** Pituitary *(p. 62)*

22. **d.** Largest organ, protects against bacteria, regulates temperature *(p. 62)*

Case Study

1. Supine is on the back (face up).

2. **a.** Large laceration to right midclavicular line (center of right clavicle) superior to (above) the right nipple. (Right = patient's right)

3. **a.** Deformity to the proximal (nearest the torso) end of the left (patient's left) humerus (upper arm bone).

4. **b.** Bilateral (to both legs) femoral region (are around and including the thigh bone) deformity with puncture wound to the left (patient's left) lateral thigh (toward the outside of the thigh, away from the body's midline which runs between the legs) proximal to (nearer the torso in relation to) the patella (kneecap).

5. Trendelenburg position is supine with lower body elevated approximately 12 inches. (It is sometimes called "shock position," but its use for shock patients is controversial.)

CHAPTER 5 — BASELINE VITAL SIGNS AND HISTORY TAKING

Terms and Concepts

1. **a.** 5 **b.** 1 **c.** 3 **d.** 4 **e.** 7 **f.** 2 **g.** 6 *(p. 81)*

Content Review

1. The components of vital sign assessment include breathing, pulse, skin, pupils, and blood pressure. *(p. 73)*

2. **c.** Counting the number of respirations in 30 seconds, multiplying by 2 *(p. 74)*

3. **d.** Inhalations and exhalations of about the same length *(p. 74)*

4. **d.** Shallow, labored, or noisy *(p.74)*

5. **a.** carotid **b.** brachial **c.** radial **d.** femoral **e.** posterior tibial **f.** dorsalis pedis *(p. 74)*

6. **c.** Counting the number of beats in 30 seconds, multiplying by 2 *(p. 75)*

7. **b.** Brachial *(p. 74)*

8. **d.** 120-150 beats per minute is normal range for an infant. *(p. 75)*

9. **b.** Full and regular at 60 beats per minute *(p. 75)*

10. **a.** Pale conjunctiva *(p. 76)*

11. capillary refill *(p. 77)*

12. the back of your hand *(p. 76)*

13. dry *(p. 77)*

14. less than 2 seconds *(p. 77)*

15. size, equality, reactivity *(p. 77)*

16. **b.** Arteries *(p. 78)*

17. Systolic pressure is a measure of the pressure exerted against the wall of the arteries when the left ventricle of the heart contracts. It is the first distinct sound of blood flowing through the artery as the pressure in the sphygmomanometer is released. *(p. 78)*

18. Diastolic pressure is a measure of the pressure exerted against the wall of the arteries when the left ventricle is at rest. It is assessed as the point during deflation of the sphygmomanometer when you can no longer hear the pulse beat. *(p. 78)*

19. **c.** A sphygmomanometer and a stethoscope *(pp. 78-79)*

20. The steps for measuring a patient's blood pressure in proper sequence are: *(pp. 78-79)* **2.** Apply the stethoscope to the brachial pulse and deflate the cuff at approximately 2 mmHG per second. **5.** Leave the deflated cuff in place so you can take additional readings. **3.** When you hear two or more consecutive beats, this is the systolic pressure. Record it. **4.** Continue releasing air from until you hear the last sound or until the sound changes from clear tapping to soft, muffled tapping. This is the diastolic pressure. Record it. **1.** Inflate the cuff to 30 mmHg above the point where you no longer feel the radial pulse.

21. 15, 5 *(p. 79)*

22. **a.** A **b.** L **c.** S **d.** M **e.** P **f.** S **g.** A **h.** E **i.** S **j.** L **k.** M **l.** P *(pp. 79-80)*

Case Study

1. Mr. Baker is in severe respiratory distress. His breathing rate is faster than normal at a rate of 26 breaths per minute and his breathing quality is both labored (using accessory muscles) and noisy (audible wheezing and gurgling).

2. His skin is slightly cyanotic, cool, and moist. His bluish skin color indicates that he has inadequate oxygenation and poor perfusion. Cool moist skin also indicates hypoperfusion.

3. His radial pulse is weak (thready) and irregular, which indicates that he is in shock (hypoperfusion). The rate of 50 beats per minute is slower than normal which may also point to heart problems. An auscultated blood pressure at 80/50 mmHg also indicates hypoperfusion. Your impression is that his heart is not working very efficiently and as a result his circulation is inadequate.

4. Signs and symptoms: Mr. Baker states that he can't breathe. Rapid, noisy (audible wheezing and gurgling), labored breathing. Skin is slightly cyanotic, cool, and moist. Weak, irregular pulse. Allergies: Mrs. Baker says that her husband has no allergies. Medications: Digoxin and Lasix taken daily, nitroglycerin as needed for angina. None today according to wife. Pertinent past history: Heart attack 5 years ago: Ate a bowl of soup at lunch. Did not eat supper. Events leading to illness: Shoveled snow this morning and since then has been increasingly short of breath but denied having chest pain.

5. Mr. Baker should have his vital signs reassessed every 5 minutes because he is an unstable patient, in severe respiratory distress and showing signs of inadequate oxygenation and perfusion.

CHAPTER 6 — PREPARING TO LIFT AND MOVE PATIENTS

Terms and Concepts

1. **a.** Body mechanics involves use of the most effective methods of gaining a mechanical advantage when lifting or moving; use of lifting and moving techniques that help prevent injury. **b.** Power grip means the palm and all fingers are in contact with the object, all fingers bent at the same angle. **c.** Power lift is done with feet apart, knees bent, back and abdominal muscles tightened, back straight, lifting force driven through feet and ankles, upper body rising before hips. (p. 90)

Content Review

1. **a.** Reaching a great distance to lift a light object (p. 83)
2. **a.** Leg, hip, and gluteal muscles (avoid lifting with your back muscles; avoid reaching) (p. 83)
3. **b.** Keeping your shoulders, hips, and feet in vertical alignment (p. 84)
4. Flexibility training, cardiovascular conditioning, strength training, and nutrition. (p. 84)
5. **c.** Always try to lock the back. Lifting the upper body first reduces movement of the back (pp. 86-87)
6. **b.** Place the weaker leg slightly forward of the good leg. (p. 87)
7. **a.** Leaning to the opposite side (p. 87)
8. **d.** Place a spotter to direct and navigate (pp. 87-88)
9. **c.** 20 inches (p. 88)
10. **b.** Push rather than pull; keep the load between hip and shoulder.

Case Study

1. **b.** Keep their backs locked and stay as close to the stretcher as possible, avoiding leaning
2. **c.** Lower the stretcher onto its wheels so the stretcher does part of the work, with the rescuers at the back pushing it along the boardwalk
3. All of the above
4. **a.** (The power lift is recommended for *all* patients, especially heavy patients.)

CHAPTER 7 — AIRWAY MANAGEMENT, VENTILATION, AND OXYGEN THERAPY

Terms and Concepts

1. **a.** 3 **b.** 1 **c.** 17 **d.** 2 **e.** 5 **f.** 18 **g.** 21 **h.** 20 **i.** 19 **j.** 8 **k.** 15 **l.** 9 **m.** 12 **n.** 7 **o.** 6 **p.** 13 **q.** 14 (pp. 127-129)

Content Review

1. **d.** All are correct. (pp. 96-97)
2. **a.** mandible **b.** thyroid cartilage **c.** trachea **d.** cricoid cartilage **e.** nasal cavity **f.** nasopharynx **g.** soft palate **h.** oropharynx **i.** tongue **j.** epiglottis **k.** vocal cords **l.** larynx **m.** esophagus (p. 94)
3. **a.** Diaphragm (p. 95)
4. **c.** Sweep the mouth with your GLOVED index finger. (p. 97)
5. To perform the head-tilt, chin-lift maneuver, place one hand on the patient's forehead, apply firm backward pressure, tilt the head backward, place the tips of the fingers of the other hand under the bone of the chin, and lift the chin. (p. 98)
6. **a.** Jaw-thrust maneuver (p. 99)
7. **d.** Neutral (p. 98)
8. **d.** All of these (p. 100)
9. **c.** Hard catheter. (p. 100)
10. **c.** 15 seconds for the adult; 5 seconds for the infant or child (p. 101)
11. **c.** Suction for 15 seconds, provide positive pressure ventilation for 2 minutes, repeat. (p. 101)
12. **c.** Measure the airway from the corner of the patient's mouth to the tip of the earlobe. (p. 102)
13. **c.** The flange rests on the flare of the nostril (p. 104)
14. In a patient who is breathing adequately **a.** The rate will be within normal limits. **b.** The rhythm will be a regular pattern, inhalations and exhalations about equal in length. **c.** The quality will include breath sounds that are equal and full bilaterally, chest rising and falling adequately and equally with each breath, and no excessive accessory muscle use (children normally use abdominal muscles in breathing more than adults do). **d.** The depth, or tidal volume, will seem adequate as you feel and hear the breath with your ear next to the patient's mouth and nose and as you see the chest rise and fall. (pp. 106-107)
15. Normal ranges are: adult 12 to 20; child 15 to 30; infant 25 to 50 respirations a minute (p. 106)
16. **a.** Bilateral chest rise (p. 107)
17. **c.** Provide positive pressure ventilation (p. 108)
18. **c.** 4, 3, 1, 2 (mouth-to-mask; two-person BVM; flow-restricted, oxygen-powered ventilation device; one-person BVM) (p. 108)

19. **b.** Inhale oxygen from a cannula or oxygen mask between ventilations. *(p. 109)*
20. **b.** (The rescuer must breathe into the mask; ventilations are not delivered automatically.) *(pp. 110-111)*
21. **a.** Ventilate adults every 5 seconds, infants and children every 3 seconds. *(p. 109)*
22. **a.** face mask **b.** nonrebreathing patient valve **c.** bag **d.** intake valve/oxygen reservoir valve **e.** oxygen reservoir **f.** oxygen supply connecting tube
23. **c.** 21% (the same atmospheric air) *(p. 111)*
24. **a.** Allows a single operator to easily maintain a tight mask seal (A disadvantage of the bag-valve mask is that it is very difficult for a single operator to squeeze the bag, maintain an open airway, and also maintain mask seal.) *(pp. 111-112)*
25. **c.** Establish in-line stabilization and perform a jaw-thrust maneuver, then ventilate *(pp. 108, 114)*
26. **b.** It is recommended for children and infants. (The flow-restricted, oxygen-powered ventilation device is designed to be used only on adult patients.) *(p. 115)*
27. **a.** As soon as the chest begins to rise *(p. 115)*
28. **c.** Reevaluate the position of the head, chin, and mask seal *(pp. 115-116)*
29. **b.** Consult with medical direction. *(p. 116)*
30. **b.** Approximately 2,000 pounds per square inch *(p. 116)*
31. **d.** All of the above *(p. 117)*
32. **c.** High pressure regulator *(p. 117)*
33. **c.** Quickly open and shut the valve on the cylinder *(p. 119)*
34. **b.** Remove the mask from the patient's face, then disconnect the tubing from the nipple *(p. 120)*
35. **d.** 15 liters per minute (A lesser flow may not inflate the reservoir bag and may cause hypoxia.) *(p. 120)*
36. **c.** Have someone familiar with the child hold the mask close to the patient's face. *(p. 120)*
37. **a.** When the patient will not tolerate a nonrebreather mask *(p. 120)*
38. **a.** 1-6 liters per minute *(p. 121)*
39. **c.** Nonrebreather mask *(pp. 120, 122)*
40. **d.** Leave them in the mouth for a better mask seal

Case Study 1

1. Answers should include at least three of these indications: her position (upright, tripod position); that she is obviously anxious; her gasping breaths; her statement, "I can't breathe."
2. **d.** The nonrebreather mask at 15 lpm. (The Venturi and simple face masks are not recommended for prehospital use, and the nasal cannula only if the patient will not tolerate the nonrebreather mask.)
3. **a.** Rigid catheter (with large bore), insert without suction, suction for 15 seconds (more time risks hypoxia).
4. **c.** Nasopharyngeal airway (responsive patient can't tolerate oral airway), bevel first (the other is upside down).
5. **b.** Continue to ventilate and suction as before. (She has a pulse, so CPR is not appropriate.

Suctioning must be done so ventilations are effective. Check pulse often. If pulse becomes absent, begin CPR or defibrillation if available.)

Case Study 2

1. **c.** In-line stabilization with jaw-thrust. (This patient has a suspected spinal injury from the fall.)
2. **d.** Suction, using the rigid or hard catheter. (Turning the head or performing back blows may compromise the spine. Finger sweeps and soft French catheter are inadequate.)
3. **d.** Any or all of these could be the cause of the chest failing to rise with ventilations (as well as BVM failure or operator error).

CHAPTER 8 — SCENE SIZE-UP

Terms and Concepts

1. **a.** medical emergency – a problem brought on by illness or a condition that affects the body (Examples: heart attack, drug overdose, diabetic emergency) **b.** trauma emergency – physical injury or wound caused by external force or violence. (Examples: burns, gunshot wounds, lacerations, fractures) *(p. 145)*
2. **a.** 5 **b.** 1 **c.** 2 **d.** 4 **e.** 3 *(p. 145)*

Content Review

1. **a.** EMT-Bs, patients, and bystanders *(p. 131)*
2. **d.** While receiving dispatch information *(p. 132)*
3. **c.** Protective gloves *(p. 132)*
4. **a.** Ask some bystanders to hold up a sheet *(p. 139)*
5. **d.** Call for additional resources *(p. 143)*
6. **a.** Consider all power lines to be energized until a power company representative advises you they are not. *(p. 134)*
7. **b.** Notify your dispatcher and wait for a rescue crew *(p. 135)*
8. **d.** Enter the scene only after it has been secured by police *(p. 136)*
9. **c.** Knock while standing off to the knob side. *(p. 137)*
10. **b.** A large laceration to the head (A mechanism of injury is what caused the injury. A laceration is the result of a mechanism of injury.) *(p. 141)*

Case Study 1

1. **d.** Stage your vehicle outside the scene, no lights and siren, until scene safety is confirmed
2. **b.** Immediately call for additional transporting and ALS units
3. **c.** Not touch the gun but notify the police (The gun is not interfering with treatment so there is no need to attempt to move it.)
4. **c.** Retreat temporarily until the police can give you support

Case Study 2

1. Answers may include any three of the following: The address of the call gives a clue about whether this is or is not generally a safe neighborhood; "elderly" helps you to anticipate a geriatric patient; "cough for months" indicates a medical condition and alerts you to take BSI precautions; a husband calling about his wife may mean a relatively safe domestic environment; the fact that no one is

presently answering the phone may indicate that the emergency is severe or that the caller is also ill.

2. **d.** Before entering the house, both EMT-Bs should put on gloves, eye protection, and a HEPA respirator.

3. **a.** Because the patient presents signs of TB, you continue to wear the respirator and advise the hospital of the precaution.

CHAPTER 9 — PATIENT ASSESSMENT

Terms and concepts

1. a. 15 b. 2 c. 9 d. 6 e. 8 f. 4 g. 13 h. 14 i. 7 j. 11 k. 12 l. 10 m. 1 n. 5 o. 3 *(pp. 217-218)*

Content Review

1. **d.** All of these *(p. 148)*
2. **c.** The other three are the main components of the scene size-up. *(p. 151)*
3. **b.** Get to the patient! Make the transition as you are treating the patient. *(p. 152)*
4. **b.** Any of these techniques might be useful, but given the overt physical threats, the best course is to leave until the scene is controlled. *(p. 153)*
5. **b.** Establish in-line stabilization *(p. 158)*
6. **c.** Until the patient is fully immobilized to a backboard *(pp. 158-159)*
7. **c.** Every patient must receive an initial assessment. *(p. 154)*
8. **c.** The initial assessment is always performed in this sequence: Form a general impression, assess mental status, assess airway, assess breathing, assess circulation, establish patient priorities. *(p. 154)*
9. **a.** General impression *(p. 155)*
10. **d.** "Why did you call the ambulance?" (or "What seems to be the problem?") elicits the patient's own statement without suggesting an answer. *(p. 157)*
11. **d.** The patient is not alert but does make some response to a verbal stimulus. *(p. 159)*
12. **c.** This patient responds to a verbal stimulus. Patients a and b respond only to a painful stimulus, patient d is completely unresponsive. *(pp. 159-161)*
13. **a.** If the patient is talking to you, he is moving air in and out. Observing the speaking pattern also helps in assessing breathing status. *(p. 161)*
14. **b.** Relaxation of upper airway muscles. The tongue and other soft tissues tend to fall back and cover the opening to the trachea. *(p. 161)*
15. **c.** Both crowing and stridor are signs of possible airway swelling that is too deep to be corrected by manual maneuvers or airway adjuncts. Positive pressure ventilation may be needed to force air past the obstruction. *(p. 162)*
16. **a.** A slightly fast respiration rate is not considered life-threatening if the patient is responsive, but is considered life-threatening if the patient is unresponsive. *(p. 163)*
17. **c.** Positive pressure ventilation is any method that forces air into the patient's lungs. A nonrebreather mask provides oxygen that the patient breathes in on his own. *(pp. 163-164)*

18. **b.** Capillary refill is considered a reliable indication of adequate perfusion (circulation) only in children under 6 years of age. In older patients, other factors commonly affect capillary refill rates. *(p. 166)*
19. **a.** The exact heart rate. The initial assessment is performed to detect life-threatening conditions, for which an approximate heart rate is sufficient. An exact pulse reading will be taken later, during the focused history and physical exam. *(p. 165)*
20. **d.** Capillary bleeding is not immediately life-threatening, and time should not be taken to control it during the initial assessment. *(p. 165)*
21. **b.** The nail beds. Problems associated with environmental temperature, medical illnesses, and smoking can affect the color of the nail beds. *(p. 165)*
22. **b.** Blood loss would cause a pale or mottled skin color. Red color is commonly associated with an increase in blood circulation in the skin, for example as a result of heat exposure when the body attempts to lose heat through the skin surface. *(p. 166)*
23. **d.** Cool, clammy skin is one of the major signs of shock (hypoperfusion). *(p. 166)*
24. **b.** Greater than 2 seconds (Two seconds can be counted by saying "One one-thousand, two one-thousand" or the words "capillary refill.") *(p. 166)*
25. All require rapid transport except 3 and 5. Your supervisor is impressed with your work. *(p. 167)*
26. **b.** Properly performed, the rapid trauma assessment takes only moments and should always be completed before moving the patient to the stretcher. *(p. 167)*
27. All are considered significant mechanisms of injury except 2 and 4. Keep up the good job. You might just get that promotion! *(pp. 170-171)*
28. **b.** A fall while running is unlikely to be a significant mechanism of injury. However, maintain "a high index of suspicion. Children's less-developed bones and muscles offer less protection to internal organs. Children have a smaller blood supply so even minor bleeding can be dangerous. And their bodies compensate for shock longer than in adults, so that by the time a child displays signs of shock, he is already in severe difficulty. Err to benefit the patient; take even minor mechanisms of injury seriously. *(p. 171)*
29. **b.** For a trauma patient with a significant mechanism of injury, perform the focused history and physical exam in this sequence: rapid trauma assessment, baseline vital signs, SAMPLE history. *(p. 170)*
30. **d.** For a trauma patient with no significant mechanism of injury, perform the focused history and physical exam in this sequence: focused trauma assessment, baseline vital signs, SAMPLE history. *(p. 170)*
31. **b.** Rapid transport and hyperventilate at 24-30 per minute. This patient's deteriorating mental status indicates a possible head injury. Ventilation at twice the normal rate is indicated. Immobilize the spine, transport immediately, and continue to monitor his mental status. *(p. 173)*

32. **d.** Use your senses of sight (inspection), touch (palpation), hearing (auscultation), and smell to pick up all possible clues to your patient's condition. *(p. 173)*

33. Deformities, contusions, abrasions, punctures/penetrations, burns, tenderness, lacerations, swelling. *(p. 173)*

34. **b.** During the rapid trauma assessment, the head is examined quickly to determine if there is a possible head injury. A more detailed examination of the head may be conducted during the detailed physical exam. *(p. 174)*

35. **d.** Inspect the neck for tracheal deviation or tugging, jugular vein distention, subcutaneous emphysema (can also be palpated), large lacerations or punctures. *(p. 178)*

36. **c.** Determine both presence and equality of breath sounds. *(p. 180)*

37. **a.** Palpate the abdomen for tenderness, distention, and rigidity. *(p. 180)*

38. **c.** Ordinarily palpate the pelvis, but assume pelvic injury if the patient complains of pain or there is obvious deformity and do not aggravate the injury or condition by palpating. *(p. 181)*

39. **a.** "PMS" refers to indicators that circulation and nerve function to the extremities are intact: pulses, motor function, and sensation. *(p. 181)*

40. **a.** Log-roll the patient while maintaining in-line stabilization. *(p. 181)*

41. **c.** Apply the CSID after the neck has been assessed. (You can't fully assess the neck with a collar on, although most have holes on the anterior surface to allow later inspection.) Remember that the CSID does not fully immobilize the head and neck; therefore, manual in-line stabilization must continue to be maintained after CSID is in place until the patient is fully immobilized to the long spine board. *(p. 179)*

42. **d.** Vital signs should be reassessed every 5 minutes in an unstable patient (every 15 minutes in a stable patient). This applies to both trauma and medical patients. *(pp. 182, 193)*

43. Signs and symptoms, allergies, medications, pertinent past history, last oral intake, events leading to the incident. *(pp. 183-184)*

44. **c.** If there is a suspicion of other injuries, always perform a head-to-toe rapid trauma assessment. *(p. 187)*

45. **d.** The focused history and physical exam in the responsive medical patient should be performed in this sequence: SAMPLE history, focused medical assessment (focused on the area of the patient's complaint), vital signs. *(p. 189)*

46. **b.** The focused history and physical exam in the unresponsive medical patient should be performed in this sequence: rapid medical assessment (head to toe), vital signs, SAMPLE history. *(p. 189)*

47. **d.** In the rapid medical assessment, palpate the abdomen for tenderness, rigidity, distention, and pulsating masses. *(p. 190)*

48. **b.** In the rapid medical assessment, assess the extremities for swelling and for PMS (pulses, motor function, sensation). Also look for a medical identification device (often a wrist or ankle bracelet). *(p. 192)*

49. **a.** The vital signs are respiration, pulse, skin, pupils, and blood pressure. *(p. 193)*

50. Onset, provocation, quality, radiation, severity, time. *(p. 195)*

51. **c.** The lateral recumbent position permits fluids to drain from the mouth of the unresponsive patient and helps prevent airway blockage or aspiration. Placing the patient on his left side assures that he will be facing the EMT-B who is riding with him in the back of the ambulance. *(p. 193)*

52. **b.** Gather both prescription and over-the-counter medications to bring to the hospital with the patient. Both will be important clues for hospital personnel. *(p. 194)*

53. **c.** If the patient doesn't have a specific complaint on which you can focus the physical exam, perform a head-to-toe rapid assessment. *(p. 196)*

54. **b.** If a patient is one who required a head-to-toe rapid assessment, he should also receive a head-to-toe detailed assessment if time and the patient's condition permit. *(p. 198)*

55. **d.** The purposes of the ongoing assessment are to detect any change in the patient's condition, to identify any injuries or conditions that were missed earlier in the assessment, and to adjust the emergency care as needed. *(p. 211)*

Case Study 1

1. **c.** Positive pressure ventilation at 24-to-30 per minute (hyperventilation) while maintaining in-line stabilization.

2. **a.** Rapid trauma assessment and, if possible, detailed physical exam

3. **c.** The presence of a carotid pulse indicates that the patient has a blood pressure of AT LEAST 60 mmHg.

Case Study 2

1. Answers should include at least three of these: The wife couldn't wake the patient; the patient was blue; the patient was unresponsive to verbal stimulus; the patient was unresponsive to painful stimulus; snoring sound; pillow behind head.

2. **c.** Head-tilt, chin-lift

3. **c.** 8/24

4. **c.** Rapid medical assessment

Case Study 3

1. **b.** Suggest a task for the girlfriend.

2. Apply direct pressure, then a pressure dressing.

3. **c.** Focused trauma assessment (focused on the injury), vitals, SAMPLE

Case Study 4

1. **b.** SAMPLE, including OPQRST to get a full description of the pain.

2. **d.** Ask an open-ended question.

3. **a.** A focused medical assessment

4. **b.** The patient is responsive and has adequate breathing, so CPR and positive pressure ventilation would be inappropriate. The patient did not refuse treatment but gave consent by saying, "As long as you're here, you may as well check me out." If he had refused, you would try to persuade him to accept treatment and transport.

Case Study 5

1. **b.** Capillary refill should be checked in a child under 6.
2. **b.** His symptoms are too generalized to permit a focused assessment.
3. **b.** The patient displays classic signs of shock (hypoperfusion), including a weak, rapid pulse and a pale, cool, and clammy skin. A child with these signs is likely to deteriorate quickly. He is a high priority for rapid transport.
4. **b.** Oxygen by nonrebreather mask.

CHAPTER 10 — ASSESSMENT OF THE GERIATRIC PATIENT

Terms and Concepts
1. **a.** 7 **b.** 4 **c.** 3 **d.** 5 **e.** 1 **f.** 6 **g.** 8 **h.** 2 *(p. 235)*

Content Review
1. **b.** False *(p. 221)*
2. **b.** All except increased arterial elasticity *(p. 222)*
3. **b.** Blunted sensitivity to hypoxia *(p. 222)*
4. **d.** Osteoporosis *(p. 222)*
5. **a.** Degeneration of nerve cells *(p. 222)*
6. **c.** Malnutrition *(p. 223)*
7. **d.** All of these *(p. 223)*
8. **d.** All of these *(pp. 223-224)*
9. **d.** All except swollen lips *(p. 224)*
10. **a.** True *(p. 225)*
11. **d.** All of these *(p. 226)*
12. **b.** Lying on her side (the best way to protect the airway in a patient with an altered mental status) *(p. 227)*
13. **c.** Immobilized with blankets (to accommodate his spinal curvature) *(p. 227)*
14. **d.** Any of these *(p. 228)*
15. **b.** Fowler's position (sitting up) (usually helps support breathing in the CHF patient) *(p. 228)*
16. **c.** Fowler's position (sitting up) (usually helps support breathing in the COPD patient) *(p. 230)*
17. **a.** Administering oxygen by nonrebreather mask (Mr. Herbert's sudden onset of breathing difficulty and pain that does not radiate may indicate a pulmonary embolism, not a heart attack with pain that usually radiates.) *(p. 229)*
18. **c.** An elderly patient can easily become fatigued from labored breathing and lose the ability to sustain it. In this case, provide positive pressure ventilation to sustain respiration and expedite transport. *(p. 230)*
19. **b.** False (Assuming that "senility," or an altered mental status, is normal or expected in the elderly is a common error.) *(p. 230)*
20. Causes for altered mental status in the geriatric patient include dementia, heart attack, head injury, decreased blood sugar level, environmental emergencies (hypothermia or hyperthermia), hypoxia or respiratory disorders, decreased blood volume, or medication-related problems. *(p. 230)*
21. **a.** A stroke patient requires aggressive oxygenation to prevent further deterioration of brain tissue. *(p. 231)*
22. **b.** False (The first priority in a case of drug toxicity is to treat the patient for the adverse effects of the drug.) *(p. 232)*
23. **d.** All of these are common injuries resulting from falls. *(p. 233)*
24. **c.** In elderly patients, falls are often caused by dizziness, which indicates a medical problem underlying the trauma. *(p. 233)*
25. All except b (The ability to control body temperature is decreased, not enhanced, in the elderly.) *(p. 233)*
26. **1.** Protect the airway; **2.** Maintain breathing and circulation; **3.** Remove the patient from the environment; **4.** Remove wet clothing; **5.** Wrap in a dry blanket. *(p. 232)*
27. **d.** All are signs of elder abuse. *(p. 234)*
28. **c.** Your first priority is to provide medical treatment. Do not confront the family or caretakers, but do report suspected abuse according to your state or local laws or protocols. *(p. 234)*

Case Study
1. Establish and maintain manual stabilization of the head and neck. Provide oxygen at 15 lpm by nonrebreather mask. (Mrs. Walter's breathing is adequate, so positive pressure ventilation is not required, but oxygen is likely to be helpful whenever there is trauma.) Conduct a focused history and physical exam, beginning with a SAMPLE history, a medical assessment focused on the injured shoulder and adjacent areas (arm, neck, chest), and vital signs measurements. Mrs. Walter's mental status is good and she does not appear to be a high priority for rapid transport, so there is probably time to apply a sling and swathe to immobilize her injured shoulder and arm* before immobilizing her to a backboard and initiating transport to the hospital. (*Methods of immobilizing injured extremities will be taught in Chapter 32, Musculoskeletal Injuries. The student is not responsible for knowing this information for Chapter 9.)
2. Although the mechanism of injury is not significant and her injury would not seem to be critical in a younger patient, given Mrs. Walter's age and her complaint of pain you should monitor her status carefully as you continue your assessment and care. Remember to keep a high index of suspicion because any complaint of pain in the elderly is considered to be a symptom of a serious injury. Also, since her skin is slightly pale and moist, this may be an early sign of shock (hypoperfusion).

CHAPTER 11 — COMMUNICATION

Terms and Concepts
1. **a.** 3 **b.** 1 **c.** 4 **d.** 2 *(p. 248)*

Content Review
1. **d.** All of these *(p. 239)*
2. **a.** Allow communications over a wide area *(p. 240)*
3. The benefits associated with the use of cellular telephones within an EMS system include excellent sound quality, availability of channels, easy maintenance and often, increased communications privacy, which is why many EMS systems use them as a back-up system. The disadvantage is

that since cellular phone systems are part of the public phone system they can easily be overwhelmed during multiple-casualty disaster situations. *(p. 241)*
4. **b.** License base stations *(p. 241)*
5. **a.** Radio use must be brief, efficient, and professional – NOT as if talking on the telephone. *(pp. 241-243)*
6. **c.** Provide instructions about what to do till help arrives *(p. 243)*
7. **1.** Announce arrival on scene; **2.** announce departure from scene and ETA; **3.** announce arrival at hospital; **4.** announce you are clear and available for another call; **5.** announce arrival back at base.
8. **d.** All of these *(pp. 243-244)*
9. **b.** Repeat instructions word for word *(p. 244)*
10. **a.** Question the order *(p. 244)*
11. **a.** It is not necessary to obtain permission from police and fire personnel before beginning patient care. *(p. 245)*
12. **b.** Talking and loudly and slowly does not help if the person doesn't understand English – although talking slowly might help if the person has limited English. *(p. 246)*

Case Study
1. Report on arrival at the scene: Unit 3 to Dispatch. We are on the scene at the playground at 1031 Bruce Road. Over.
2. Report en route to the hospital: Washington Memorial, this is Green County BLS Unit 3 en route to you with an ETA of 12 minutes. We have a 3-year-old male with a 1-inch laceration to his chin due to a fall on the playground. He is alert and oriented. Mother reports no allergies. His vital signs are blood pressure 80/68 mmHg, pulse strong at 80, respirations 28 and of good quality. His skin is flushed, warm, and moist. Capillary refill is less than 2 seconds. Pupils are normal. The wound has been dressed and bandaged. The bleeding is controlled. Patient reports injury "hurts bad." Over.
3. Report to the hospital personnel when transferring care: This is Mikey Smith. He has a 1-inch laceration to his chin. Mrs. Smith reports that he has no allergies. We applied a dressing and a bandage. The bleeding is controlled. Current vitals: blood pressure is 80/68 mmHg, pulse 80, respirations 28, skin normal, pupils normal.

CHAPTER 12 — DOCUMENTATION

Terms and Concepts
1. a. 4 b. 2 c. 1 d. 3 *(p. 288)*

Content Review
1. **c.** To insure the continuity of patient care. *(pp. 250-251)*
2. Documentation is governed by two basic rules: "If it wasn't written down, it wasn't done," and "If it wasn't done, don't write it down." The first rule reinforces the concept that the patient care report must be a complete and accurate record of the patient encounter. Without a written record of our actions, we cannot prove that anything was done. The second rule is a reminder that recording

things that were not done as if they were done constitutes falsification of information, which is unethical and may compromise patient care. *(p. 252)*
3. **a.** True *(p. 253)*
4. **b.** Pertinent information about the scene (Include only objective and pertinent subjective information.) *(pp. 253-254)*
5. **c.** The patient denies back and neck pain. (These are symptoms that would be expected in this kind of accident, so the denial is a pertinent negative.) *(p. 254)*
6. **b.** False (Write in a simple, direct style. Avoid codes unless they are standard and commonly used in your service.) *(p. 25)*
7. **b.** Patient information must not be given out to friends, reporters or others who are merely curious. *(p. 255)*
8. **d.** All of these *(p. 255)*
9. **b.** False (Not all states would impose penalties such as these. However, your certification may be suspended or revoked if you have falsified information.) *(p. 255)*
10. **c.** Draw a single line through the incorrect entry and initial it. *(p. 256)*
11. **a.** Triage tags *(p. 257)*
12. **c.** Patient care is documented on the PCR, not on a special report form. *(p. 257)*

Case Study
1. Patient care report narrative section for this call:

    50-year-old male complains that his right ankle is "a little sore" after slipping on a wet floor approximately one half hour ago. Patient found to be alert and oriented, having no apparent difficulty breathing, and in no apparent distress. No signs of bleeding. Pulse is strong and regular. Skin is pink, warm, and dry. Focused physical exam reveals right ankle is markedly swollen, discolored, and very tender to gentle palpation. Pedal pulse is present. Good motion and sensation in injured extremity. Foot is slightly pale, but warm to touch. Denies any other injuries. Vital signs: BP 138/78 mmHg, pulse 68, respirations 18 and adequate. Pupils normal. No allergies or medications. Patient denies any medical problems. Last meal (soup and a sandwich) about one half hour earlier. States he felt fine all day but slipped on some water on the floor and twisted his ankle. Patient advised ankle should be splinted for transport to the hospital for evaluation and x-rays. Patient refuses, stating that his wife is already en route to take him to the doctor. Advised against weight-bearing on injured ankle until evaluated by doctor. Encouraged to call 9-1-1 should any problems arise. B. Jones, EMT-B
2. Before leaving the scene, you should have Mr. Henderson read your patient care report and sign the form acknowledging his refusal. If possible, ask any bystanders who witness his refusal to also sign the report. Notify dispatch and/or medical direction of refusal per local protocol.

CHAPTER 13 — GENERAL PHARMACOLOGY

Terms and Concepts
1. a. 2 b. 1 c. 3

Content Review
1. c. Identified in local protocols *(p. 261)*
2. b. Carried on the unit or prescribed for the patient *(p. 261)*
3. a. Epinephrine *(p. 261)*
4. c. Ask a family member to retrieve the medication. (Never ask a patient to retrieve his medication. This activity could aggravate his condition.) *(p. 261)*
5. a. The brand name is also known as the trade name *(p. 262)*
6. b. Isoetharine is also known by the trade names Bronkosol and Bronkometer *(p. 262)*
7. b. Glucose is also known by the trade names Glutose and Insta-glucose *(p. 262)*
8. d. The sublingual route *(p. 262)*
9. a. Shaken (The solids in a suspension will settle to the bottom) *(p. 263)*
10. b. Contraindications *(pp. 264-265)*
11. a. The six essential items of information are indications, contraindications, dose, administration, actions, and side effects. *(pp. 264-265)*
12. b. Epinephrine is given by injection with a spring-loaded auto-injector. (Be careful to avoid a needle stick.) *(p. 263)*
13. g. It is not necessary to contact the patient's own physician. (Verify the prescription by reading the label. Obtain the order to administer from medical direction.) *(pp. 265-267)*
14. c. It's the American Hospital Formulary Service, not Wilson's Formulary Service. *(p. 267)*
15. Oxygen *(p. 262, Table 13-1)*
16. Oral glucose *(p. 262, Table 13-1)*
17. Altered mental status with diabetic history *(p. 262, Table 13-1)*
18. Poisoning, overdose *(p. 262, Table 13-1)*
19. Chest pain *(p. 262, Table 13-1)*
20. Nitroglycerin spray *(p. 262, Table 13-1)*
21. Chest pain *(p. 262, Table 13-1)*
22. Adrenalin *(p. 262, Table 13-1)*
23. Proventil, Ventolin *(p. 262, Table 13-1)*
24. Alupent, Metaprel *(p. 262, Table 13-1)*
25. Breathing difficulty associated with respiratory conditions *(p. 262, Table 13-1)*
26. Isoetharine *(p. 262, Table 13-1)*
27. Breathing difficulty associated with respiratory conditions *(p. 262, Table 13-1)*
28. Serevent *(p. 262, Table 13-1)*

Case Study
1. c. Never administer medication unless prescribed to the patient and/or you are ordered to do so by medical direction.
2. b. False. The medications should not be administered to a patient who has an altered mental status.
3. c. Chest pain

CHAPTER 14 — RESPIRATORY EMERGENCIES

Terms and Concepts
1. a. 2 b. 7 c. 3 d. 6 e. 9 f. 1 g. 5 h. 8 i. 4 j. 10 *(p. 291)*
2. Apnea and respiratory arrest *(p. 291)*

Content Review
1. d. All of the above *(p. 272)*
2. c. Bronchoconstriction *(p. 272)*
3. c. Either of the above *(p. 272)*
4. a. Severe respiratory distress *(p. 272)*
5. d. Respiratory rate of 50 in infants *(p. 273)*
6. Crowing, gurgling, snoring, stridor *(p. 276)*
7. a. Immediately begin positive pressure ventilation (14 is below the normal respiratory range for children of 15 to 30 breaths per minute) *(p. 273)*
8. c. Apply oxygen by nonrebreather mask at 15 lpm. *(p. 273)*
9. a. Following the initial assessment *(p. 273)*
10. c. The patient is working so hard to breathe that the tissues are being pulled inward. *(p. 275)*
11. d. All of the above. Immediate and aggressive treatment is required. *(p. 275)*
12. c. Paradoxical motion (can cause ineffective ventilation) *(p. 276)*
13. c. When in doubt, provide positive pressure ventilation with supplemental oxygen. Delays can permit rapid deterioration and adversely affect the patient's outcome. *(p. 276)*
14. For the patient with adequate breathing but who is experiencing breathing difficulty; (1) provide oxygen first; (2) assess vitals signs which may reveal signs of severe respiratory distress such as elevated pulse or blood pressure; (3) pursue administration of a prescribed MDI, if the patient has one, to alleviate symptoms; (4) complete the focused history and physical exam; (5) place the patient in a position of comfort (most patients will find breathing is easiest in a sitting position) and transport to the hospital. *(p. 277)*
15. b. Don't delay transport. Perform the ongoing assessment en route. *(p. 277)*
16. a. Since the medication will be aimed into the mouth, the patient must breath through the mouth, not the nose, to take the medication into the lungs. *(p. 281)*
17. Any of these: Use of accessory muscles, retractions during inspiration, grunting, tachypnea, tachycardia, nasal flaring, grunting, prolonged exhalation, frequent coughing, cyanosis in the extremities, anxiety *(p. 282)*
18. b. Increased muscle tone (loss of muscle tone or a limp appearance is associated with respiratory failure in infants and children) *(p. 282)*
19. c. Immediately initiate positive pressure ventilation and transport, This is a dire emergency *(p. 282)*
20. c. Position of comfort to reduce the work of breathing and maintain an open airway *(p. 282)*
21. d. Do NOT perform foreign body airway obstruction maneuvers if epiglottitis or other disease is suspected. These may seriously aggravate the

338

CHAPTERS ANSWER KEY

condition. Foreign body maneuvers should be performed only if there is clear evidence that the child is choking and has not seemed to be ill. *(p. 283)*

22. **d.** Croup *(p. 283)*

Case Study

1. **b.** Breathing is adequate, although respiration rate is at the high end of the normal range. However, patient is experience breathing difficulty and so should receive high-flow oxygen.
2. **a.** Provocation (what provokes the illness; what makes it better or worse).
3. **b.** The body attempts to make up for inadequate oxygenation. (Asthmatic attacks are usually sporadic with no symptoms between attacks; the range of normal respiration rates is the same for all adults; Albuterol should reduce a rapid breathing rate by improving oxygenation.)
4. **c.** Beta agonist, which relaxes the smooth muscle and dilates the airway.
5. The indications for administration of an MDI are: (1) The patient exhibits signs and symptoms of breathing difficulty; (2) the patient has a physician-prescribed metered dose inhaler; and (3) approval has been given by medication direction to administer the medication.
6. **b.** Consult medication to consider re-administering.
7. **d.** Fowlers or semi-Fowlers (sitting up with back straight or at a slightly reclining angle). This is usually the "position of comfort" for the patient, permitting the greatest ease of breathing.

CHAPTER 15 — CARDIAC EMERGENCIES

Terms and Concepts

1. **a.** 2 **b.** 10 **c.** 12 **d.** 7 **e.** 4 **f.** 9 **g.** 11 **h.** 1 **i.** 6 **j.** 3 **k.** 5 *(p. 307)*

Content Review

1. **a.** pulmonary artery **b.** lung capillaries **c.** pulmonary vein **d.** veins **e.** venules **f.** bronchi **g.** alveoli **h.** arteries **i.** arterioles **j.** body capillaries *(pp. 294-295)*
2. The heart (pumps the blood); the blood vessels (carry the blood); the blood (the fluid within the system) *(p. 294)*
3. **d.** Any of the above *(p. 299)*
4. **b.** Assess airway, breathing, circulation, skin (Memorize these steps in this sequence. You will use them all through your career.) *(p. 299)*
5. **c.** Administer oxygen at 15 lpm by nonrebreather mask. *(p. 291)*
6. **c.** Severity *(p. 300)*
7. **d.** A silent heart attack *(p. 300)*
8. **a.** Sublingual *(p. 301)*
9. **b.** 2, 3, and 5 (Nitroglycerin should not be given if the systolic blood pressure is below 100, the patient has a suspected head injury, or three doses have already been taken.) *(p. 302)*
10. **b.** The EMT-B's assessment and care will not change no matter what the cause of the patient's chest pain. (The EMT-B should not spend time trying to diagnose the cause of chest pain. Administer oxygen, reassure the patient, consult

medical direction regarding administering physician-prescribed nitroglycerin if the patient has it, consider requesting ALS backup, initiate early transport. Be alert for the occurrence of cardiac arrest and, should this occur, be prepared to perform CPR and defibrillation as appropriate.) *(pp. 301, 304)*

Case Study

1. **c.** Nonrebreather mask at 15 lpm
2. **b.** Mr. Hansen is experiencing cardiac compromise, and early transport is necessary.
3. **a.** Reassure him that this is a common side effect of nitroglycerin and the headache pain should pass.
4. **b.** Continue to evaluate him and to update the receiving facility (ongoing assessment).

CHAPTER 16 — AUTOMATED EXTERNAL DEFIBRILLATION

Terms and Concepts

1. **a.** 2 **b.** 4 **c.** 3 **d.** 1 *(p. 326)*

Content Review

1. **a.** (The requirements for placement of the AED are: adult [over the age of 12 and greater 90 pounds] who is in cardiac arrest [no breathing, no pulse and unresponsive to verbal or pain stimuli]. The AED is not intended for trauma patients.) *(p. 315)*
2. **a.** (The first link is early access to EMS.) *(pp. 310-312)*
3. **c.** Defibrillation *(p. 311)*
4. **c.** (The AED, not the operator, analyzes the rhythm.) *(p. 312)*
5. **c.** The age of the patient (This is the same question as item 2 about the links in the chain of survival, asked another way. The age of the patient is not a factor. Which link in the chain is missing here?) *(pp. 310-312)*
6. **a.** A patient complaining of severe chest pain. (To utilize the AED, the patient must be unresponsive and pulseless.) *(p. 315)*
7. **d.** No emergency care actions should take precedence over shock delivery. *(p. 316)*
8. **c.** There are two methods of placement for the AED electrodes: anterior-anterior and anterior-posterior. Anterior-anterior placement positions the (-) sternum electrode on the right upper anterior chest wall, on the right upper border of the sternum. The (+) apex electrode is positioned over the left lower ribs on the anterior axillary line below and to the left of the nipple. *(p. 318)*
9. **a.** 6, 3, 2, 1, 5, 4, 7 (BSI and initial assessment; CPR and prepare AED; attach cables and pads; turn on power; begin narrative; stop CPR, clear, press button to begin analysis; press button to deliver shock if indicated. *(pp. 316-319)*
10. **c.** 3, 1, 2, 5, 4, 6 (Initial assessment; verify unresponsiveness, no breathing, and no pulse; attach cables and pads; turn on AED and begin narrative; initiate rhythm analysis; deliver shocks as indicated.*(p. 320)*

11. b. (The allowance of six shocks begins again if the patient regains a heartbeat, then goes back into cardiac arrest. The vehicle should be stopped and the engine turned off.) *(pp. 320-321)*

12. d. (The EMT-B is not permitted to provide ALS treatments.) *(p. 321)*

13. d. Battery failure. *(p. 321)*

14. b. Refresher training and practice is recommended every 90 days or 3 months. *(p. 323)*

15. d. Contact with water, metal, and nitroglycerin patches are all safety hazards during AED operation. *(p. 321)*

16. d. The checklist should be completed at the beginning of each shift to ensure that your AED will work when you need it. Completing the checklist also provides documentation of AED maintenance. *(p. 321)*

Case Study 1

1. b. Stop CPR, perform an initial assessment, and verify the absence of pulse/breathing.

2. b. Resume CPR and prepare for AED operation.

3. d. After any "no shock" message, check the pulse and, if no pulse, resume CPR for 1 minute, then initiate re analysis.

Case Study 2

1. d. You must ensure that the patient has a patent airway prior to the use of the AED. Make sure that the problem is not due to an airway obstruction by ventilating the patient once.

2. d. If you are working alone, call for help from EMS after delivering three shocks.

3. b. If the pulse returns, immediately check the breathing. Continued positive pressure ventilation may be required for a time after the heartbeat has returned.

Case Study 3

1. c. If, before ALS arrives, the patient regains a pulse, or you have given a total of six shocks, or if you the AED has given three consecutive "no shock" messages, transport. Do not wait for ALS arrival.

2. c. Either 1 or 2 (Medical direction may request additional shocks or may direct that CPR and transport continue. Note that additional shocks beyond the six shocks may NOT be given without orders from medical direction, unless the patient has regained pulse, then gone into cardiac arrest again.)

3. d. All of these are important for quality improvement of AED operations.

CHAPTER 17 ALTERED MENTAL STATUS — DIABETIC EMERGENCIES

Terms and Concepts

1. a. 4 b. 6 c. 2 d. 1 e. 5 f. 3 *(p. 338)*

Content Review

1. d. Any of these *(pp. 328, 330)*

2. d. Any of these *(p. 330)*

3. c. A medical illness (An altered mental status may be caused by either traumatic injury or a medical illness, but a patient in bed with no evident mechanism of injury is likely to be suffering a medical illness.) *(p. 329)*

4. b. Decorticate or decerebrate posturing is commonly associated with trauma. The others are signs commonly associated with non-trauma or medical illness. *(p. 330)*

5. b. 1, 2, and 4. (Do not administer oral glucose unless the patient meets all three criteria for this medication: altered mental status, history of diabetes controlled by medication, and ability to swallow. This patient met only the first and third criteria. Your suspicion that he is suffering a diabetic emergency could not be confirmed. Assure an open airway, provide oxygen, place him in a lateral recumbent position, and transport. This is the recommended care for a patient with an altered mental status and no known history of diabetes controlled by medication.) *(pp. 334, 335)*

6. Type I – commonly acquired in childhood; no insulin produced; must inject insulin daily. Type II – usually developed in adulthood; some insulin still secreted; usually controlled by diet, exercise, oral medication, or in severe cases controlled by insulin *(p. 331)*

7. d. Any of these may be true of the diabetic patient. Choice 4 includes the other three. *(pp. 330-331)*

8. Did the patient take his medication the day of the episode? Did the patient eat (or skip any) regular meals on this day? Did the patient vomit after eating a meal on that day? Did the patient do any unusual exercise or physical activity on that day? *(p. 332)*

9. c. A diabetic emergency with signs and symptoms that mimic a stroke is a frequent occurrence in elderly patients. *(p. 332)*

10. Answers may include: A medical identification device indicating diabetes; the presence of medications commonly prescribed to control diabetes; information provided by the patient, family, or bystanders that the patient is a diabetic who takes medication to control his condition. *(pp. 331-332)*

11. b. Determine if the patient can swallow. (Never give anything orally to a patient whose mental status is altered severely enough that he cannot swallow or protect his airway.) *(pp. 334, 335)*

12. b. Improvement after administration of oral glucose may happen quickly or may take 20 minutes or more. However, also be prepared for further deterioration of the patient's condition, and continually monitor the airway and breathing. Never insert anything in the mouth of a seizing patient. If oral glucose was administered with a tongue depressor and the patient seizes, immediately remove the tongue depressor. *(p. 335)*

Case Study

1. Probably a rapid onset if it occurred during jogging, anxious, speaks with inappropriate words, medical identification bracelet (insulin-dependent diabetic), episode follows a period of physical exercise, tachycardia (heart rate 104), skin cool and moist.

2. b. Nonrebreather mask at 15 lpm (Her breathing is adequate so positive pressure ventilation is not necessary at this time. Simple face mask and nasal cannula are not recommended for prehospital use.

3. The three criteria for administration of oral glucose are: (1) The patient must have an altered mental status. (2) The patient must have a history of diabetes controlled by medication. (3) The patient must be able to swallow.

4. In some jurisdictions, off-line medical direction allows the EMT-B to administer oral glucose without direct consultation with medical direction, on the basis of standing orders or protocols. Some jurisdictions require on-line medical direction for the administration of oral glucose: approval given by radio or phone.

CHAPTER 18 — ALTERED MENTAL STATUS WITH LOSS OF FUNCTION

Terms and Concepts
1. a. 4 b. 3 c. 2 d. 1 *(p. 348)*

Content Review
1. d. Any of the above *(p. 340)*
2. a. A stroke (which is a nontraumatic, or medical, brain injury) may result from any disruption of blood flow to the brain, for example from a rupture to or blockage of a blood vessel in the brain. *(p. 344 – with further explanation in the Enrichment section on pp. 345-346.)*
3. b. Nausea or vomiting, a common sign of nontraumatic brain injury (An ice pack may signal a headache, another common sign of nontraumatic brain injury.) *(p. 341)*
4. Muscles of the throat may be paralyzed, preventing the patient from clearing his airway of any secretions. (Be prepared to provide immediate suctioning.) *(p. 341)*
5. If the patient is able to understand you, have him answer yes-and-no questions by blinking his eyes or squeezing your finger, once for no and twice for yes. *(p. 341)*
6. b. Paralysis to both right and left legs (Paralysis to both sides of the body is most likely to occur below the site of a spinal injury.) *(p. 341)*
7. a. Administer positive pressure ventilation with supplemental oxygen. *(p. 343)*
8. c. Lateral recumbent position. (This will allow secretions to drain from the patient's mouth and help prevent aspiration when the patient cannot protect his airway. If the patient is responsive, place him in a supine position with head and chest elevated.) *(p. 343)*
9. d. Perform an ongoing assessment every 5 minutes, paying close attention to airway, breathing, circulation, and mental status. *(p. 344)*
10. b. Osteoporosis. Elderly patients with a history of heart disease, hypertension (high blood pressure), or atherosclerosis (plaque build-up in the arteries) are likely candidates for stroke. *(p. 344)*
11. a. Approximately one-third of those who suffer a transient ischemic attack (TIA) will go on to have a stroke. *(p. 345)*
12. d. The elderly patient who has signs and symptoms of a stroke may, instead, be a diabetic who is suffering hypoglycemia. (As detailed in Chapter 17, this patient may be a candidate for administration of oral glucose. The history of diabetes will also be important information for the hospital staff.) *(p. 341)*

Case Study
1. a. Place her on oxygen at 15 lpm by nonrebreather mask.
2. The victim of a nontraumatic brain injury may be suffering paralysis of the throat muscles which will cause her to be unable to protect her airway, even if the airway is open. Vomiting is also a frequent consequence of a nontraumatic brain injury. Suctioning may be required to remove secretions or vomitus that the patient might aspirate.
3. d. Administer positive pressure ventilation at greater than 24 ventilations per minute with the highest possible concentration of supplemental oxygen. (Extra oxygen can help prevent further deterioration of the injured brain. Since the patient is unresponsive with inadequate breathing, she cannot breathe on her own through a nonrebreather mask; positive pressure ventilation is required to force the oxygen into her lungs.)

CHAPTER 19 ALTERED MENTAL STATUS — SEIZURES AND SYNCOPE

Terms and Concepts
1. a. 1 b. 5 c. 4 d. 2 e. 6 f. 7 g. 3 *(p. 359)*

Content Review
1. d. Any of these *(pp. 355-356)*
2. Aura – sensory perception that warns a patient a seizure is about to occur, sometimes described as a sensation that rises from the stomach toward the chest. Tonic phase — loss of responsiveness, followed by muscle contraction and rigidity. Clonic phase — convulsions; jerky muscle activity. Postictal phase — recovery phase; confusion or disorientation to complete unresponsiveness, exhaustion, possible headache and weakness. *(pp. 354-355)*
3. d. Postictal *(p. 351)*
4. b. Move objects away; guide the patient's movements. (Never place anything in the patient's mouth, which could break and cause airway obstruction. Do not attempt to restrain the patient, which could cause injury.) *(p. 351)*
5. d. All are at risk. *(p. 352)*
6. b. Positive pressure ventilation and immediate transport are required for the status epilepticus patient. *(p. 352)*
7. c. High fever *(pp. 352, 357)*
8. c. The patient who has regained responsiveness between seizures. (This patient still should be transported for evaluation at a medical facility but is not a high priority for immediate transport.) *(p. 352)*
9. The extremities can be injured from the fall to the ground, by striking objects while seizing, or from the severe muscle contractions. *(p. 353)*

10. The nasopharyngeal airway is soft and can be inserted when the teeth are clenched. A rigid oropharyngeal airway could break the teeth or be bitten off, risking airway obstruction. *(p. 355)*

11. **b.** Lateral recumbent *(p. 355)*

12. The lateral recumbent position permits secretions to drain from the mouth and helps protect the airway and prevent aspiration. *(p. 355)*

13. **b.** (The skin of a syncope patient is usually pale and moist.) *(p. 356)*

Case Study

1. **d.** All are correct.

2. **d.** Positive pressure ventilation with a nasopharyngeal airway in place and rapid transport. (If Karl is in status epilepticus, positive pressure ventilation is required. A nasopharyngeal airway cannot be bitten off as an oropharyngeal airway can.)

3. The blood could have come from an injury from a fall or other mechanism; however, it often results when a seizing patient bites the tongue or cheek. Treat by suctioning.

4. **c.** Postictal

5. **d.** Now that Karl is responsive, and since no head or spinal injury is suspected, place in a lateral recumbent position and administer oxygen by nonrebreather mask at 15 lpm.

CHAPTER 20 — ALLERGIC REACTION

Terms and Concepts

1. a. 8 b. 2 c. 5 d. 4 e. 6 f. 3 g. 1 h. 7 *(p. 372)*

Content Review

1. **d.** All of these are true for anaphylaxis. *(p. 362)*

2. **c.** Medications *(pp. 362, 363)*

3. **b.** Excretion (Ingestion, injection, and contact are routes by which allergens may enter the body.) *(p. 362)*

4. **c.** 1, 2, 4, and 5 (Venom, foods, pollen, and medications are common causes of allergic reaction and anaphylaxis. Metals are not.) *(pp. 362, 363)*

5. **a.** Stridor or crowing indicates significant swelling to the upper airway, requiring positive pressure ventilation. *(p. 363)*

6. **a.** Deactivate the pop-off valve or cover it with your thumb in order to achieve adequate pressure to force air past swollen airway structures. *(p. 363)*

7. **c.** Hives and itching are the hallmark signs of an allergic reaction. *(pp. 363-364)*

8. **d.** 20 minutes *(p. 364)*

9. **b.** Respiratory compromise and/or shock must be present for an allergic reaction to be severe enough to be considered anaphylaxis. (Respiratory compromise is characterized by partial or complete airway occlusion, breathing difficulties, wheezing. Shock, or hypoperfusion, may be indicated by absent or weak pulses, rapid heartbeat, decreased blood pressure, and deteriorating mental status.) *(pp. 364, 366)*

10. **d.** Never underestimate the severity of an allergic reaction. Because death can occur within minutes, immediate intervention is imperative.

Do not mistake anaphylaxis for conditions with similar signs and symptoms such as hyperventilation, anxiety attacks, alcohol intoxication and hypoglycemia. *(p. 366)*

11. **d.** All of these (A severe allergic reaction, or anaphylaxis, requires aggressive treatment and swift transport. Because a mild allergic reaction can deteriorate into anaphylaxis rapidly, the patient with a mild allergic reaction must be monitored closely.) *(p. 366)*

12. **d.** All of these *(p. 366)*

13. **c.** Signs and symptoms of severe allergic reaction including respiratory distress and/or shock. *(pp. 367, 369)*

Case Study

1. **d.** Although she looks well and is not having difficulty breathing, the patient's skin is flushed, she feels a "lump" in her throat, and her stomach "feels upset" – all early signs of anaphylaxis.

2. **d.** Airway and breathing compromise and poor perfusion

3. **d.** Excessive mucus in the lower airways

4. **d.** All of these signs may develop as the anaphylactic reaction develops.

CHAPTER 21 — POISONING EMERGENCIES

Terms and Concepts

1. a. 5 (or 6) b. 3 c. 1 d. 2 e. 6 f. 4 *(p. 389)*

Content Review

1. **d.** All of these *(p. 375)*

2. **c.** Request assistance from a trained "hazmat" team *(p. 375)*

3. **b.** Open chemical containers, empty pill bottles, and chewed-up plants near a child are all possible indicators of a poisoning. The presence of a hazardous material warning label on a locked cabinet door is not necessarily an indicator that a poisoning has taken place. *(p.375)*

4. **c.** While all of these things might eventually be done at the scene of a poisoning emergency, the medical priority is to maintain the patient's airway. *(p. 375)*

5. **d.** Any of these may affect the airway. *(p. 375)*

6. Questions listed may include any five of these: Was any substance ingested? When did the exposure (or ingestion) take place? Over what time period did the exposure (or ingestion) take place? How much of the substance was taken? Has anyone attempted to treat the poisoning? Does the patient have a psychiatric history that may indicate this is a suicide attempt? Does the patient have an underlying medical illness, allergy, drug use, or addiction? How much does the patient weigh? *(p. 376)*

7. **b.** False. (Most assessment findings – signs and symptoms – in a poisoning patient may also be found in other types of emergencies. This underscores the importance of scene size-up and obtaining a good history, as well as the need to provide treatment based on your assessment findings rather than searching for an antidote for a specific poison.) *(p.376)*

8. **d.** Any of these *(pp. 378, 379)*

9. **b.** Prevent further injury by rinsing the substance from his mouth and lips. *(p. 379)*
10. **c.** Activated charcoal inhibits the absorption of poisons. *(pp. 380, 381)*
11. **a.** Activated charcoal is indicated for ingested poisons, when ordered by medical direction. *(p. 381)*
12. **b.** (Activated charcoal is contraindicated for all patients who have an altered mental status, have ingested acids or alkalis, or are unable to swallow.) *(p. 381)*
13. **c.** The usual adult dosage of activated charcoal is 25 to 50 grams. *(p. 381)*
14. **b.** False. (Activated charcoal is not an effective binding agent against alcohol, kerosene, gasoline, caustics, or metals, such as iron.) *(p. 381)*
15. **a.** True *(p. 381)*
16. **a.** Blackened stool (Common side effects of activated charcoal include blackened stool, nausea, and vomiting. Other side effects are rare.) *(p. 381)*
17. **c.** Fire-related incidents. *(p. 380)*
18. **b.** Difficulty breathing *(p. 382)*
19. **c.** Activated charcoal will have no effect on substances that have not been ingested. *(pp. 382-383)*
20. **d.** All of these *(pp. 383-386)*

Case Study

1. If you are not wearing a self-contained breathing apparatus or have not been properly trained for a hazardous materials rescue, withdraw and request assistance. If you are properly trained and equipped, remove Mr. Johnson from the workshop and into the fresh air as quickly as possible.
2. Maintain spinal immobilization that would have been established by the rescue team. Assure a patent airway and start positive pressure ventilation with supplemental oxygen immediately. Loosen tight clothing.
3. Perform a rapid trauma assessment to determine if there are any potentially life-threatening injuries. Obtain baseline vital signs and a SAMPLE history. Send someone who is wearing a self-contained breathing apparatus to retrieve any containers of chemicals that might have been in use by Mr. Johnson in the workshop. It would also be a good idea to have that person open the workshop window.
4. Continue to maintain an open airway and provide positive pressure ventilation with supplemental oxygen. Perform an ongoing assessment at least every 5 minutes en route to the receiving facility.

CHAPTER 22 — DRUG AND ALCOHOL EMERGENCIES

Terms & Concepts

1. a. 3 b. 1 c. 2 *(p. 402)*

Content Review

1. **b.** The goals at the scene of a drug or alcohol emergency are the identification and treatment of potential life threats, such as airway or breathing compromise. Treatment should never be delayed to identify the substance. *(pp. 391-392)*

2. Potential dangers at the scene of a drug or alcohol emergency include infectious disease, violent behavior, and weapons. It may be prudent to call for police backup because of the potential for harm. *(p. 392)*
3. **b.** Keep them with the patient as a source of information for the hospital staff *(p. 393)*
4. **a.** True. This is why finding evidence in the patient's environment, such as empty pill or alcohol containers, may be the only way to determine that this may be a drug- or alcohol-related emergency and why these containers will be important to the hospital staff who will need to diagnose the condition. *(p. 393)*
5. **d.** All of these *(p. 394)*
6. Six signs and symptoms that indicate a life threatening drug or alcohol emergency are: unresponsiveness, respiratory difficulties, fever, abnormal pulse rate (high, low or irregular), vomiting (with an altered mental status), seizures. *(p. 395)*
7. **c.** Scene size-up and patient history *(pp. 395-396)*
8. The emergency care steps for the disoriented patient who reports overdose (or, in general, for any drug or alcohol emergency patient) are: (1) Establish and maintain a patent airway. (2) Administer oxygen at 15 lpm by nonrebreather mask or positive pressure ventilation with supplemental oxygen. (3) Monitor vital signs, maintain body temperature, prevent shock. (4) Gather medications (or empty medication or alcohol containers) to bring to the hospital. (5) Transport. *(p. 396)*
9. Hallucinogenic substances often produce a psychological emergency that may present as intense anxiety or panic ("bad trip"), depression, mood changes, disorientation, or an inability to differentiate fantasy from reality. *(p. 396)*
10. **b.** Touch can be comforting, but invading the drug- or alcohol-abuse patient's "personal space" can trigger a violent response. Always establish rapport and obtain the patient's permission before touching him. *(pp. 396-397)*
11. Elements of the "talk-down" technique for the potentially violent patient who is suffering a "bad trip" include: (1) Make the patient feel welcome; remain relaxed and sympathetic. (2) Identify yourself clearly and establish rapport before touching the patient. (3) Reassure the patient that his condition is caused by the drug and will not last forever. (4) Help the patient verbalize what is happening to him. (5) Make simple statements to help orient the patient to time and place. Help him feel more secure by helping him identify where he is and what is happening. (6) Forewarn the patient about what he may experience as the drug wears off. (7) Transport the patient after he has been calmed. *(pp. 396-397)*
12. **a.** A patient you know has used PCP (The talk-down technique can aggravate this patient.) *(p. 397)*

Case Study

1. Establish an airway. Use a head-tilt, chin-lift if spinal injury is not suspected or a jaw-thrust if spinal injury is suspected. (Since the patient is on the floor, consider that she may have fallen from a

standing position with possible spinal injury.) If spinal injury is suspected, maintain in-line spinal stabilization until the patient is fully immobilized to a long spine board. Suction mouth and nose as necessary. Place an oral or nasal airway if the patient will tolerate it. Begin positive pressure ventilation with supplemental oxygen (because this patient's breathing is inadequate). Cover the patient to maintain body temperature.

2. This patient should not receive activated charcoal because she is unresponsive and cannot swallow or protect her airway.

3. This is a life-threatening situation. Your patient is a high priority for transport. Remember to take the pill bottles and wine bottle and a sample of the vomitus with you to the medical facility. Complete the physical exam and the baseline vital signs. Perform an ongoing assessment every 5 minutes en route, closely monitoring the airway and breathing.

CHAPTER 23— ACUTE ABDOMINAL PAIN

Terms and Concepts

1. a. 7 b. 4 c. 5 d. 6 e. 2 f. 3 g. 1 h. 8 *(p. 413)*

Content Review

1. a. diaphragm b. umbilicus c. right upper quadrant (RUQ) d. right lower quadrant (RLQ) e. left upper quadrant (LUQ) f. left lower quadrant (LLQ) *(p. 405)*

2. a. All except the heart and lungs *(pp. 404-406)*

3. b. 1 or 2 (Acute abdominal pain, acute abdomen, or acute abdominal distress are terms that are used interchangeably.) *(p. 405)*

4. b. Consider the abdominal pain patient to have a life-threatening condition until proven otherwise. *(p. 406)*

5. d. The position with knees drawn up is called a guarded position and is typically assumed by a patient with abdominal pain. *(p. 407)*

6. A criterion for priority transport of the acute abdomen patient is ANY of the following: (1) poor general impression, (2) unresponsive with no gag or cough reflex, (3) responsive but not following commands, (4) difficulty breathing, (5) shock (hypoperfusion), (6) uncontrolled bleeding, and (7) severe pain. *(p. 407)*

7. c. Bloody vomitus is *not* always present in acute abdominal conditions. *(pp. 406-407)*

8. a. Have the patient point to the area of the pain and palpate this quadrant last. *(pp. 408-409)*

9. d. A soft abdomen, not rigid or distended, is normal. *(p. 409)*

10. d. Never give anything by mouth (which can be vomited and aspirated) to an acute abdomen patient. A supine position with legs flat is usually not comfortable for the acute abdomen patient. Ongoing assessment should be performed every 5 minutes for the unstable patient. *(pp. 409-410)*

11. d. Transport should not be delayed. (The focused or rapid medical exam may be performed en route if the patient is a priority for transport. A detailed physical exam, if any, would be

performed en route but may not be performed at all. See Chapter 9, "Patient Assessment.") *(pp. 408-409)*

12. b. A transient ischemic attack is a form of nontraumatic brain injury, not likely to cause abdominal pain. (The other choices are among the wide variety of conditions that may cause acute abdominal pain.) *(pp. 410- 412)*

Case Study

1. d. Remember the indicators of a serious medical emergency. This patient is displaying a poor general impression, a diminished mental status (slow to respond to questions, does not look at you when you enter), signs of hypoperfusion (rapid weak pulse, cool clammy skin, diminished mental status, nausea), and the patient is in severe pain.

2. c. Ask her to point to the area which is the most painful. Then start with the area that is least painful. Palpate each abdominal quadrant of the abdomen, the most painful quadrant last.

3. a. Emesis (vomitus) should be saved for possible testing at the hospital.

4. c. This patient is an unstable patient who requires careful monitoring. Ongoing assessment should be performed at least every 5 minutes.

CHAPTER 24 — ENVIRONMENTAL EMERGENCIES

Terms and Concepts

1. a. 1 b. 5 c. 2 d. 7 e. 9 f. 4 g. 11 h. 3 i. 10 j. 12 k. 6 l. 8 *(p. 437)*

Content Review

1. c. Consolidation (Mechanisms of heat loss are radiation, convection, conduction, evaporation, and respiration.) *(pp. 416-417)*

2. b. Generalized hypothermia (also called generalized cold emergency) and local cold injury. *(p. 417)*

3. d. Middle age (Extreme youth and old age are risk factors for hypothermia.) *(p. 418)*

4. c. (The stages of hypothermia are, in this order, shivering, apathy and decreased muscle function, decreased level of responsiveness, decreased vital signs, and death.) *(p. 419)*

5. c. Having the patient walk briskly. (In the hypothermia patient even minor physical activity or rough handling can cause heart dysrhythmia, resulting in cardiac arrest.) *(p. 424)*

6. b. The body temperature should be increased no more than 1°F per hour. (Active rewarming must be attempted only if the patient is alert and responding appropriately. The patient should never be immersed in hot water or a hot shower, which will raise the temperature too abruptly. It is dangerous to warm the extremities before the core body.) *(pp. 424-425)*

7. a. 10 minutes. (Make sure you familiarize yourself with normal spring, summer, and fall river and lake temperatures in your community! Body temperatures can drop rapidly in what you THINK is relatively warm water.) *(p. 419)*

8. **a.** (The patient should be lifted horizontally to prevent vascular collapse.) *(p. 425)*
9. **b.** The stages of local cold injury are early (superficial) and late (deep). *(p. 420)*
10. **b.** Never remove clothing if it is frozen to the skin. This will cause further injury. *(p. 426)*
11. **d.** (Rapid rewarming is recommended only when transport will be delayed or extremely long and upon consultation with medical direction.) *(p. 426)*
12. **b.** Hyperthermia. *(p. 427)*
13. **b.** Inactive lifestyle. (Although an inactive lifestyle may not be healthful in general, it is physical exertion in a hot environment that is a predisposing factor for hyperthermia.) *(p. 427)*
14. **d.** Hot skin – either moist or dry – signals a dire medical emergency in a patient who has been exposed to heat. (In early stages of hyperthermia, the skin will be cool to the touch. If the skin is hot, hyperthermia is in an advanced and life-threatening stage. In about half the cases, the patient with hot skin will still be sweating. In the remainder of cases, sweat mechanisms will have shut down.) *(p. 430)*
15. **c.** Shivering produces heat. If the patient begins to shiver the cooling method should be slowed. *(p. 430)*
16. **b.** If the patient is unresponsive or is vomiting do not give fluids orally. *(p. 430)*
17. **d.** Most often the only time a hyperthermic patient with moist, pale skin that is normal-to-cool in temperature needs transport is if the patient is unresponsive, vomiting, has a history of medical problems, the body temperature is above 101°F or the patient's temperature is rising. *(p. 430)*
18. **c.** The first step for any heat emergency patient, with cool or hot skin, is to move the patient to a cool place such as the back of an air-conditioned ambulance or at least out of the sun and into the shade. *(p. 430)*
19. **c.** A rapid increase or decrease in the pulse with a decline in the patient's mental status is a grave finding. *(p. 431)*
20. **a.** Snakebites are relatively uncommon and the number of people who die from snakebite each year is extremely small. *(pp. 431-432)*

Case Study 1
1. **b.** Remove as much clothing as possible as quickly as possible.
2. **c.** Begin to cool the patient by one or a combination of the following methods: pour cool water over the patients body, place cold packs on the patient's groin, side of the neck, armpits, and behind each knee; wrap the patient in a wet sheet; fan the patient; keep the skin wet. Use slower cooling if the patient begins to shiver.
3. **d.** Be alert for seizures and the potential for aspiration of vomitus in the hyperthermia patient.

Case Study 2
1. **c.** Cold packs for insect bites and stings, but not for snakebites or marine animal stings.
2. **a.** Lower the injection site slightly below the level of the heart and closely watch for signs of anaphylaxis. Cutting and suctioning of the site is not recommended. Epinephrine would not be administered unless the patient had a current prescription for the epinephrine, the patient was showing signs and symptoms of anaphylaxis, and you have authorization from medical direction to administer the medication.

Case Study 3
1. **c.** (Take longer than normal to assess pulse in a hypothermia patient; the pulse may be present but extremely slow.)
2. **b.** This patient is unresponsive, so passive (not active) rewarming should be utilized. Seek medical direction and follow local protocols.
3. **d.** Handle the patient gently. Keep the patient supine to improve blood flow to the brain. Ventilation of the patient is indicated at a normal rate; hyperventilation can cause cardiac complications.

Case Study 4
1. **c.** The signs and symptoms of early or superficial local cold injury include; blanching of the skin, loss of feeling or sensation, continued softness of the skin in the injured area, tingling sensation during any rewarming. Swelling and blisters would indicate later or deep cold injury.
2. **d.** NEVER rub or massage the affected area. This can cause injury to frozen tissues.
3. **b.** You must prevent the occurrence of refreezing of the tissue. Significant tissue loss can occur if the tissue is subjected to refreezing. All the other items are true except for using a moist sterile dressing. Use a dry sterile dressing.

CHAPTER 25 — DROWNING, NEAR-DROWNING, AND DIVING EMERGENCIES

Terms and Concepts
1. **a.** 4 **b.** 3 **c.** 1 **d.** 2
Content Review
1. **a.** (Recent studies demonstrate that one-fourth of all infants who drown do so in five-gallon buckets; others drown in bathtubs and toilets.) *(p. 439)*
2. **c.** Wearing a personal flotation device *(p. 440)*
3. **c.** Sustained head, neck, or spine injuries *(p. 441)*
4. **a.** (Near-drowning is defined as survival for at least 24 hours from near-suffocation due to submersion. Death before 24 hours is classified as drowning.) *(p. 440)*
5. **b.** EMT-B training is not a criterion. (See the criteria listed for answer 6.) *(p. 441)*
6. **c.** Rescue attempts near shore should be tried in this safest-to-riskiest sequence: Reach (by holding out an object), throw (something that floats), row (get a boat), go (wade or swim). Wade or swim only if you meet ALL of these criteria: You are a good swimmer, you are specially trained in water rescue, you are wearing a personal flotation device, and you are accompanied by other rescuers. *(pp. 441-442)*
7. **a.** An unresponsive patient found in shallow water should be suspected to have a spinal injury. (The other choices are also possible, but spinal injury should be your primary suspicion.) *(p. 442)*

8. c. Attempt resuscitation with full efforts. (Patients submerged in cold water for 30 minutes or longer have been resuscitated. Some experts advise resuscitation for every drowning patient regardless of water temperature. Resuscitation efforts should always be performed in an "all-or-none" manner. Resuscitate the patient fully or don't resuscitate the patient. So-called "show codes" or "slow codes" are not appropriate. *(p. 443)*

9. c. A detailed physical exam is appropriate for a near-drowning patient and should be performed, if time and the patient's condition permit, to discover any injuries that may have been overlooked. *(p. 446)*

10. c. Mammalian diving reflex. *(p. 443)*

Case Study 1

1. d. Let's hope you didn't have to think much about this one! Begin resuscitation at once!

2. b. All the clues to possible spinal injury are present. You found the patient at the shallow end of the pool. The patient has a laceration on her forehead. These are signs that she may have dived into the pool and struck her head. Observed bleeding is minor. Checking for gastric distention may be necessary if positive pressure ventilations are noted to be ineffective. This patient is not breathing on her own, so oxygen by nonrebreather is not appropriate.

3. d. Gastric distention occurs when the stomach fills with water (during a near-drowning) or air (during artificial ventilation). The air or water in the stomach may put enough pressure on the diaphragm and lungs to interfere with the ability to ventilate the patient. Position the patient on her side and – with suction equipment immediately available, because the patient is likely to regurgitate stomach contents – gently press on the epigastric region to relieve the distention. Suction the mouth and nose and then resume ventilation efforts.

Case Study 2

1. d. Complications from near-drowning can occur up to 72 hours after the incident. Even though this patient looks well now, he must be transported for evaluation by a physician.

2. b. Administer oxygen, monitor carefully, and transport on his left side to allow drainage in case he vomits.

CHAPTER 26 — BEHAVIORAL EMERGENCIES

Terms and Concepts
1. a. 4 b. 1 c. 5 d. 3 e. 2 *(p. 463)*

Content Review
1. Clues or indicators that a behavioral emergency may be due to a physical cause include: a relatively sudden onset of symptoms; or the patient exhibits memory loss, visual hallucinations, incontinence, or excessive salivation. Your physical examination may reveal abnormal pupils or pupilary response. *(p. 452)*

2. Anxiety *(p. 452)*

3. Depression *(p. 453)*
4. Schizophrenia *(p. 435)*
5. d. 35-year-old married male who recently had gall bladder surgery. (Characteristics that indicate a high suicide risk include being a male over 40 years of age who is single, widowed or divorced; a history of previous suicidal attempts; recent diagnosis of a serious or debilitating illness; or a history of chronic depression. The availability of a suicide device or the formulation and communication of a highly lethal plan all point to a high risk of suicidal behavior.) *(p. 454)*

6. d. Any of these. *(pp. 452-454)*
7. Documentation (which is careful and complete) *(p. 460)*
8. b. Never attempt restraint until you have sufficient help and an appropriate plan. (Effective teamwork is more important than strength. Use only the amount of force needed. Metal cuffs should not be used. Act quickly; surprise is a key element.) *(pp. 459-460)*

9. c. The first priority in dealing with a behavioral emergency is to protect yourself and others from harm. Safety is of the utmost importance. *(p. 456)*

10. b. Do not "play along" with auditory and visual hallucinations. Reassure the patient that the hallucinations are only temporary. *(p. 455)*

Case Study
1. Scan the scene for potential hazards. Then, speaking quietly and calmly, identify yourself by name as an EMT-Basic who is here to help him. Ask if you can come closer to him so that you can talk about what's going on. If Jim allows you to come closer, move slowly but confidently.

2. Maintain eye contact. Encourage him to tell you more about the situation. Ask him if this has ever happened before. Ask if he has any medical problems or has been injured. Ask if he has eaten today. Reassure him that he is safe and that you are here to help him.

3. Your partner should keep you in his line of sight and be alert to any signs that Jim may become violent. At the same time, he should try to get more information about Jim and the situation from bystanders. He should also try to disperse the onlookers if possible.

4. En route to the hospital you should explain what you're going to do and seek his permission, then obtain baseline vital signs and complete your focused assessment. Continue talking quietly with Jim and answer his questions honestly but do not create false expectations.

CHAPTER 27 — OBSTETRIC AND GYNECOLOGICAL EMERGENCIES

Terms and Concepts
1. a. 3 b. 5 c. 4 d. 1 e. 2 *(p. 466)*

CONTENT REVIEW
1. c. Vagina *(p. 466)*
2. Labor *(p. 467)*

3. The three stages of labor are: dilation, expulsion, and placental. Dilation occurs as the contractions begin and ends when the cervix becomes fully dilated. Expulsion ends with the delivery of the infant. The placental stage ends with the passage of the placenta (afterbirth). *(pp. 467-468)*

4. **d.** All of these. When performing a focused history on any female in the childbearing years, you should always include questions related to pain, menstrual period, vaginal discharge or bleeding and pregnancy. *(p. 470)*

5. **c.** Headache with numbness in arms (Abdominal pain or trauma, vaginal bleeding or discharge, altered mental status, seizures, nausea, vomiting, weakness, dizziness, swelling of face or extremities, or shock may signal a pre-delivery emergency. (p. 470)

6. Supine hypotensive syndrome *(p. 470)*

7. **c.** (Transporting the patient on her left side will minimize compression of the vena cava and improve her cardiac output.) *(pp. 470-471)*

8. **a.** (You should never pack the vagina to control bleeding.) *(p. 471)*

9. **c.** A pregnant women should be transported on her left side. *(p. 471)*

10. **c.** The passage of a slight amount of blood and mucus usually marks on the onset of the first stage of labor, not the imminent delivery. *(p. 472)*

11. (1) Support the bony part of the infant's skull and exert gentle pressure against the perineum as the head delivers. Determine the position of the umbilical cord. (2) Suction the infant's mouth and nose. Support the body as it delivers, then again suction the mouth and nose. Dry and wrap the infant. (3) Keep the infant level with the vagina. Have your partner assume care of the infant. When the pulsations cease clamp, tie, and cut the umbilical cord. (4) Observe for the delivery of the placenta. As it delivers, grasp it gently and rotate. Place in a towel and bag it for transport to the hospital. (5) Place sanitary napkin at the vaginal opening. Record the time of delivery and transport. Keep mother and infant warm en route. *(pp. 473-475)*

12. **b.** Emergency care for the patient with excessive post-delivery bleeding should include the administration of oxygen and firm massage of the uterus. If the mother appears to be in shock (hypoperfusion), transport immediately and initiate uterine massage en route. *(p. 475)*

13. **b.** It is not abnormal for strong contractions to cease after delivery of the infant. Continued contractions indicate multiple births. *(p. 476)*

14. **d.** All of these *(p. 476)*

15. Prolapsed cord *(p. 476)*

16. **b.** Insert a gloved hand into the vagina to relieve pressure on the cord. The mother should be transported immediately in a knee-chest position. *(p. 476)*

17. **c.** Meconium staining of the amniotic fluid should be managed by suctioning mouth and nose before infant takes his first breath. It is critical to clear the airway before the infant begins to breathe to prevent aspirating the meconium into the lungs. *(p. 478)*

18. **d.** In addition to the usual care for a newborn, care of the premature infant requires vigilant attention to prevent heat loss or contamination. Suctioning should be done very gently and oxygen should be administered using a "blow by" technique. *(p. 478)*

19. Apgar scoring is a method to assess the newborn's overall condition at 1 minute and 5 minutes after delivery. Components of the Apgar assessment include appearance, pulse, grimace, activity, and respirations. *(pp. 478-479)*

20. **b.** Purple or blue extremities are normal immediately after delivery. However, a cyanotic core body, as well as cyanotic extremities, indicates a severely depressed newborn. *(pp. 478, 479)*

21. **b.** Emergency care for a newborn with shallow, gasping respirations and a heart rate that is less than 100 beats per minute should include assisting ventilations with a bag-valve mask and reassessing in 30 seconds. If there is no improvement, continue ventilations and again reassess in 30 seconds. *(p. 480)*

22. **c.** After taking appropriate BSI precautions and completing the initial assessment of the sexual assault victim, your focused history and physical exam should include tactfully questioning the patient about other potential injuries. *(p. 481)*

23. Emotional care and reassurance *(p. 482)*

24. **d.** Emergency management of the sexual assault victim should include maintenance of airway, breathing, and circulation, control of bleeding from the vagina with a sanitary napkin, and treatment of any other signs and symptoms as you would any other patient. *(p. 482)*

CASE STUDY

1. Stabilize the cervical spine and open the airway using a jaw thrust. Place an oral or nasal airway if tolerated. Assist respirations with positive pressure ventilation and supplemental oxygen. Perform a rapid trauma assessment paying particular attention to evidence of injuries to her abdomen, back, and pelvis. Secure to long spine board for transport. Cover with a blanket to help maintain body heat.

2. Place pillows under the edge of the right side of the backboard to help tilt your patient to the left, thereby relieving pressure on the inferior vena cava during transport.

3. Check for vaginal bleeding or possible rupturing of membranes and loss of amniotic fluid, while being careful to not touch the vagina. Continue to monitor and record vital signs. Complete a detailed physical exam and an ongoing assessment every 5 minutes. Establish radio contact with medical direction.

4. Start CPR immediately. CPR must be continued throughout transport and until the infant is surgically delivered at the hospital. Vigorous resuscitation of the mother to save the fetus is acceptable and appropriate.

CHAPTER 28 — MECHANISMS OF INJURY: KINETICS OF TRAUMA

Terms and Concepts
1. a. 1 b. 7 c. 4 d. 6 e. 3 f. 8 g. 5 h. 2 *(p. 506)*

Content Review
1. **d.** Mass and velocity *(p. 488)*
2. **c.** Velocity is the most significant factor. (Review the formula for calculating kinetic energy. Notice that if you double the mass, you double the amount of kinetic energy. However, if you double the speed, the kinetic energy produced is four times as great.) *(pp. 488-489)*
3. **d.** Acceleration (Deceleration is the rate at which a body in motion decreases its speed.) *(p. 489)*
4. **c.** The typical vehicular collision involves three impacts: the vehicle collision (it strikes an object), the body collision (it strikes the inside of vehicle), and the organ collision (they strike the inside surface of the body). *(p. 490)*
5. **b.** Falls are the most common mechanism of injury and account for over half of all trauma incidents. *(p. 490)*
6. **a.** Vehicular collisions account for over one-third of all deaths due to trauma. *(p. 490)*
7. Have a high index of suspicion for severe injury when (a) the vehicle collided at a high speed, (b) one passenger dies, or (c) when a passenger is unresponsive or has an altered mental status. *(p. 490)*
8. Frontal impact (The "up and over" pathway can cause injuries to the head, neck, chest, and abdomen. The "down and under" pathway can cause injuries to the knees, hips, femurs, acetabulum, and spine.) *(p. 491)*
9. "Spider web" (This is the term frequently used to describe the crack pattern caused by a vehicle occupant's head striking the windshield.) *(p. 494)*
10. **b.** A rear-end impact. *(p. 495)*
11. **c.** A lateral impact *(pp. 495-496)*
12. **a.** True. An unrestrained occupant can impact any and every surface inside the vehicle or be ejected. *(pp. 496-498)*
13. **c.** Children turn toward the vehicle; adults turn away. *(p. 498).*
14. **b.** Femur, chest, abdomen, and head (Because a child is small and has a low center of gravity, he is likely to be struck high on the body, then thrown in front of the vehicle and run over.) *(p. 497)*
15. **d.** (The reverse is true. Manufacturers recommend that rescuers lift the deployed airbag to check for deformity indicating impact with the steering wheel.) *(p. 498)*
16. **a.** True *(p. 500)*
17. **c.** A severe fall for an adult is 15 feet; for a child, 10 feet. *(p. 500)*
18. **b.** Three times his height *(p. 500)*
19. **a.** Between the nipple line and the waist *(p. 502)*
20. **b.** Blasts and explosions *(pp. 503-504)*

Case Study 1
1. **c.** An occupant of the same car was killed! Significant forces are involved in this accident.

After the initial assessment, immobilize the patient and begin a rapid trauma assessment.
2. **b.** Along with high speed and death of another vehicle occupant, altered mental status is one of the factors that call for a high suspicion of significant mechanism of injury. You need to assess her mental status and monitor it carefully.

Case Study 2
1. **d.** Knowing how the patient struck the ground will help you determine how the energy dissipated and what potential injuries resulted. The severity of trauma depends on the distance of the fall, the type of surface, and the body part that impacted first.
2. **b.** In a feet-first fall with knees locked, energy will travel all the way up the skeleton. When the patient is thrown forward it may also cause a Colles' fracture — a fracture of the wrist that occurs when the patient tries to break his fall.

Case Study 3
1. **d.** Any information that can obtained about the kind of gun, bullets, distance (since velocity decreases with distance), and number of wounds is important if it can be obtained.
2. **a.** It is critical to look for an exit wound and treat it if there is one. Obviously, the wound should not be probed and nothing should be poured into the wound. Nothing in this case study indicates that the patient's breathing is inadequate. Provide oxygen by nonrebreather mask, but not postiive pressure ventilation.

CHAPTER 29 — BLEEDING AND SHOCK

Terms and Concepts
1. *Shock (hypoperfusion)* is the insufficient supply of oxygen and other nutrients to the body's cells, which results from inadequate circulation of blood.
2. The medical term for a nosebleed is *epistaxis*.
3. By compressing an artery at a *pressure point*, arterial blood flow can be reduced in an extremity. *(p. 526)*

Content Review
1. The role of the circulatory system is to provide the body with blood and a continuous supply of nutrients. *(p. 509)*
2. The three main components of the circulatory system are: (a) the heart, (b) blood vessels: arteries, capillaries, and veins, (c) the blood *(p. 509)*
3. **c.** Pulse and blood pressure *(p. 509)*
4. **a.** 2 **b.** 3 **c.** 1 *(pp. 509-510)*
5. **b.** False. Severe external bleeding should be controlled only after (or simultaneously with) ensuring an adequate airway and breathing. *(p. 511)*
6. **c.** The first step in controlling severe bleeding is to apply direct pressure and elevate the extremity. (Tourniquet or sling and swathe are inappropriate for this kind of injury. Compressing an artery at a pressure point may be necessary if direct pressure and elevation have not completely controlled major bleeding in an extremity.) *(p. 512)*

7. **a.** Brachial pressure point **b.** Femoral pressure point (*Figure 29-5, p. 514*)
8. **b.** Tourniquets are used only as a last resort to control bleeding of an amputated extremity when all other methods have failed. (*p. 514*)
9. Mechanisms of injury that can cause internal bleeding include falls, motor vehicle collisions, pedestrian impacts, blast injuries, and penetrating injuries. (*p. 517*)
10. Emergency medical care of internal bleeding includes: Take BSI precautions. Establish and maintain an open airway and adequate breathing. Administer high-flow oxygen. Control external bleeding, and splint painful, swollen, or deformed extremities. Provide immediate transport of critical patients with signs of shock. Provide care for shock. (*p. 518*)
11. **d.** Shock (hypoperfusion) should be suspected in any patient who has suffered or may have suffered trauma. (*p. 519*)
12. Restlessness, anxiety, and other signs of altered mental status are early signs of shock. (*p. 519*)
13. Shock (hypoperfusion) generally progresses in the following sequence: (*Figure 29-10, p. 518*) **1.** Blood loss causes rapid heart rate and weak pulse. **2.** Blood vessels constrict in extremities to conserve blood causing cold, clammy skin. **3.** Low oxygen levels to breathing control centers of the brain make respirations rapid and shallow; nervous system reaction results in profuse sweating. **4.** Vasoconstriction fails, and blood pressure drops. **5.** Leaking capillaries cause loss of vital blood plasma; unresponsiveness and death may result.
14. Emergency care of shock includes: Take all BSI precautions. Maintain an open airway, and administer oxygen. Control any external bleeding. Apply and inflate the PASG when appropriate and as directed by local protocols and if approved by medical direction. Position the patient according to local protocol. Splint suspected bone or join injuries. Cover the patient with a blanket to prevent loss of body heat. Transport immediately. (*p. 520*)

Case Study

1. If you have not already done so, take BSI precautions (because blood is spurting, include eye protection and a mask as well as gloves). Since this patient has both venous and arterial bleeding, this is a potentially life-threatening situation. Place a sterile gauze over the large wound and apply fingertip pressure to the site. Due to the number of lacerations, have your partner apply a sterile pressure dressing to both hands and the other arm. Both extremities should be elevated above the level of the heart to slow the blood flow and aid in clotting.
2. His increasing agitation may be an early sign of shock. You should assess for other signs of shock and begin administration of oxygen via a nonrebreather mask at 15 lpm, and then expedite transport.
3. As long as you take BSI precautions, no other precautions are necessary. Remember to document the patient's health history on your patient care report, and dispose of bloody dressings or equipment appropriately in biohazard containers. Later follow appropriate procedures for cleaning and disinfecting the ambulance, equipment, and your clothing.
4. En route to the hospital, assess your patient for changes in mental status and vital signs throughout the focused history and physical exam (which will be conducted en route since you made an early transport decision based on the signs of shock), detailed physical exam, and ongoing assessment. Be sure to prevent heat loss by covering the patient with a blanket during transport.

CHAPTER 30 — SOFT TISSUE INJURIES

Terms and Concepts

1. **a.** 8 **b.** 6 **c.** 5 **d.** 1 **e.** 10 **f.** 2 **g.** 4 **h.** 7 **i.** 9 **j.** 3 (*p. 546*)

Content Review

1. **d.** Epidermis, dermis, subcutaneous layer (*p. 529*)
2. **c.** The white blood cells are produced by bone marrow. (*p. 529*)
3. **b.** An amputation is an open injury. Contusions and hematomas are closed injuries. A crush injury may be either open or closed. (*pp. 529-530*)
4. **b.** False. Always take BSI precautions. The potential for the presence of blood and body fluids is present with every patient. (*p. 530*)
5. **c.** Take BSI before approaching any patient. Assess the airway, breathing, and circulation. Assure open airway and adequate breathing. Treat for shock, if necessary. Then splint painful, swollen, or deformed extremities. (*pp. 530-531*)
6. **d.** Occlusive (*p. 536*)
7. **b.** On three sides only to allow air to escape as the patient exhales. (*p. 536*)
8. (a) Take BSI precautions. (b) Assure an open airway and adequate breathing. (c) Expose the wound. (d) Control the bleeding. (e) Prevent further contamination. (f) Dress and bandage the wound. (g) Keep patient calm and quiet. (h) Treat for shock. (i) Transport. (*pp. 534, 536*)
9. **a.** 2, 4, 3, 1 Manually secure the object. Expose the wound area. Control bleeding. Use a bulky dressing to help stabilize the object. (An impaled object should never be removed in the field, unless it is through the cheek.) (*p. 537*)
10. **a.** Never immerse the part in water or in sterile saline since this may cause damage. (*p. 538*)
11. **a.** True. (In addition to severe bleeding, there is the danger of air being sucked into a neck vein and carried to the heart, which can be lethal.) (*p. 539*)
12. To apply a pressure dressing: (a) Cover the wound with several sterile gauze dressings. (b) Apply hand pressure until bleeding is controlled. (c) Bandage firmly to create enough pressure to maintain control of bleeding. Check distal pulses to be sure the bandage is not too tight. (d) If blood soaks through, apply additional dressings and bandage over the original ones. (*p. 541*)

13. **c.** Distal to proximal. *(p. 541)*
14. **c.** Distal pulses, motor function, and sensory function. (Bandages should be snug, not tight. To be sure the bandage is not interfering with circulation, always check distal pulses and motor and sensory function before and after bandage application.) *(p. 541)*
15. **a.** Sterile, moist gauze, then an occlusive dressing. (Avoid absorbent materials that could adhere to organs.) *(p. 537)*
16. **c.** It reduces the tension on the abdominal muscles and will make the patient more comfortable. *(p. 537)*

Case Study 1
1. **c.** Venous bleeding (The bleeding from the patient's neck is dark red and flows steadily. If it were a combination of venous and arterial, you would expect some spurting from the wound.)
2. **a.** For a large open neck wound, place your gloved hand over the wound, then an occlusive dressing, and finally a pressure dressing.

Case Study 2
1. **b.** With any penetrating chest injury, also suspect a spinal injury.
2. **d.** Given the number of shots fired, and in any case of a shooting, you need to look for additional entry and exit wounds.

CHAPTER 31 — BURN EMERGENCIES

Terms and Concepts
1. a. 5 b. 3 c. 2 d. 1 e. 6 f. 4 *(p. 562)*

Content Review
1. Functions of the skin include (a) providing a barrier against infection, (b) providing protection from harmful agents in the environment and injury, (c) aiding in the regulation of body temperature, (d) sensation transmission (hot, cold, pain, touch), (e) aiding in elimination of some body wastes, (f) containing fluids necessary to the functioning of other organs and systems. *(p. 549)*
2. **a.** Body surface area *(p. 551)*
3. **a.** Superficial burn *(pp. 549-550)*
4. **b.** Partial thickness burn *(p. 550)*
5. **c.** Burns to the face are considered critical because of the potential for respiratory compromise or injury to the eyes. *(p. 552)*
6. **b.** In a child, partial thickness burns of 10% to 20% BSA are considered moderate. *(pp. 553-554)*
7. **c.** Children under 5 and adults over 55 have less tolerance for burn injuries. Because of relatively larger skin surfaces, children have the potential for greater fluid loss. Older adults have prolonged and possibly impaired healing processes. *(pp. 552, 554)*
8. Emergency care for burn injuries includes (a) Remove patient from source of burn and stop the burning process. (b) Assess airway, breathing, and mental status. (c) Classify the severity of the burn, and transport immediately if critical. (d) Cover the burned area with a dry sterile

dressing. (e) Keep patient warm and treat other injuries as needed. (f) Transport to the appropriate facility. *(pp. 555-556)*
9. **b.** Separate burned fingers or toes with dry sterile dressings to prevent adherence of burned areas. *(p. 556)*
10. **b.** Always apply a dry sterile dressing to BOTH eyes because the eyes move simultaneously, and if the patient moves the unburned eye, the burned eye will move, too. (Reassure the patient and keep him informed about what is going on.) *(p. 556)*
11. **b.** Dry chemicals should be brushed off before flushing with water. *(p. 558)*
12. **c.** All tissue between entry and exit wounds is suspect for injury even if not readily visible. *(p. 559)*

Case Study
1. **b.** Cut around the area. Do not attempt to remove the adhered portion, since this may cause further damage to the soft tissues.
2. **c.** Singed nasal hair may be an indication of a compromised airway. Provide oxygen via nonrebreather mask at 15 lpm. If breathing becomes inadequate, use positive pressure ventilations. (The child's loud crying indicates that breathing is still adequate.)
3. **c.** Using the rule of nines, approximately 14% of the child's body surface area is affected by the burn. Any partial thickness burn affecting from 10% to 20% of the body surface area should be considered critical in a child.
4. **b.** Use dry sterile dressings on the burn, and keep the patient warm. (Remember that the heat regulation function of burned skin is impaired.)

CHAPTER 32 — MUSCULOSKELETAL INJURIES

Terms and Concepts
1. a. 6 b. 1 c. 3 d. 2 e. 5 f. 4 *(p. 582)*

Content Review
1. **b.** Produces platelets. (This is a function of the circulatory system) *(p. 564)*
2. The six basic components of the skeletal system are (a) skull, (b) spinal column, (c) thorax, (d) pelvis, (e) lower extremities, and (f) upper extremities. *(p. 565)*
3. **c.** Direct, indirect, and twisting. *(p. 566)*
4. **d.** Pulselessness and cyanosis *(p. 566)*
5. The additional steps should be performed in this order of priority: *(p. 566)*
   1. Immobilize the patient to a spine board.
   2. Initiate transport. 3. Perform further management of the life-threatening injuries and ongoing assessments every 5 minutes. 4. Splint the injured extremity.
6. **b.** An open injury *(p. 567)*
7. Signs and symptoms of bone and joint injury include: deformity or angulation, pain and tenderness, grating or crepitus, swelling, disfigurement, severe weakness and loss of function, bruising, exposed bone ends, joint locked into position. *(p. 567)*

8. c. When in doubt, splint! *(pp. 568, 569)*
9. c. Check distal pulses, motor function, and sensation before and after splinting and during the ongoing assessment. *(p. 568)*
10. a. The joints above and below the injury site. *(p. 569)*
11. b. Make one attempt at aligning the extremity (follow local protocol). If pain, resistance, or crepitus increase, stop. *(p. 569)*
12. b. Never intentionally replace protruding bones or push them back below the skin. *(p. 569)*
13. d. The improvised splint should be padded so that the inner surfaces are not in contact with the skin. It should also be light in weight, firm and rigid; long enough to extend past the joints above and below the site; and as wide as the thickest part of the injured limb. *(p. 569)*
14. b. An improperly applied splint can compress the nerves, tissues, and blood vessels under the splint, aggravating the existing injury and causing new injury. *(p. 571)*
15. b. Shoulder injury (The sling supports the arm, and the swathe holds the it against the side of the chest.) *(p. 571)*
16. d. The position of function for a hand is fingers curled as if holding a ball. A roll of bandage in the hand can support this position. *(p. 571)*
17. d. Use a traction splint if the thigh is painful, swollen, or deformed. You do not have to be certain the femur has actually been fractured. However, do not apply a traction splint if there is injury to the hip, pelvis, or knee or within 1 to 2 inches of the knee because the traction could aggravate these injuries. *(p. 574)*
18. c. It pulls on the thigh and realigns the broken femur. This helps relieve pain and reduces movement of the broken bone ends. *(pp. 573-574)*

Case Study 1
1. b. Remember, check pulses, motor function, and sensation before and after splinting. (Apply a sling and swathe after checking PMS.)
2. c. Sensation is intact if the patient can tell you, without looking, which finger or toe you are touching.
3. b. The energy from the impact of this patient's hand with the ground travels up the arm and causes an injury to the collarbone (clavicle). This is a classic example of an injury caused by indirect force.

Case Study 2
1. c. Do not release traction until after the splint has been applied.
2. a. Assess the pedal or posterior tibial pulse for a lower extremity, and assess the radial pulse for an upper extremity.

Case Study 3
1. a. Paresthesia or tingling may indicate some loss of sensation.
2. b. The position of function is with the foot bent at the normal angle to the leg, not pushed downward or upward toward the shin or otherwise manipulated into an unnatural position.

3. c. If the injury involves a lower extremity, motor function is intact if the patient can tighten the kneecap and move the foot up and down as if pumping a gas pedal.

CHAPTER 33 — INJURIES TO THE HEAD

Terms and Concepts
1. a. 4 b. 1 c. 6 d. 2 e. 5 f. 3 *(pp. 596-597)*

Content Review
1. d. Elevated oxygen levels will not further injure the brain in the prehospital setting. *(p. 586)*
2. c. While pupillary changes are often a sign of head injury, they will not be observed as part of the scene size-up. *(p. 587)*
3. The first step in the initial assessment of the patient with a possible head injury is to manually stabilize the cervical spine. *(p. 587)*
4. b. Jaw-thrust maneuver (This maneuver is done without tilting the patient's head, which might aggravate any possible head or spine injury) *(p. 587)*
5. d. The lowest level on the AVPU scale is unresponsiveness; that is, the patient does not respond to any stimulus indicating the most serious injury. *(p. 587)*
6. c. Immediate transport and monitoring. *(p. 590)*
7. When there is possible head injury, pay particular attention to examination of the head, eyes, ears, and nose and to motor/sensory assessment. *(p. 591)*
8. When a patient is unresponsive and has a breathing rate above or below the normal range or any other sign of inadequate breathing, you should administer positive pressure ventilation with supplemental oxygen and hyperventilate at 24 to 30 breaths per minute. *(p. 593)*
9. b. Although you should always ask about a history of allergies, it is not likely to be pertinent to a possible head injury. (Prior head injury and any pattern of altered mental status or unresponsiveness are critical factors when head injury is suspected.) *(p. 592)*
10. c. While it is always important to control bleeding, you should never apply a pressure dressing to an open skull injury since doing so may drive pieces of fragmented bone into the brain tissue. *(p. 593)*

Case Study
1. Insure BSI precautions. Establish in-line spinal stabilization while maintaining a patent airway using the jaw-thrust technique. Suction as necessary to clear the airway. Begin hyperventilation at a rate of 24 to 30 breaths per minute with supplemental oxygen. *(p. 593)*
2. The bruising on the mastoid area (Battle's sign) indicates a basilar skull fracture. The bruising around both eyes (raccoon sign) is an indication of intracranial bleeding with skull fracture. Both signs may appear as early as one-half hour following injury or as late as one day following injury. *(p. 591)*

3. The vital signs are typical of those seen in a head-injured patient who has intracranial bleeding and/or increased intracranial pressure. You should continue the treatment you have already started, expedite transport, and try to obtain a SAMPLE history from her nephew. *(pp. 591-592)*

CHAPTER 34 — INJURIES TO THE SPINE

Terms and Concepts

1. a. 4 b. 3 c. 1 d. 2 *(p. 632)*
2. a. cervical spine (first seven vertebrae which form the neck); b. thoracic spine (the next twelve vertebrae, which form the upper back); c. lumbar spine (the next five vertebrae, which form the lower back); d. sacral spine or sacrum (the next five vertebrae, which are fused together to form the rigid part of the back side of the pelvis); e. coccyx (the four fused vertebrae that form the lower end of the spine) *(pp. 601, 632)*

Content Review

1. Be especially alert to the possibility of spine injury when called to these scenes: (a) motorcycle crashes; (b) motor vehicle crashes; (c) pedestrian-vehicle collisions; (d) falls; (e) blunt trauma; (f) penetrating trauma to the head, neck, or torso; (g) hangings; (h) diving accidents or near-drownings; (g) gunshot wounds; (h) unresponsive trauma patient; (i) electrical injuries. *(p. 602)*
2. b. Maintain a high index of suspicion for spinal injury (regardless of the lack of obvious trauma and based solely on a scene size-up of mechanism of injury and unresponsive patient). *(pp. 602, 604)*
3. c. Never place a patient with a suspected spinal injury in a lateral recumbent position. Instead, maintain manual stabilization and suction to clear the airway. *(p. 604)*
4. Major complications of spinal injury may include: (a) impaired breathing effort due to paralysis of the respiratory muscles, (b) paralysis below the level of spinal-cord damage, and (c) inadequate circulation. *(pp. 607-608)*
5. a. Assess the pulse, motor function, and sensation of the suspected spine-injured patient during the rapid trauma assessment, after immobilization on a long backboard, and during the detailed physical exam — not during the initial assessment. *(pp. 604, 609)*
6. c. In manual spinal stabilization the patient's nose is aligned with the navel with the head neither flexed nor extended. *(p. 608)*
7. d. Two rescuers are needed to apply a cervical spine immobilization collar — one to stabilize the neck manually while the other applies the device. *(p. 610)*
8. d. The spinal immobilization devices indicated for the seated spine-injured patient include a cervical spine immobilization collar and a short spinal immobilization device applied while the patient is in the seated position, followed by transfer to a long backboard. *(pp. 616-617)*
9. b. False. Patients must be secured to the backboard with straps or cravats in a manner that does not interfere with the patient's breathing but tight enough to prevent the patient's torso from moving during transport. The head and extremities must also be immobilized. *(p. 611)*
10. Log rolling is the maneuver used to position the supine or prone patient onto a long backboard while maintaining in-line stabilization. *(pp. 611-613)*
11. 1. Establish and maintain in-line manual stabilization. 2. Apply a cervical spine immobilization collar. 3. Log roll the patient onto the long spine board. 4. Place pads in the spaces between the patient and the board. 5. Immobilize the patient's torso to the board with straps. 6. Immobilize the patient's head to the board. 7. Secure the patient's legs to the board. *(pp. 611-613)*
12. b. Immobilize the patient from a standing position while maintaining alignment. *(pp. 613-615)*
13. a. Never use a chin strap to help maintain neutral spinal alignment. This will prevent your patient from opening his mouth if he needs to vomit. *(p. 617)*
14. Indications for the use of rapid extrication are: (a) an unsafe scene; (b) patient's condition is too unstable to delay treatment; or (c) the patient blocks your access to a second, more seriously injured patient. *(p. 617)*
15. a. Safe and effective rapid extrication requires constant cervical spine stabilization. *(p. 617)*
16. Criteria for leaving the helmet in place on a patient with suspected spinal injury are: (a) helmet fits well with little or no movement of the head within the helmet; (b) no impending airway or breathing problems; (c) removal would cause further injury; (d) possible to immobilize spine with helmet in place; (e) helmet doesn't interfere with ability to assess airway and breathing. *(p. 619)*
17. a. Removing the helmet while leaving the shoulder pads in place may aggravate the injury due to the hyperextension of the neck. *(p. 623)*
18. 1. Apply manual in-line stabilization. 2. Assess for life-threatening injuries or other reasons for removal from car seat. 3. Support the head in a neutral position using towel rolls and tape. 4. Determine if padding is required between infant's body and seat. 5. Transport in the normal seated position after securing car seat to ambulance seat. *(pp. 626-627)*

Case Study

1. Begin by taking BSI precautions. Establish and maintain manual in-line stabilization, bringing the head into neutral in-line position. Perform an initial assessment.
2. During the initial assessment, use a jaw-thrust maneuver to open and maintain the airway. If necessary, insert an oropharyngeal or nasopharyngeal airway, suction, and provide positive pressure ventilation or oxygen via nonrebreather mask.
3. To prepare the patient for transport, apply a cervical spine immobilization collar and immobilize the patient to a long backboard. Reassess, record, and document pulses and motor and sensory function in all extremities. Load the patient into the ambulance and transport.

CHAPTER 35— EYE, FACE, AND NECK INJURIES

Terms and Concepts

1. a. 3 b. 1 c. 8 d. 6 e. 7 f. 4 g. 2 h. 5 i. 9 (p. 652)
2. Labels on the left of the drawing, top to bottom: cornea, conjunctiva, pupil, aqueous humor. Labels in the center, top to bottom: iris, lens, vitreous humor. Labels on the right, top to bottom: retina, sclera. (pp. 635, 652)
3. a. The orbits are the bony structures that surround the eyes. (p. 652)

Content Review

1. You may need to treat both the patient and family or friends for emotional trauma because of their fears of blindness and permanent disfigurement. (p. 637)
2. b. Stabilize the head and neck of the patient with facial trauma before doing anything else. (p. 637)
3. d. Suspect significant damage to the eye if there is unusual sensitivity to the light. Also suspect significant damage if the patient has loss of vision that does not improve with blinking, loses part of the field of vision, has severe pain in the eye, or has double vision. (p. 638)
4. d. Every patient with an eye injury must be transported (in a supine position) for evaluation by a physician. (p. 638)
5. a. Attempt to remove foreign objects from the conjunctiva only. All of the rest should be removed by a physician. (pp. 633-639)
6. d. Apply cold compresses to decrease swelling, not warm ones. (pp. 640-641)
7. a. True (p. 641)
8. a. Begin treatment of a chemical burn to the eye immediately. Further delay will increase the injury. (p. 641)
9. d. Flush for at least 20 minutes. Remember to remove contact lenses, which can trap chemicals (p. 642)
10. c. Place the patient with an impaled or extruded eye injury in a supine position with the head immobilized. (p. 642)
11. d. Hard lenses show up as shadows over the iris; soft lenses show up as shadows over the outer portion of the eye. (p. 642)
12. a. Pinch the soft lens between your thumb and index finger, allowing air to get underneath it. (If the lens has dehydrated, run sterile saline across the eye surface, slide the lens off the cornea, and pinch it up.) (pp. 643-644)
13. b. False (The dentures can help support the structures of the mouth. Remove the dentures if they are broken.) (p. 646)
14. a. Cover the exposed nerves and tendons with a moist sterile dressing. Any other type of dressing may dry out the nerves and tissues. (p. 646)
15. b. Rinse an avulsed tooth with saline to remove debris. Never scrub. Transport the tooth in a cup of saline or wrapped in gauze soaked in sterile saline. (p. 647)
16. c. Push or pull it out in the same direction in which it entered. (If not removed, it could fall into the mouth and obstruct the airway.) (p. 647)
17. c. Tape it to the outside of the mouth and monitor closely. (Don't insert your fingers; the patient may bite you, and you need your hands for other procedures. Don't have the patient hold the dressing; he may forget or lose responsiveness and let the dressing fall into the airway.) (p. 647)
18. b. Apply cold compresses to reduce the swelling, and then transport. (p. 648)
19. d. Clear or bloody fluid draining from the ear may indicate a skull fracture. Place a loose clean dressing across opening to absorb the fluids. Do not exert any pressure. (pp. 648-649)
20. b. False. (When treating bleeding wounds to the neck, do not probe the wound, but also never use circumferential bandages. They can interfere with blood flow to the brain on the uninjured side of the neck and can also impair respiration. Instead, make a figure-eight wrap of bandage over the dressing, across one shoulder and the back, under the opposite armpit, and anchor at the shoulder.) (pp. 649-650)

Case Study

1. Yes, paramedic back up should be considered; the patient may need advanced airway procedures.
2. d. This is a high priority patient. Transport immediately, and provide emergency care and meet the paramedics en route.
3. a. Immediately begin flushing the eyes with saline. At the same time, place a gloved hand over the neck wound to control bleeding and administer high flow oxygen.

CHAPTER 36 — CHEST, ABDOMEN, AND GENITALIA INJURIES

Terms and Concepts

1. a. 2 b. 4 c. 1 d. 3 e. 5 (p. 673)

Content Review

1. Chest cavity: aorta, heart, lungs, superior vena cava, trachea. Abdominal cavity: intestines, liver, spleen, stomach, urinary bladder. (pp. 655, 663)
2. An open chest injury is the result of a penetrating chest wound caused by a mechanism of injury such as a knife, bullet, nail, screw driver, or post. A closed chest injury is the result of blunt trauma, which may cause severe damage to the ribs and internal organs; it is typically caused by a fall, vehicle crash, and/or blow to the chest. (p. 655)
3. a. Initial assessment. (Chest injury is potentially life threatening.) (p. 657)
4. b. It is an attempt to reduce pain. (Shallow, rapid breathing can be inadequate and can easily lead to hypoxia.) (p. 657)
5. c. Gravity pulls fluids and other heavier matter downward, forcing air to flow upward. (p. 658)

6. c. In tension pneumothorax, breath sounds will be absent on the injured side and decreased on the uninjured side. (The air on the injured side forces the mediastinum to shift, compressing the cavity on the uninjured side, interfering with inflation of the lung on the uninjured side.) *(p. 659)*

7. d. When there is no suspected spinal injury, place the open chest wound patient on the injured side so the uninjured lung can inflate more fully. *(p. 660)*

8. b. False. (The hollow organs include the stomach, gallbladder, urinary bladder, and intestines. The liver, spleen, pancreas, and kidneys are solid organs.) *(p. 663)*

9. a. True (A solid organ may bleed into the capsule that surrounds it for some time before the capsule ruptures and allows the blood to spill into the abdominal cavity.) *(p. 663)*

10. c. Mechanism of injury. (Because signs and symptoms may be subtle, the other choices are less reliable indicators.) *(p. 664)*

11. d. Start palpating farthest from the pain. *(p. 665)*

12. c. Supine, legs flexed at knees. *(p. 665)*

13. c. Dressings for an abdominal evisceration are a dressing soaked in saline or sterile water, then an occlusive dressing, then an additional dressing over the occlusive dressing. *(pp. 666-667)*

14. d. The best care for any amputated part is to wrap it in saline-moistened sterile dressing, put it in a plastic bag, and place the bag on a cold pack or ice that has been wrapped in a towel. (Placing directly on ice may cause tissues to freeze.) Label the bag and transport the part with the patient. *(p. 667.)*

15. a. Apply direct pressure with a moistened sterile compress such as a sanitary napkin. *(p. 667)*

Case Study

1. c. Immediately seal the open chest wound with a gloved hand. Any delay will worsen the patient's condition.

2. c. Only the occlusive dressing on an open chest wound needs to have an open side to allow air to escape from the chest cavity with breathing. An occlusive dressing on an abdominal evisceration should be sealed on all sides.

3. d. Lift the corner of the occlusive dressing on the chest wound to release air that is trapped and building up in the chest cavity.

CHAPTER 37 — AGRICULTURAL AND INDUSTRIAL EMERGENCIES

Content Review

1. Hazards at the scene of an agricultural or industrial accident include toxic gases, chemicals, unstable equipment, and livestock. *(p. 675)*

2. b. The best approach to a tractor accident is to have at least two rescue teams at the scene–one to handle the potential fire hazard and one to provide patient extrication and treatment. *(p. 675)*

3. c. Never attempt rescue alone or without a lifeline at scenes involving agricultural storage areas. *(pp. 675, 677)*

4. d. Once the scene is safe, all of these actions will be accomplished. However, your first action is to establish a patent airway while maintaining in-line manual spinal stabilization. If your patient was exposed to chemicals or manure, also remove all exposed clothing and flush the patient with copious amounts of water before transport. *(p. 677)*

5. a. True. (Preserve all avulsed body parts, however mangled their appearance, and transport them with the patient.) *(p. 677)*

6. a. 4 b. 5 c. 2 d. 1 e. 3 *(p. 679)*

7. c. Appropriate ways to stabilize agricultural equipment include blocking or chocking the vehicle, tying it to another vehicle, and setting the parking brake. When the equipment is stabilized, attempt to shut it down. *(p. 679)*

8. a. If the patient's life is threatened and other attempts to shut down the engine have failed, you should discharge a fire extinguisher into the air intake. (Note that this can cause extensive damage to the engine.) *(p. 679)*

9. b. Assume that a patient who has been buried in a grain tank is hypothermic. For that reason, always assume a patient is alive, even if he has been trapped for a long period of time. *(p. 681)*

10. Signs of silo gas include bleach-like odor; yellowish or reddish vapor; red, yellow, or brown stains on surfaces touched by the gas; dead birds or insects near the silo; signs of illness in nearby livestock. *(p. 682)*

11. c. Never enter a livestock building or livestock area until all the animals have been secured. *(p. 683)*

12. Guidelines for any industrial rescue include: check with the staff to determine potential hazards; never assume any machine is locked and secured; if the patient is in a confined space or has been exposed to chemicals, wait for specialized hazardous material personnel for rescue and decontamination. *(p. 683)*

Case Study

1. Administer oxygen by nonrebreather mask at 15 lpm. Apply dressings as needed to control bleeding. Further assess the situation, and evaluate the need for additional assistance. You might consider having Mr. Wilson help you, depending on his emotional status.

2. Do not remove the impaled tine. It probably is controlling hemorrhage, so it should be stabilized with dressings in the position found to minimize movement and transported with John.

3. Continue manual in-line spinal stabilization and oxygen therapy. Stabilize the tine while Mr. Wilson removes the bolts holding it in place. Once that is done, have the forklift moved out of the way. Perform standing backboard procedures and immobilize John to the board.

4. Treat for shock and transport. En route, complete a detailed physical exam and ongoing assessment.

CHAPTER 38 — INFANTS AND CHILDREN

Terms and Concepts

1. **a.** Neonate, 0 to 4 weeks: has total dependence on others; birth defects and unintentional injuries are common emergencies; no special assessment challenges. **b.** Infant, 0 to 1 year: recognizes the caregiver's face and voice; older infants are stressed by separation; start assessment from a distance and allow caregiver to hold infant for exam; frightened by initial stimulation around face, so begin exam with heart and lungs and end with the head. **c.** Toddler, 1 to 3 years: "do not like..." stage, so limit touch, avoid separation, limit clothing removal or involve caregiver; fear of pain/needles but comforted by security objects; try toe-to-head exam. **d.** Preschooler, 3 to 6 years: concrete thinkers and literal interpreters, so explain simply and slowly before any action is taken; modest and resistant to attempts to unclothe, so involve caregiver; fear of pain, blood, and permanent injury but comforted by security objects; believe illness or injury is their fault and view it as punishment; allow them to see and "check out" equipment first; be sensitive, since stress may cause bladder or bowel accidents. **e.** School age, 6 to 12 years: cooperative and curious; usually have some understanding of EMS system; maturity levels are highly individualized; honesty very important, so seek their cooperation; modesty and body image issues are common, so explanations are critical; fear of blood, pain, death, and permanent injury. **f.** Adolescent, 12-18 years: have concrete and abstract thinking skills, but believe nothing bad can happen to them; respect their privacy; obtain history when alone; peer influence strong; body conscious; may overreact. *(pp. 687-689)*

Content Review

1. **b.** Involve the caregivers if you can; it helps to calm them and acknowledges them as "experts" for this child. *(p. 687)*
2. **a.** The diameter of a newborn's trachea is only about 4 mm to 5 mm, compared to the 20 mm diameter of the adult trachea. This means that inhalation of steam or toxic fumes can cause life-threatening airway swelling not only faster but with less exposure. *(pp. 689-91)*
3. **c.** Hypothermia *(p. 690)*
4. **b.** Metabolic rates. (Infants and children use oxygen from the bloodstream faster, making respiratory difficulties more dangerous.) *(p. 691)*
5. **c.** Respiratory system problems. *(p. 691)*
6. Signs of early respiratory distress in infants and children include an increased respiratory rate, nasal flaring, intercostal retractions on inspiration, neck muscle retractions, audible breathing noises, and "see-saw" respirations. *(p. 691)*
7. **c.** Decompensated respiratory failure. (Provide positive pressure ventilation with supplemental oxygen and prompt transport.) *(p. 692)*
8. **c.** Respiratory arrest. (Treat the patient aggressively with oxygenation and positive pressure ventilation. Transport immediately.) *(p. 692)*
9. Causes of rapid breathing in infants and children include oxygen deficiency, head injury, fever, diabetes emergencies, aspirin overdose or other poisonings, and stress or fear. *(p. 693)*
10. In partial airway obstruction some air is still getting through; indications include a patient who is alert (possibly crying), pink, with peripheral perfusion; stridor; retractions; noisy respirations; forceful cough may still be present. Indications of complete airway obstruction include no crying or talking; ineffective or absent cough; altered mental status; cyanosis. *(pp. 692-693)*
11. **b.** Urinary output *(p. 694)*
12. **1.** Support in prone head-down position. **2.** Deliver 5 sharp back blows. **3.** Transfer to supine position and deliver 5 chest thrusts using 2 fingertips. **4.** Look in mouth, sweep out visible object. **5.** Attempt to ventilate; if unsuccessful, repeat sequence. *(p. 699)*
13. Common causes of seizure in infants and children include fever, epilepsy, head injury, meningitis, oxygen deficiency, drug overdose, and low blood sugar. *(p. 702)*
14. The general emergency care procedures for an infant or child suffering a seizure include: Assure airway position and patency; position the patient on his side if there is no possibility of spinal injury and make sure he will not injure himself; be prepared to suction; provide oxygen or ventilate as appropriate; transport. *(p. 703)*
15. **b.** Never sponge with alcohol; the body may absorb it and cause hypothermia. *(p. 704)*
16. **b.** False (When infants and children deteriorate because of hypoperfusion, they deteriorate faster, not slower, and more severely than adults.) *(p. 704)*
17. The emergency medical care of an infant or child with possible shock includes: Assure an open airway and provide oxygen; be prepared to provide positive pressure ventilation with supplemental oxygen if necessary; control hemorrhage if present; if possible, place patient in supine position with legs raised; keep patient warm and calm; transport to the hospital quickly. *(p. 704)*
18. **a.** True *(p. 706)*
19. **b.** False (If possible, the SAMPLE history of a SIDS patient should include both what you can observe at the scene and information from the parents or other caregivers, including circumstances concerning discovery of the unresponsive patient, time the baby was put to bed or fell asleep, problems at birth, general health, any recent illnesses, date and result of last physical exam. Be careful, however, not to convey by the wording of your questions or your manner that you feel the parents may be responsible for the child's condition.) *(p. 706)*
20. **a.** 3 **b.** 1 **c.** 4 **d.** 2 *(p. 707)*
21. **d.** Hypoperfusion is not usually associated with closed head injuries. If signs of hypoperfusion are present with a closed head injury, be suspicious of other internal injuries. *(p. 707)*
22. **b.** False (The flexibility and pliable nature of the child's rib cage cause rib fractures to be uncommon, but internal damage is more likely.) *(pp. 707-708)*

23. **a.** Interference with diaphragm movement and lung inflation may compromise respiratory effort. *(p. 708)*
24. **a.** True. *(p. 708)*
25. **b.** Fluid loss *(p. 708)*
26. General indications of child abuse include multiple abrasions, lacerations, bruises, broken bones; multiple injuries or bruises in various stages of healing; injuries on both the front and back or on both sides of the child's body; unusual wounds; fear; injuries to the genitals; injuries to the central nervous system; situations in which signs of trauma on the patient do not match the reported mechanism of injury; lack of adult supervision; untreated chronic illness; malnourishment and unsafe living environment; delay in reporting injuries. *(p. 709)*
27. **c.** Objectively record your observations, follow local reporting protocols, and maintain total confidentiality. *(p. 711)*
28. **a.** True *(p. 713)*
29. **b.** A suction catheter that is half the diameter of the tube. *(p. 711)*
30. **a.** Request a meeting with the CISD team for everyone involved. If you are having some trouble, others probably are too. *(p. 713)*

Case Study
1. This baby is in decompensated respiratory failure. Without immediate intervention, respiratory arrest may occur.
2. Establish and maintain a patent airway. Gently suction any secretions, but no longer than 5 to 10 seconds at a time. Insert an oropharyngeal airway, and initiate positive pressure ventilation with supplemental oxygen. Position infant to prevent aspiration. Initiate rapid transport.
3. Reassure her that she did the right thing to call 9-1-1 and that although the baby is very sick you are doing everything you can to help him. Thank her for her helpfulness in providing information that will better enable you to care for her son.

CHAPTER 39 — MOVING PATIENTS

Terms and Concepts
1. **a.** 3 **b.** 1 **c.** 2 *(p. 738)*

Content Review
1. **b.** Lift an object as CLOSE to your body as possible. *(Table 39-1, p. 723)*
2. **d.** A motor vehicle collision patient with a critical head injury would require an urgent move. The other choices require emergency moves. *(p. 723)*
3. **a.** The armpit-forearm drag *(p. 723)*
4. **c.** The shirt drag *(pp. 723-724)*
5. **a.** Direct ground lift *(p. 726)* **b.** Extremity lift *(pp. 727)*
6. **a.** Direct carry *(p. 727)* **b.** Draw sheet method *(p. 728)*
7. **1.** Hold in-line stabilization of the head and neck, and apply a cervical-spine immobilization collar. **2.** Support the patient's thorax as another rescuer frees the legs from the pedals. **3.** Rotate the patient in several coordinated moves until the patient's back is in the doorway. **4.** Place the long

backboard next to the patient's buttocks, and lower the patient onto the board. *(pp. 724-725)*
8. **a.** The direct ground lift should NOT be used for the heavier patient. *(p. 725)*
9. **c.** 400 pounds *(p. 730)*
10. **d.** A scoop stretcher is NOT recommended for spine-injured patients. *(p. 731)*
11. **c.** When a wheeled stretcher cannot traverse narrow corridors. *(p. 731)*
12. **a.** Stokes basket. *(p. 733)*
13. **a.** Wheeled-stretcher *(Figure 39-9b, p. 731)* **b.** portable ambulance stretcher *(Figure 39-12a, p. 733)* **c.** Scoop stretcher *(Figure 39-16, p. 735)* **d.** Basket stretcher *(Figure 39-18a, p.736)* **e.** Short wooden backboard *(Figure 39-15b, p. 734)* **f.** Vest-type immobilization device *(Figure 39-15c, p. 734)*

Case Study
1. **d.** Given that the patient has osteoporosis, the least traumatic method of moving her would be the draw sheet method. This patient must be handled very gently.
2. **a.** Never have a patient walk to the stretcher if the patient is dizzy or lightheaded, sweaty when sitting or standing, having chest pains, respiratory problems, or an injured lower extremity.
3. **b.** When moving this patient on the wheeled stretcher to the awaiting ambulance, the EMT at the head pushes and the EMT at the foot guides.

CHAPTER 40 — AMBULANCE OPERATIONS

Content Review
1. Privileges associated with the operation of emergency vehicles include exceeding posted speed limits, driving the wrong way down a one-way street, turning in any direction at any intersection, parking anywhere, leaving the ambulance standing in the middle of a street or intersection, going through red lights or red flashing signals, and passing other vehicles in a no-passing zone. In executing any of the above listed, you must first signal, ensure that the way is clear, and avoid endangering life and property. *(p. 742)*
2. **b.** Driving the wrong way down a one-way street without using any warning devices *(p. 742)*
3. **c.** Know the "high-traffic" areas and times for your community. *(p. 743)*
4. **c.** The use of escorts doubles the hazards associated with emergency driving; they should only be used as a last resort. *(p. 744)*
5. **b.** Debriefing is, at times, an important activity, but it is not a phase of an ambulance call. *(p. 745)*
6. Benefits of an emergency vehicle maintenance and inspection schedule include decreased vehicle down time, improved response times, safer emergency and non-emergency responses, improved transport times to the medical facility, and safer patient transports to the medical facility. *(p. 746)*

7. Six points of information you should receive from the dispatcher are (a) the location of the call, (b) the nature of the call, (c) the name, location, and callback number of the caller, (d) the location of the patient, (e) the number of patients and severity of the problem, and (f) any other special problems or circumstances that may be pertinent. (Do not hesitate to ask the dispatcher to repeat or restate information if anything is unclear.) *(p. 746)*

8. **a.** Determine and clarify the responsibilities of each team member *(pp. 746-747)*

9. **c.** "Jaws of Life" and an assortment of small hand tools (Tools may be carried on an ambulance, especially in a jurisdiction in which EMS may at times perform extrication. However, they are not considered basic ambulance supplies.) *(Table 40-2, p. 748)*

10. **a.** In front of or behind the collision *(p. 748)*

11. **b.** Stay a minimum of 100 feet from wreckage or a burning vehicle and 2000 feet from hazardous materials spills. *(p. 748)*

12. **d.** All of the above *(p. 750)*

13. **c.** Every 15 minutes for a stable patient, every 5 minutes for an unstable patient *(p. 750)*

14. **c.** Review patient priorities and check interventions (Be sure to keep the driver informed of the patient's condition.) *(p. 752)*

15. **a.** Ensure proper continuity of care *(p. 752)*

16. **d.** Should be left at the emergency department (Some EMS systems also may require you to leave a copy with the patient.) *(p. 752)*

17. Once you have completed a call, prepare for a return to service by cleaning and inspecting the ambulance, patient care equipment, reusable supplies, and the patient care compartment before notifying dispatch of your availability. *(p. 752)*

18. **a.** Sterilize *(p. 753)*

19. 1:10 solution of household bleach and water. *(p. 753)*

20. **a.** 3 **b.** 1 **c.** 4 **d.** 2 *(pp. 753-754)*

21. **d.** All of these *(p. 755)*

Case Study

1. En route to the scene of "an unknown emergency involving school bus," anticipate potential hazards at the scene and review with your partner what environmental hazards the call location might present. Be sure to determine and clarify responsibilities of the team members. *(pp. 746-747)*

2. As the designated patient attendant, you follow the child to the driver to begin your initial assessment. Your partner should contact dispatch and request law enforcement personnel assistance and ask that dispatch contact the school bus company to send another driver. Then he should check on the well-being of the school children and make sure that they are staying out of harm's way. *(pp. 747-750)*

3. En route you should complete the detailed physical exam, if appropriate, begin an ongoing assessment, check interventions and patient security, and review patient priorities. Meanwhile your partner should notify dispatch of your destination, number of patients being transported, and anticipated time of arrival. You should also communicate with the hospital to provide them with pertinent information about Mr. Michaels. *(pp. 750-752)*

CHAPTER 41 — GAINING ACCESS AND EXTRICATION

Content Review

1. **a.** When receiving dispatch information *(p. 762)*
2. **b.** Motor vehicle collisions *(p. 763)*
3. **c.** Binoculars can help you assess the scene from a safe distance. *(p. 763)*
4. **a.** Full protective turnout gear. (This includes coat, pants, steel-toed boots, helmet with ear flaps and wide brim and a face shield, eye protection, and heavy leather gloves over disposable gloves.) *(p. 763)*
5. **c.** ALWAYS assume downed power lines are alive. (Call the electric service company for assistance.) *(p. 764)*
6. **b.** Stop all traffic and reroute it to different roads. (Remember, however, that special prior training in traffic direction and control is necessary.) *(p. 764)*
7. A child may have been involved. (This clue should prompt you to ask questions and complete a thorough search of the area.) *(p. 764)*
8. **c.** A vehicle is stable when it can no longer move, rock, or bounce. *(p. 765)*
9. **d.** Simply turns off the ignition *(pp. 765-766)*
10. Before disconnecting the power to the vehicle, you should try to move the seat backward, lower power windows, and unlock power door locks. This will give you greatest access to the patient. *(p. 766)*
11. **a.** Remove the negative battery cable first. *(p. 766)*
12. (a) Simple access is access that does not require tools. (b) Complex access requires tools and specialized equipment. *(p. 766)*
13. **a.** Breaking a window *(p. 766)*
14. **c.** From the front (Approach facing the patient to keep him from moving his head.) *(p. 767)*
15. **d.** Start your request by saying "Without moving your head or neck." (If you wait until the end of your sentence to say this, the patient may move before you can finish.) *(p. 767)*
16. **c.** Against the lower corner of the window *(p. 767)*
17. **b.** Patient care always precedes removal from the vehicle EXCEPT when delay would endanger the patient or rescue personnel. *(p. 768)*
18. **d.** Use blankets, a tarp, or a spine board *(p. 768)*
19. **b.** Explain the activities, noises, and movements *(pp. 768-769)*
20. The only exception to the rule that the spine must be stabilized and, if possible, immobilized before removing a patient from a vehicle is when there is an immediate threat to your patient's life or your own. *(p. 769)*

Case Study

1. **a.** Secure an area that is more than 80 feet in all directions. Yell instructions to the patient to stay in the vehicle. Do not approach the car, because power can be automatically restored. Trust only the power company or specialized teams trained in electrical hazards to tell you when it is safe.

2. **c.** Tell the patient to focus and keep his attention on an object directly in front of him.
3. Make the patient aware of how long the process may take, explain the activities and movements around him, explain the noises that will be present, ask the patient if he is ready to have the door opened, stay with the patient at all times, and reassure him constantly.

CHAPTER 42 — HAZARDOUS MATERIALS EMERGENCIES

Terms and Concepts
1. **a.** 3 **b.** 2 **c.** 4 **d.** 1 *(p. 792)*

Content Review
1. **b.** Rescuer, public, and patient safety (Accidental exposure to hazardous materials may be limited to a few victims, but an accident also may cause widespread destruction and loss of life.) *(p. 776)*
2. **a.** Dose, concentration, and time exposed *(p. 776)*
3. **c.** A four-sided diamond shape (Many are red or orange. A few are white or green. The placard contains a four-digit identification number and a legend that indicates whether the material is flammable, radioactive, explosive, or poisonous.) *(p. 780)*
4. **a.** A health hazard. (The NFPA 704 system identifies potential danger with the use of background colors and numbers ranging from 0-4. Blue identifies a health hazard, red a fire hazard, yellow a reactivity hazard; the higher the number the greater the hazard.) *(p. 780)*
5. **a.** The Chemical Transportation Emergency Center, or CHEMTREC (CHEMTREC may be reached at 1-800-424-9300 around the clock. for advice on how to handle any emergency involving hazardous materials.) *(p. 780)*
6. Visual clues to the probable presence of a hazardous material include: smoking or self-igniting materials, extraordinary fire conditions, boiling or spattering of materials that have not been heated, wavy or unusually colored vapors over a container of liquid material, characteristically colored vapor clouds, frost near a container leak, unusual condition of containers. *(p. 780)*
7. **b.** False (ALWAYS assume that the area surrounding a spill or leak is dangerous.) *(p. 780)*
8. Hazardous Materials: Emergency Response Guidebook *(p. 780)*
9. OSHA and the EPA levels of training for those dealing with hazardous materials emergencies are First Responder Awareness, First Responder Operations, Hazardous Materials Technician, and Hazardous Materials Specialist. *(p. 783)*
10. **c.** Presents an environmental hazard (By carrying toxins and particles of hazardous materials through the air, smoke from a hazardous materials fire not only threatens the immediate safety of victims and rescuers, it also may threaten long-term health, in some cases causing cancer and chronic poisoning affecting the brain, liver, lungs, and kidneys.) *(p. 784)*
11. **a.** True *(p. 784)*

12. **a.** 3 **b.** 1 **c.** 2 *(p. 784)*
13. **b.** False (AVOID risking your life or your health. Specially trained environmental workers will clean up the hazard. *(p. 784)*
14. **b.** Decontaminate the patient fully (A contaminated patient in a closed, tight space could affect the breathing or vision of the air transport team.) *(p. 788)*
15. **c.** Keep uphill, upwind, and away from the danger *(p. 786)*
16. If you are accidentally exposed to hazardous materials, (a) wash with mild detergent or green soap and plenty of running water, (b) irrigate exposed skin for at least 20 minutes, (c) seek medical attention, (d) document the emergency, (e) report the emergency to your employer, and (f) get a thorough medical examination and medical surveillance. *(p. 788)*

Case Study 1
1. **d.** Quickly call for additional assistance.
2. **c.** Keep uphill, upwind, and protect yourself and the patient. (Prevent others from approaching the accident site until specialized help arrives.)

Case Study 2
1. **c.** Under the arms and in the groin. (Contamination occurs most easily in areas of your body where skin is thin or moist.)
2. **a.** Wash with green soap and plenty of running water. Irrigate exposed skin for at least 20 minutes.
3. **b.** Cover exposed areas of the vehicle with plastic sheeting. (Take precautions to protect your vehicle and equipment prior to transport.)

Case Study 3
1. **a.** Remove the bystander, evacuate the area, contact dispatch. (Do not attempt or allow other untrained persons to attempt to put out the fire. Do not remain near the building. Because toxic fertilizers may be burning at this fire, evacuate to a safe area until specialized help arrives.)

CHAPTER 43 — MULTIPLE-CASUALTY INCIDENTS

Terms and Concepts
1. **a.** 13 **b.** 4 **c.** 7 **d.** 10 **e.** 5 **f.** 9 **g.** 2 **h.** 12 **i.** 6 **j.** 3 **k.** 11 **l.** 1 **m.** 8 *(p. 807)*

Content Review
1. **b.** A unified command system involves collaborative decision-making among the response agencies. *(p. 796)*
2. **d.** In a safe area near where patients will be loaded for transport *(p. 796)*
3. **a.** The senior EMT assumes responsibility as the EMS incident manager until relieved by a predesignated officer or other senior officer. *(p. 796)*
4. **c.** Wears a reflective vest (The incident manager and each sector officer must be easily recognizable from a distance.) *(p. 796)*
5. **a.** To assess and assign a priority to each patient *(p. 798)*

6. **d.** Perform a quick initial assessment (Check for airway, breathing, circulation, and severe bleeding.) *(p. 798)*
7. **a.** Priority 1 patients are transported first followed by Priority 2, then Priority 3 patients. *(p. 798)*
8. **c.** Low priority (Cardiac arrest patients are classed in the lowest class when there are limited numbers of rescuers available.) *(p. 798)*
9. **a.** Red indicates high priority. (Tagging helps arriving EMT-Bs to quickly and efficiently identify treatment and transport priorities.) *(p. 798)*
10. **d.** Triage or priority level (Color flags or ribbons should be erected at the ends of each row to designate the respective treatment areas. Place the patient in the appropriate row according to the color or level triaged.) *(p. 799)*
11. **c.** Provide plenty of nourishing food and drinks. (Rest every 1 to 2 hours; rapidly remove any rescue worker who becomes hysterical and transport to the hospital; encourage rescuers to talk among themselves.) *(p. 802)*

Case Study
1. **b.** Request additional help and assistance EARLY in the MCI. It's better to call too many rescuers than too few.
2. **c.** The senior EMT on the scene should assume responsibility until the arrival of a predesignated officer.
3. **c.** Position arriving rescue vehicles. (This will help with the smooth transport of patients and prevent accidents and injuries. Moving the dead to the morgue area and transporting the walking wounded are low priorities. Communicating with the media is an even lower priority.)
4. **a.** H **b.** H **c.** S **d.** L **e.** H

CHAPTER 44 — ADVANCED AIRWAY MANAGEMENT

Terms and Concepts
1. **a.** 7 **b.** 10 **c.** 9 **d.** 1 **e.** 5 **f.** 6 **g.** 3 **h.** 2 **i.** 4 **j.** 11 **k.** 8 *(pp. 845-846)*

Content Review
1. **a.** vallecula **b.** epiglottis **c.** tongue, **d.** glossoepiglottic ligament *(p. 811)*
2. **a.** epiglottis **b.** false vocal cords **c.** aryepiglottic fold **d.** true vocal cords **e.** glottis **f.** cuneiform cartilage **g.** corniculate cartilage *(p. 811)*
3. **d.** The right mainstem bronchus is almost in line with the trachea (Choices a and b refer to the bronchioles, which branch from the bronchi, not the trachea.) *(p. 812)*
4. **a.** Place a small folded towel under the child's shoulders. *(p. 812)*
5. If the patient's airway is not patent, it is essential to quickly open the airway using basic measures and provide oxygen, hyperventilating the patient, before inserting an endotracheal tube. Air cannot enter the lungs during the intubation procedure, and attempting intubation before basic airway measures will cause or exacerbate hypoxia. (In a few situations, such as anaphylaxis or upper airway

burns, swelling of the larynx may require immediate insertion of an endotracheal tube.) *(pp. 813, 819)*
6. **d.** Gurgling indicates fluid that needs to be removed prior to using advanced airway techniques *(p. 813)*
7. Advantages of endotracheal intubation include: (a) provides complete control of the airway (a direct route for ventilation and oxygenation, prevents the tongue from blocking the airway so manual maneuvers such as a head-tilt, chin-lift are not necessary); (b) isolates the trachea, lessening the risk of aspiration; (c) permits better ventilation and oxygen delivery (the bag-valve device can be connected directly to the endotracheal tube); (d) allows for deeper suctioning through the endotracheal tube. *(p. 814)*
8. Indications for endotracheal intubation include: (a) inability to ventilate the apneic patient effectively with standard methods; (b) inability of the patient to protect his own airway (is unresponsive to any type of stimulus; has no gag reflex). *(p. 814)*
9. **b.** You are able to insert an oropharyngeal airway without the patient gagging. (Don't insert your fingers; the patient may bite you.) *(p. 814)*
10. **d.** All of these (Remember, your face will be very close to the patient's mouth.) *(p. 814)*
11. **d.** Hold the tongue out of the way *(p. 815)*
12. **b.** Pressing on the glossoepiglottic ligament to lift the epiglottis indirectly (The curved blade is inserted into the vallecula, which presses on the glossoepiglottic ligament.) *(p. 816)*
13. Check if the blade is securely locked, the bulb tightly screwed into the socket, if the bulb or the batteries need to be changed. *(p.816)*
14. **b.** 7.5 mm i.d. *(p. 816)*
15. **a.** 15 mm adapter **b.** centimeter marker **c.** pilot balloon **d.** inflation port **e.** cuff **f.** bevel **g.** Murphy eye *(p. 817)*
16. **a.** Permits airflow if the tube is obstructed *(p. 817)*
17. **b.** Distal tip of tube should be in the trachea, midway between the carina and the vocal cords. *(p. 817)*
18. **c.** Never extend the stylet past the end of the tube; it may cause severe trauma to the patient's airway. *(p. 817)*
19. **b.** Inflate the cuff with 10 cc of air. *(p. 817)*
20. The purpose of the cuff is to seal the trachea (not to secure the tube in place). *(p. 818)*
21. Place the index finger and thumb of one hand on the anterior aspect of the throat just lateral to the midline of the cricoid cartilage, then apply pressure backward to close off the esophagus. (Decreases the chance of vomitus coming up the esophagus and into the airway. Also pushes the glottic structures into the visual field during intubation.) *(p. 818)*
22. **b.** Most laryngoscope blades are designed to be held in the left hand and to sweep the tongue to the left. *(p. 820)*

23. The three landmarks that identify the glottic opening are: (a) the cartilaginous structures surrounding the glottic opening, (b) the glottic opening is round, not oval like the esophageal opening; (c) the glottic opening contains the vocal cords through which the tube will pass *(p. 822)*

24. To verify correct endotracheal tube placement (in addition to watching the tube pass through the vocal cords): (a) Auscultate over the epigastrium (gurgling or breath sounds over the stomach indicate improper tube placement in the esophagus — deflate and remove the tube at once). (b) Watch for chest rise and fall during ventilations (assures tube placement in the trachea). (c) Auscultate breath sounds at the apex and base of the right and left lungs (presence of equal sounds in both lungs assures that the tube has not advanced into the right mainstem bronchus, depriving the left lung of air). (In addition, you might use an end-tidal carbon dioxide detector to measure the concentration of exhaled carbon dioxide or a pulse oximeter to measure the blood oxygen level. Also observe the patient for signs of deterioration, combativeness, cyanosis.) *(pp. 822-823)*

25. **d.** 1, 2, 3, 4, and 5. All may occur in the adult patient who has been intubated. (The most common complications in an adult are hypertension, tachycardia, and dysrhythmias. Bradycardia and hypotension are more commonly seen in infants and children but may be experienced by some adults. Additional potential complications of intubation are hypoxia and trauma to the lips, tongue, gums, teeth and airway structures.) *(p. 823)*

26. **b.** The patient must be unresponsive and in severe respiratory distress. *(p. 824)*

27. **d.** The straight blade lifts the epiglottis directly. The curved blade is placed into the vallecula to lift the epiglottis indirectly. *(pp. 815, 816, 825)*

28. **a.** Refer to a sizing chart or resuscitation tape. (Other methods include matching the outisde diameter of the tube to the child's little finger and using this formula: Tube size = 16 + the patient's age in years divided by 4.) *(p. 825)*

29. **a.** A deactivated pop-off valve (A pop-off valve that has *not* been deactivated may cause inadequate lung expansion or tidal volume during orotracheal intubation, especially in children with poor lung compliance or high airway resistance.) *(p. 827)*

30. Two indications for nasogastric intubation in infants and children are: (a) You are unable to provide positive pressure ventilation due to gastric distention, or (b) the patient is unresponsive and at risk of vomiting or developing gastric distention. *(p. 827)*

31. Contraindications for nasogastric intubation in infants and children (situations in which the NG tube should not be inserted) are: (a) The patient has suffered major facial, head, or spinal trauma (the tube could exacerbate the trauma or be pushed through a basilar skull fracture into the brain; do not insert an NG tube in such patients without consulting medical direction). (b) Airway disease such as epiglottitis or croup is suspected (the NG tube can cause spasms or exacerbate swelling to the point of occluding the airway). *(pp. 827-828)*

32. **b.** Measure the NG tube from the tip of the nose, around the ear extending doward, until the distal end is past the xophoid process. (Don't forget to mark the length with tape; when inserting the tube, you will stop when the tape is at the nostrils.) *(pp. 828, 829)*

33. Possible complications of orotracheal suctioning are: (a) hyopxia caused by removing residual air and interrupting ventilations; (b) cardiac dysrhythmias, possibly lethal; (c) coughing, which can dangerously increase pressure within the skull and decrease blood flow to the brain; (d) trauma to the mucosa; and (e) bronchospasms if the catheter is inserted past the carina. *(pp. 830, 832)*

Case Study

1. **b.** Always provide basic airway management before attempting intubation: Perform a jaw thrust, insert an oropharyngeal airway, and hyperventilate.

2. Yes. This patient should be intubated because the patient is unresponsive and cannot protect his own airway.

3. **c.** Suction the patient before performing any advanced airway techniques.

4. **d.** 24 breaths per minute for at least 1 minute (This will help saturate the blood with oxygen, which is necessary because there will be no ventilations while the endotracheal tube is being inserted.)

5. Because this patient has a suspected spinal injury, you must maintain in-line stabilization. Have Jill stabilize the head and neck from below while you secure the head with your thighs. Jill should apply Sellick's maneuver to help push the glottic structures into the visual field.

6. **b.** 30 seconds (Intubation attempts longer than 30 seconds can cause hypoxia.)

7. **a.** Half an inch to one inch past the cords. (This will place the tip approximately halfway between the carina and vocal cords.)

8. **b.** The tube is past the carina and in the right mainstem bronchus. Deflate the cuff and pull back enough to restore lung sounds on the left. When equal lung sounds are confirmed, reinflate the cuff.

The number(s) following each question refer to the textbook page(s) where the answer can be found or supported.

CHAPTER 1

1. d. *(p. 3)*

CHAPTER 8

2. b. *(pp. 131-132)* 3. a. *(pp. 134-135)* 4. d. *(p. 136)*

CHAPTER 9

5. b. *(p. 152)* 6. c. *(p. 154)* 7. b. *(p. 163)* 8. a. *(p. 168)*
9. b. *(p. 178)* 10. a. *(p. 183)* 11. c. *(p. 190)* 12. d. *(p. 197)*
13. b. *(p. 203)* 14. b. *(p. 210)* 15. c. *(p. 209)*

CHAPTER 13

16. d. *(pp. 264-265)* 17. b. *(p. 262)*

CHAPTER 6

18. b. *(p. 86)* 19. a. *(p. 89)*

CHAPTER 39

20. d. *(p. 723)* 21. d. *(p. 731)* 22. a. *(p. 737)*

CHAPTER 27

23. a. *(p. 466)* 24. b. *(p. 468)* 25. d. *(p. 466)* 26. d. *(p. 472)*
27. b. *(p. 473)* 28. c. *(p. 480)*

CHAPTER 7

29. c. *(pp. 96-97)* 30. b. *(p. 97)* 31. d. *(p. 102)* 32. c.
(pp. 103-104) 33. b. *(p. 106)* 34. a. *(p. 107)* 35. a. *(pp. 108, 110)*
36. d. *(pp. 111-112)* 37. c. *(p. 115)* 38. d. *(p. 116)* 39. b. *(p. 117)*
40. c. *(p. 120)*

CHAPTER 17

41. b. *(p. 332)* 42. b. *(pp. 334, 335)*

CHAPTER 5

43. c. *(p. 75)* 44. a. *(p. 80)* 45. c. *(pp. 74, 75, 78)*

CHAPTER 2

46. a. *(p. 18)* 47. c. *(p. 20)* 48. b. *(p. 22)*

CHAPTER 29

49. b. *(p. 511)* 50. c. *(p. 513)* 51. b. *(pp. 519, 520)*

CHAPTER 38

52. c. *(p. 687)* 53. a. *(p. 691)* 54. b. *(p. 692)* 55. d. *(p. 692)*
56. a. *(p. 693)* 57. d. *(p. 705)* 58. c. *(p. 705)* 59. b. *(p. 712)*

CHAPTER 43

60. b. *(p. 798)* 61. b. *(p. 799)*

CHAPTER 14

62. b. *(pp. 272-273)* 63. b. *(p. 276)* 64. c. *(p. 276)*
65. a. *(p. 282)* 66. c. *(p. 274)* 67. a. *(p. 273)*

CHAPTER 30

68. c. *(p. 532)* 69. a. *(p. 537)* 70. c. *(p. 538)*

CHAPTER 18

71. d. *(p. 342)* 72. d. *(p.343)*

CHAPTER 3

73. a. *(p. 33)* 74. d. *(p. 35)*

CHAPTER 15

75. c. *(p. 294)* 76. b. *(p. 301)* 77. b. *(pp. 301, 303)*

Course Review Self Test Answer Key

MEDICATION CARDS

In addition to oxygen, there are five medications the EMT-Basic can administer or assist the patient in administering, with on-line or off-line approval from medical direction. They are activated charcoal, epinephrine by auto-injector, metered dose inhaler, nitroglycerin, and oral glucose. Detailed information on each of these medications (as listed in the U.S. Department of Transportation's 1994 *Emergency Medical Technician-Basic: National Standard Curriculum*) is provided on the next pages in a format that you may cut from the book and carry with you for reference.

ACTIVATED CHARCOAL

Medication Name: Activated charcoal, SuperChar, InstaChar, Actidose, LiquiChar

Indications: Patients who have ingested poisons by mouth, administer after receiving orders from medical direction or the poison control center.

Contraindications: (1) Altered mental status (not fully conscious) (2) Swallowed acids or alkalis (3) Unable to swallow

Medication Form: 12.5 grams premixed in water; powder form should be avoided.

Dosage: 1 gram of activated charcoal per kilogram of body weight; usual adult dose 25 to 50 grams, infants and children 12.5 to 25 grams.

(see over)

EPINEPHRINE AUTO-INJECTOR

Medication Name: Epinephrine, Adrenalin, EpiPen®, EpiPen® Jr.

Indications: (1) Signs and symptoms of a severe allergic reaction (anaphylaxis).(2) Medication is prescribed to the patient. (3) EMT-B has received an order from medical direction.

Contraindications: None, when used in the life-threatening allergic reaction

Medication Form: Liquid drug contained within an auto-injector

Dosage: Auto-injectors deliver a single dose, Adult dose 0.3 mg, Infant and child 0.15 mg

(see over)

Activated Charcoal (continued)

Administration: Consult medical direction; shake container; encourage patient to drink through a straw; record time and response; if patient vomits notify medical control for repeat dose.

Actions: Binds with poisons in the stomach and prevents their absorption into the body

Side Effects: Blackening of the stools, possible vomiting

Reassessment: (1) Check for abdominal pain or distress upon administration. (2) Watch for vomiting; position the patient and be prepared to suction.

Epinephrine Auto-Injector (continued)

Administration: Push the uncapped tip of the auto-injector firmly against the lateral aspect of the thigh until the needle is deployed and the medication delivered.

Actions: Mimics the response of the sympathetic nervous system:
(1) Constricts blood vessels to improve the blood pressure. (2) Relaxes smooth muscles in the lungs to improve breathing. (3) Stimulates the heartbeat. (4) Reverses swelling and hives.

Side effects: Increased heart rate, pale skin (pallor), dizziness, chest pain, headache, nausea and vomiting, excitability and anxiousness

Reassessment: (1) Reassess for decreasing mental status, decreasing blood pressure, increased breathing difficulties. (2) If condition worsens you may have to call medical direction for second dose, treat for hypoperfusion, may need CPR and use of the AED

METERED DOSE INHALER

Medication Name: Albuterol, Metaproterenol, Isoetharine, Proventil®, Ventolin®, Metaprel®, Alupent®, Bronkosol®, Bronkometer®

Indications: (1) Exhibits signs and symptoms of breathing difficulty. (2) Patient has a physician-prescribed MDI. (3) EMT-B has received medical direction approval.

Contraindications: (1) Patient is not responsive enough to use the MDI. (2) MDI is not prescribed for the patient. (3) Maximum dose allowed is reached prior to your arrival. (4) Permission denied by medical direction.

Medication Form: Aerosolized medication in a metered dose inhaler

(see over)

NITROGLYCERIN

Medication Name: Nitroglycerin, Nitrostat®, Nitrobid®, Nitrolingual® Spray

Indications: (1) Patient exhibits signs and symptoms of chest pain. (2) Patient has physician-prescribed nitroglycerin. (3) EMT-B has approval from medical direction.

Contraindications: (1) Baseline blood pressure below 100 mmHg systolic. (2) Suspected head injury. (3) Patient is a child or infant. (4) Three doses have already been taken.

Medication Form: Tablet or sublingual spray

Dosage: One tablet or one spray under the tongue; may be repeated in 3 to 5 minutes if (1) Patient experiences no relief. (2) Blood pressure remains above 100 mmHg systolic. (3) Medical direction gives approval.

(see over)

ORAL GLUCOSE

Medication Name: Oral glucose, Glutose®, Insta glucose®

Indication: (1) Altered mental status with, (2) history of diabetes controlled by medication and (3) ability to swallow the medication

Contraindications: (1) Unconscious (2) Unable to swallow the medication

Medication Form: Gel, in a toothpaste-type tube

Dosage: Typical dose is one tube.

Administration: Oral, squeeze or place a portion between the cheek and gum.

(see over)

Metered Dose Inhaler (continued)

Dosage: Each depression of the MDI delivers a precise dose. The number of times the medication can be delivered is determined by medical direction.

Administration: (1) Ensure the medication is the patient's and the patient is alert; determine number of doses administered prior to your arrival. (2) Obtain order from medical direction. (3) Assure the MDI is at room temperature, shake for 30 seconds. (4) Administer while the patient is inhaling; encourage him to hold breath.

Actions: Beta agonist, relaxes the bronchiole smooth muscles, dilates the lower airway

Side Effects: Tachycardia, tremors, shakiness, nervousness, dry mouth

Reassessment: Perform an ongoing assessment, reassess vital signs, question patient about effect, focused history and physical exam, monitor airway, record and document.

Nitroglycerin (continued)

Administration: (1) Assure medication is the patient's, blood pressure greater than 100 mmHg systolic, approval from medical direction. (2) Assure patient is alert; check expiration date; ask patient when he took his last dose. (3) Place or spray medication under the tongue; keep mouth closed. (4) Reassess the blood pressure in 2 minutes; record your actions.

Actions: Relaxes blood vessels, decreases workload of the heart

Side Effects: Vessel dilation may cause headache, drop in blood pressure, pulse rate changes.

Reassessment: (1) Monitor blood pressure. (2) Question patient about effect. (3) Obtain approval from medical direction before re-administering. (4) Record and document all findings and reassessment.

Oral Glucose (continued)

Action: Increases blood and brain sugar levels

Side effects: May cause an airway obstruction in the patient without a gag reflex

Reassessment: Reassess the mental status to determine if the drug has had an effect.